Advance Praise

Social medicine has the power to transform how we understand health and practice medicine. This book is an excellent introduction to the history and underlying philosophy of social medicine, but most importantly it points to the future, showing how a better understanding of social medicine can actually improve the health of populations.
— *Sandro Galea, Dean & Robert A. Knox Professor, Boston University School of Public Health*

This is the first comprehensive text on social medicine that portrays its emergence and the ways in which capitalist development has produced and reproduced huge global inequalities that cause huge health disparities. The involvement of the authors in social medicine within the U.S. and in Latin America is the basis of their fertile perspective for comprehending the rise and demise of the capitalist globalization project and a hopeful basis for organizing a more humane and democratic global society.
— *Christopher Chase-Dunn, Distinguished Professor of Sociology and Director of the Institute for Research on World-Systems at the University of California, Riverside*

A provocative primer on social medicine – its histories, scope, arguments, and praxis. With an emphasis on critical contributions from Latin American Social Medicine, the authors ask health workers to grapple with how capitalism, imperialism, income inequality, racism, and sexism have harmed people's health and health care systems – and present revolutionary proposals for imagining and creating a more equitable, post-capitalist, and healthier future.
— *Nancy Krieger, Professor of Social Epidemiology, American Cancer Society Clinical Research Professor, Harvard University T. H. Chan School of Public Health*

Social Medicine and the Coming Transformation

Social medicine, starting two centuries ago, has shown that social conditions affect health and illness more than biology does, and social change affects the outcomes of health and illness more than health services do. Understanding and exposing sickness-generating structures in society helps change them.

This first introductory book in social medicine provides a critical introduction to this increasingly important field. The authors draw on examples worldwide to show how principles based on solidarity and mutual aid have enabled people to participate collaboratively to construct health-promoting social conditions. The book offers vital information and analysis to enhance our understanding about promoting health through social and individual means; the micro-politics of medical encounters; the social determination of illness; the influences of racism, class, gender, and ethnicity on health; health and empire; and health praxis, reform, and sociomedical activism.

The authors provide compelling ways to understand and to change the social dimensions of health and health care. Students, teachers, practitioners, activists, policy makers, and people concerned about health and health care will value this book, which goes beyond the usual approaches in public health, medical sociology, health economics, and health policy.

Howard Waitzkin is Distinguished Professor Emeritus of Sociology at the University of New Mexico and practices internal medicine part time in New Mexico and Illinois. For many years, he has been active in struggles focusing on social medicine in the United States and Latin America. He is the author and coordinator with the Working Group for Health beyond Capitalism of *Health Care under the Knife: Moving beyond Capitalism for Our Health* (2018), and author of *Medicine and Public Health at the End of Empire* (2011), among other books.

Alina Pérez is a community-based physician at St. Luke's Hospital in New Bedford, Massachusetts. A graduate of the University of Illinois College of Medicine at Rockford, she completed her residency at the Beth Israel Deaconess Harvard-Affiliated Medical Center in Boston. She has conducted research on health policy and is pursuing interests in global health and social medicine.

Matthew Anderson is Associate Professor in the Department of Family and Social Medicine at the Albert Einstein College of Medicine in New York City. As a family physician working in the Bronx, New York, he is a core faculty member of the Montefiore Residency Program in Social Medicine. He is Founder and Co-editor of the bilingual online journal *Social Medicine/Medicina Social*.

Social Medicine and the Coming Transformation

Howard Waitzkin,
Alina Pérez, and
Matthew Anderson

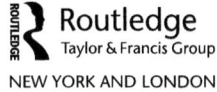
Routledge
Taylor & Francis Group
NEW YORK AND LONDON

First published 2021
by Routledge
52 Vanderbilt Avenue, New York, NY 10017

and by Routledge
2 Park Square, Milton Park, Abingdon, Oxon, OX14 4RN

Routledge is an imprint of the Taylor & Francis Group, an informa business

© 2021 Howard Waitzkin, Alina Pérez, and Matthew Anderson

The right of Howard Waitzkin, Alina Pérez, and Matthew Anderson to be identified as authors of this work has been asserted by them in accordance with sections 77 and 78 of the Copyright, Designs and Patents Act 1988.

All rights reserved. No part of this book may be reprinted or reproduced or utilized in any form or by any electronic, mechanical, or other means, now known or hereafter invented, including photocopying and recording, or in any information storage or retrieval system, without permission in writing from the publishers.

Trademark notice: Product or corporate names may be trademarks or registered trademarks, and are used only for identification and explanation without intent to infringe.

Library of Congress Cataloging-in-Publication Data
Names: Waitzkin, Howard, author. | Pérez, Alina, author. | Anderson, Matthew (Matthew R.), author.
Title: Social medicine and the coming transformation / by Howard Waitzkin, Alina Pérez, and Matthew Anderson.
Description: New York, NY: Routledge, 2020. | Includes bibliographical references.
Identifiers: LCCN 2019048092 (print) | LCCN 2019048093 (ebook) | ISBN 9781138685970 (hardback) | ISBN 9781138685987 (paperback) | ISBN 9781315542898 (ebook)
Subjects: LCSH: Social medicine—Textbooks.
Classification: LCC RA418 .W348 2020 (print) | LCC RA418 (ebook) | DDC 362.1—dc23
LC record available at https://lccn.loc.gov/2019048092
LC ebook record available at https://lccn.loc.gov/2019048093

ISBN: 978-1-138-68597-0 (hbk)
ISBN: 978-1-138-68598-7 (pbk)
ISBN: 978-1-315-54289-8 (ebk)

Typeset in Bembo
by codeMantra

eResources available at: https://www.routledge.com/9781138685987

To the memory of Doctors Salvador and Beatriz Allende.

Strengthened by their sacrifices, their vision of social medicine will prevail.

Contents

Preface   xii
Acknowledgments   xxiii

1 What Is Social Medicine?   1
   An Outbreak of Fatal Respiratory Disease – Part One 1
   An Outbreak of Fatal Respiratory Disease – Part Two 2
   Another Outbreak: Typhus in Upper Silesia 5
   Other Roots of Social Medicine 7
   Social and Economic Conditions Impacting Health, Illness, and the Practice of Medicine 8
   The Health of the Population as a Matter of Social Concern 9
   Promoting Health through Both Social and Individual Means 12
   Why Is Critical Social Medicine Relevant Now? 19

2 One and Half Centuries of Forgetting and Remembering the Social Origins of Illness   24
   How This Viewpoint Emerged 25
   Friedrich Engels 27
   Rudolf Virchow 30
   Salvador Allende 34
   Capitalism, Empire, Illness, and Early Death 39

3 The Social Determination of Illness, Part 1: Health and Social Contradictions   45
   Social Contradictions – Effects on Health 47
   Social Determinants versus Social Determination 48
   Plastic Workers' Liver Cancer 54
   Asbestos Workers' Lung Disease and Cancer 55
   Farmworkers' Back 57

Brain Disease from Mercury Poisoning 60
Leukemia and Lymphoma among Electronic Workers 62
Upstream Causes of COVID-19 and Other Epidemics to Follow 64
Levels of Analysis in Social Medicine 72

4 The Social Determination of Illness, Part 2: Inequality, Class, Race, Ethnicity, and Gender 79
Improving Research on Worsening Social Determination 79
Social Class and Classism 80
Race and Racism 89
Gender and Sexism 95
Social Origins, Social Reconstruction 99

5 Social Medicine in the United States 109
Can One Speak of a U.S. Social Medicine? 109
The First U.S. Factories, Struggles for Workers' Health, and the Labor Movement 109
Social Medicine Centered in the "Little Germany" of New York City 112
Health Initiatives during the Progressive Era 118
Experiments in Social Medicine outside New York 123
The Contested Status of Social Insurance in the United States 125
Why the Weakness of U.S. Social Insurance Compared with Those of Other Countries? 131

6 Health and Empire, Part 1: Empire's Historical Health Component 139
Imperialism, Medicine, and Public Health 139
Philanthropic Foundations 142
International Financial Institutions and Trade Agreements 145
International Health Organizations 150
Recycling Public Health Interventions at the End of Empire 154

7 Health and Empire, Part 2: Resisting Empire, Building an Alternative Future in Medicine and Public Health 158
A World without Empire 158
The Struggle against Privatization of Health Services in El Salvador 160
Resistance to Privatization of Water in Bolivia 164

*Social Medicine's Coming to Power in Mexico City
  and Mexico 167*
Sociomedical Activism toward a New Order 173

8 Social Medicine in Latin America 177
Productivity and Danger 178
Historical Roots of Latin American Social Medicine 180
*The "Golden Age" of Social Medicine in Chile and the Role of
  Salvador Allende 181*
Social Medicine versus Public Health Elsewhere in Latin America 183
The 1960s and Later 185
Political Repression and Work Challenges 188
Theory, Method, and Debate 189
Emerging Themes 191
The Future of Latin American Social Medicine 193

9 Social Medicine and the Micro-politics of Medical Encounters 199
How Society Impinges on the Medical Encounter 199
The Human Experience of Access Barriers 199
Patient–Doctor Relationships in the Era of Managed Care 204
Social Context and Patient–Doctor Communication 210
Trauma, Militarism, Mental Health, and Physical Symptoms 213

10 Health Praxis, Reform, and Sociomedical Activism 224
Contradictions of Reform 225
Struggles for National Health Programs 227
*Struggles to Address the Social Determination of
  Health and Illness 236*
*Praxis and the Health and Mental Health of Social Medicine
  Practitioners 254*

*Appendix: Organizations and Resources in Social Medicine
and Collective Health* 265
Index 277

Preface

Social Medicine versus Critical Social Medicine

Since it started about two centuries ago, social medicine has shown that the characteristics of society affect health and illness more than biology does, and social change affects the outcomes of health and illness more than health services do. This perspective becomes threatening to those who hold wealth and power in society. Why? Because the social change that would improve the lives and health of the population's great majority would reduce the power and privilege of those in society's upper tier. As a result, social medicine that brings critical attention to injustice and inequality does not win much favor in the corridors of power and has become forgotten or marginalized in each generation. Social medicine attracts praise when it does not try to threaten in any fundamental way the unjust and exploitative structures in society that contribute to ill-health and early death.

But that unthreatening approach is not what we are trying to do here. Instead, we are trying to understand those sickness-generating structures in society in order to help change them. As practitioners, teachers, and students in this sometimes threatening field of social medicine, we know that the perspectives in this book may not win praise or rewards from those who command power in medicine, public health, or the broader society. That's probably the main reason why there is no similar book on social medicine available in the English language. There are some in Spanish and other languages, spoken and read in countries mainly in the global South, where the critical traditions of social medicine have been less discouraged and marginalized than they have been in the United States and other countries of the global North. In addition to these inspiring sources, we also are adding to social medicine the perspective of "collective health," an adaptation of social medicine that Brazilian activists and scholars have promoted. Collective health emphasizes that positive health emerges from a collectivity that promotes health. Through the creation of a just society based on solidarity and mutual aid, people participate communally and collaboratively to construct health-promoting social conditions.[1]

The Context of What We Are Trying to Do

> Of all the forms of inequality, injustice in health is the most shocking and inhuman.
> – Martin Luther King, 1966

Dr. King's words followed more than half a century of failed efforts in the United States to achieve a national health program that provides universal access to health care. In 2010, a reform occurred in the United States – the Affordable Care Act (ACA), or Obamacare – that reduced the number of uninsured, increased the costs of care for many who previously held health insurance, shifted responsibility for costs away from insurance companies and to patients (leading to more "underinsurance"), and created tax-generated public subsidies for private insurance companies. Even before Donald Trump and Congress tried, or at least said they tried, to repeal and replace the ACA with policies that would assure even less access to care, the ACA was failing because the out-of-pocket costs for the average family under Obamacare were rising and were projected to equal half the average family income within the next decade.[2]

Outside the United States, countries continue to struggle as their populations seek accessible and affordable health services, as well as public health policies that promote health rather than illness. High-income countries face problems of increasing costs of care and sources of illness in social inequality and the environment that do not respond to health services alone. In lower income countries, the unequal distribution of wealth within and among countries creates continuing barriers to the construction of responsive health care systems, and inequality remains an intractable social determinant of a population's health.[3]

Social medicine offers compelling ways to understand and to change the social dimensions of health and health care. As students and as teachers, we have not been able to find another single source in English that provides a critical introduction to social medicine and collective health that could be used as a sort of introductory text. (A few books that include social medicine in the titles do not offer a consistent, critical analysis that traces the roots of illness and early death to the unjust conditions of society and also clarify ways that those illness-generating social conditions can change.) In this effort, we are trying to reach students, teachers, practitioners, activists, people who take part in policy making, and general readers who may value a book that goes beyond the usual approaches of texts in public health, medical sociology, health economics, and health policy.

Who Are We and Why Are We Doing This?

Dean Birkenkamp, esteemed editor, publisher, and activist, first recognized that a critical book on social medicine seemed missing, especially one that tried to clarify the century and a half of prior work in this field rather than largely ignoring it. In 2015, Dean asked Howard to write the book. Although Howard has spent years trying to study and to advance social medicine and collective health, the job of presenting this inspirational field alone seemed overwhelming.

So Howard approached Matt Anderson, who has worked in developing what many people consider the most effective teaching program on social medicine in the United States. Matt also initiated and still edits the most widely read online journal on social medicine in the world. Howard and Matt have collaborated on several previous projects, including a major focus on social medicine and collective health in Latin America. As teachers, Howard and Matt often have felt frustration because they could not locate a single source that presented a critical introduction for people starting out.

Still, Howard and Matt felt limited in finding ways to present these perspectives that might interest younger people with different experiences, needs, and creative energies. So Howard approached Alina, who was trying to maintain a focus on health policy and social issues in medicine during the challenging clinical years of medical school. Alina agreed to work initially as a research assistant but wound up writing or rewriting whole chapters in a unique way that she thought learners in her generation would find more engaging and less boring than the texts generated by Howard and Matt. Realizing the importance of Alina's contributions, Howard suggested that she become a co-author, and Matt and Dean agreed. The order of the authors' names, we decided, indicates the relative amounts of work we contributed.

COVID-19 and Black Lives Matter

The coronavirus disease 2019 (COVID-19) pandemic shows why social medicine is so important. Because the pandemic broke out when this book already had entered production, we had to "hold the presses" until we could address the pandemic. At the time of this writing (November 2020), knowledge about severe acute respiratory syndrome coronavirus 2 (SARS CoV-2), its biological effects, treatments, impacts on populations and population subgroups, economic effects, and suitable public health responses and prevention remains preliminary. Even the data about numbers of cases, about whom the virus has infected and whom it has spared, and about whom it has killed vary widely across communities, states, regions, and countries. These variations have emerged because of large differences in testing, diagnosis, categorization, validity, and reliability of reports in the scientific literature and popular media.

So, we cannot yet present a complete picture of COVID-19 from the standpoint of social medicine. Our discussion of COVID-19 and the evidence that supports the statements below within this preface appear in several chapters. The following part of the preface that describes how we organized the book ("Where the Path Leads") also indicates the main locations where we have placed our analyses of COVID-19 in relation to the book's core themes. These analyses appear mostly in Chapters 1 and 3, with briefer commentaries in other chapters.

Like many other diseases that we consider in this book, it is clear that the "upstream" causes of COVID-19 in society and the environment are extremely important and often overlooked. Predictions about how this current pandemic would happen have appeared regularly over past decades. COVID-19 is just one of many emerging viral epidemics that have arisen and will continue to arise until we decide to change their upstream social and environmental causes.

We, like other health professionals and scientists working in social medicine, trace the causes of COVID-19 upstream to industrial agriculture and its impact on natural environments, especially through deforestation. Forest habitats previously provided natural protections against the "zoonotic" spread of viruses and some other pathogens from wild animals to other species including humans. Especially under the procedures introduced by capitalist industrial agriculture, deforestation has destroyed these protective habitats.

In addition to deforestation, the industrial production of meat has created unsanitary, dangerous factory conditions in which animals are born, bred, reproduced, slaughtered, packaged, and shipped to consumers within environments that inevitably cause the emergence of virus mutations that affect workers in those factories and that spread quickly to other human populations. Because meat packing plants employ people who frequently are poor, immigrants, ethnic minorities, and otherwise marginalized, these plants become hotspots for the spread of infections such as COVID-19 to the vulnerable populations most at risk during epidemics.

Such upstream social and environmental conditions have caused all recent major viral epidemics and pandemics, including HIV/AIDS, multiple influenzas, swine flu, avian flu, Nipah virus, Zika, the earlier SARS pandemic, COVID-19, and predictable future pandemics with even worse effects on health and well-being. They are the same conditions that contribute to other critical challenges like global warming and the climate crisis, multi-drug-resistant bacterial infections, plastic pollution, and shortages of clean drinking water. Until we address these upstream causes through profound social and economic change, we will face recurrent pandemics, increasingly frequent and severe, as well as other worsening upstream conditions that directly impact the health and survival of human populations.

In addition to upstream causes, social medicine also illuminates the downstream effects of COVID-19. Epidemics almost always affect people in certain groups disproportionately. As noted already, the workers affected by COVID-19 in meat-packing plants come from the same population subgroups as many other high-risk "essential workers" and community residents who work and live in deprived social conditions that increase the risk of illness and early death. In several chapters, we show how patterns of disease and mortality affect poor people, racial/ethnic minorities, immigrants, indigenous peoples, and other marginalized groups more than wealthy people, those from majority racial/ethnic backgrounds, those from non-immigrant and non-indigenous groups, and those from groups that hold power in their societies. Those groups suffering most from COVID-19 also suffer most under almost all other epidemics and also from essentially all other physical and mental health problems. Social and economic inequality is the key determinant of illness and death in today's world, as it has been in the past, and COVID-19 shows the impact of inequality in a crystal-clear way.

While we were writing updates about COVID-19, the brutal killing of George Floyd took place. This event led to worldwide protests against racism and police brutality, which the United States has tolerated for generations since enslavement of peoples from Africa and genocide against indigenous peoples in the Americas began with the European invasion and conquest. Other countries also have suffered from these horrendous problems. Because racism is one fundamental cause in the social determination of health outcomes, we already had devoted substantial attention to racism in Chapter 4, which also addresses classism and sexism as fundamental causes in social determination. Because this killing and the profound reactions to it have transformed many people's understanding of social determination in medicine, public health, and social medicine, we also have added some additional comments about these crucial events during the momentous year of 2020.

Where the Path Leads

We start the book in Chapter 1 by describing two devastating epidemics of infectious diseases, two recent (one of these is COVID-19) and another a century and a half ago. These epidemics show the social conditions that play a fundamental role in physical illnesses. The epidemics also help us answer the question, "What is social medicine?" The notion that social conditions shape illness and early death first arose as a field of clinical practice, teaching, and research in the 1800s, and this history often gets overlooked in current attempts to grapple with what now are called "social determinants." With roots in Europe, the social medicine perspective spread to the Americas early in the twentieth century. We trace this history and try to explain why social medicine has flourished in many other countries but not the United States. One main question in social medicine that we address is why the United States remains the only economically developed country without a national health program that provides universal access to health services. In contrast, we describe several exciting programs in the United States and other countries that embody the core values of social medicine.

Chapter 2 focuses on three heroes of social medicine, who took risks by courageously focusing on the social causes of illness in their lives and work. Friedrich Engels, who collaborated with Karl Marx during the mid-1800s, wrote a book – *The Condition of the Working Class in England in 1844* – that became the first comprehensive study in social medicine. Based on his efforts with workers and their families in the industrial city of Manchester, Engels offered a detailed account of occupational and environmental diseases that anticipated research on these problems during the next 170 years. His analyses remain no less gripping and relevant now than they did then. Influenced by Engels, Rudolf Virchow in Germany developed the field of cellular pathology, for which he still receives wide recognition in the United States and other countries. Because of his focus on the social conditions that cause epidemics and on the social responsibilities of health professionals, Virchow also has gained recognition around the world as the "father of social medicine." However, this important component of his work has received little attention in the United States. And Salvador Allende in Chile, himself influenced by social medicine through the prior work of a pathologist in Chile, Max Westenhöfer, who was Virchow's student, became a leader of social medicine in Latin America during the 1930s. As an elected senator, Allende founded the first national health program in the Americas. Then, as president of Chile in the early 1970s, until he died in a military coup supported by the United States, Allende orchestrated a series of influential social medicine initiatives that became models throughout Latin America and the rest of the world.

Based partly on these historical examples of social medicine's focus on links between social conditions and health, we then offer two chapters on the social determination of illness. Chapter 3 clarifies unhealthy contradictions in society. We introduce the chapter with stories of three patients – a man suffering infertility from pesticide exposure, a woman whose infant dies needlessly, and a man who endures expensive and unnecessary medical procedures. Although these case histories seem quite different on the surface, they all reflect contradictions in our society that contribute to illness and death. To clarify these contradictions, we explain the theoretical approach in social medicine that emphasizes a "dialectic" relationship between social contradictions. After giving a brief overview of several contradictions, we focus on one of them, which is the contradiction between profit and safety. We then analyze how this contradiction contributes to disease and mortality in several devastating medical disorders: plastic workers' liver cancer, asbestos workers' lung disease and cancer, farmworkers' back, brain disease from mercury poisoning, cancers among electronics workers who make computers and cellphones, and the recent pandemic of COVID-19. This chapter turned out longer than we expected, because COVID-19 manifests so clearly the problem of social determination and other core themes of social medicine.

In Chapter 4, extending the focus on the social determination of illness, we analyze three categories of social conditions that profoundly impact health outcomes. First, poverty and inequality persist as the most important determinants of a population's patterns of morbidity and mortality. In clarifying "social class and classism," we discuss the astonishing recent deterioration of health in the U.S. population, where middle-age white adults show worsening life expectancy and worsening health outcomes for a variety of health problems. These problems include suicide, overdose deaths from opiates, and overall mortality rates. Geographically, the problems are concentrated disproportionately in areas with high levels of income inequality, which are the same areas where Donald Trump received his highest levels of support in the 2016 presidential election. We also try to clarify how social class is defined and how inequality could be improved by small changes in policies to redistribute wealth. Second, in the next section on "race and racism," we present the extensive scientific evidence that race is a socially constructed category that does not correspond to biological differences. From this perspective, people in different socially constructed racial groups suffer worse health outcomes and mortality not due to biology, but rather due to the damaging effects of racism. Black people's much higher risk of police brutality leading to incarceration, injury, and death, as shown in the killing of George Floyd and many others through the decades, is one key way that racism exerts its very harmful effects. We also show that it often is difficult to separate the impact of racism from the impact of social class on health outcomes. A third category of social determinants, "gender and sexism," also shapes illness and death, but again less through biology than through discrimination and unequal treatment. We emphasize especially harassment and violence as mechanisms by which sexism affects health.

Chapter 5 shifts the focus from social determination to the largely hidden story of social medicine in the United States. The story begins in the textile factories of New England during the early 1800s, when the demands of capitalist production created devastating health problems for workers, especially women workers. At about the same time as Engels and Virchow studied and agitated around such illness-generating social conditions (as noted in Chapter 2), activists like Orestes Brownson and public health practitioners like Lemuel Shattuck struggled to improve such conditions in the United States. A few years later, immigrants from

Germany, especially the pediatrician Abraham Jacobi (who had studied with Virchow), developed an influential practice of social medicine in New York City. Jacobi's partner, Mary Putnam, became one of the first women physicians in the United States and worked tirelessly to improve women's health with a vision based on social medicine. We trace this history that led to the creation of community health centers as part of the settlement house movement during the Progressive Era of the early twentieth century, as well as community development projects with social medicine components in such places as Milwaukee and Cincinnati. Social insurance emerged as a key goal of social medicine; we clarify the meaning of social insurance and clarify the early history of this approach that culminated in the creation of the Social Security System during the 1930s, as well as Medicare and Medicaid during the 1960s. The chapter concludes by showing how social medicine points the way toward a comprehensive national health program in the United States and how opposition has blocked that path, leaving this country unique among economically advanced nations in lacking universal access to health services.

In Chapter 6, we continue to emphasize the United States, but from the standpoint of that country's role in neocolonialism and imperialism. The role of the United States as an imperial power has troubled social medicine teachers, students, researchers, and activists around the world. We begin by defining imperialism and showing how public health initiatives have supported imperialism historically and now. We then focus on institutions that have mediated the relationships between imperialism and health. Philanthropic foundations have fostered empire by supporting public health measures designed to enhance the productivity of workers in poor countries affected by endemic infectious diseases. Through such programs, the Rockefeller Foundation reinforced the economic interests of Rockefeller-controlled corporations. As we show, this foundation encouraged "vertical" efforts to control specific diseases like hookworm, malaria, and yellow fever, rather than "horizontal" programs to develop a well-organized public health infrastructure of clinics and hospitals. The Bill and Melinda Gates Foundation, currently the world's largest funder in global health, has resurrected the vertical approach by emphasizing so-called magic bullets, like new vaccines and medications for infectious diseases, rather than the creation of public health systems. As a result, we report that countries with fewer economic resources cannot respond effectively when crises arise, such as HIV in Africa, Ebola, Zika, COVID-19, and other emerging epidemics. In the same chapter, we clarify how international financial institutions like the World Bank and international trade agreements like the North American Free Trade Agreement (NAFTA) have affected health, often by supporting the financial interests of multinational corporations. Similarly, international health organizations – such as the World Health Organization and Pan American

Health Organization – increasingly support the same corporate agenda as the World Bank and the Gates Foundation.

People who work in social medicine usually do not remain content simply to describe problems. Instead, we try to use our knowledge and skills to address the problems we study, that is, we try to change the world to make it less destructive and more supportive of healthy lives, and this challenge often requires a struggle with those who benefit from the oppressive conditions that lead to illness and early death. In Chapter 7, we present accounts of inspiring efforts to change the world according to principles of social medicine. These examples all involve mostly successful efforts to reduce the overall unhealthy effects of economic imperialism in the context of Latin America. First, we describe the long-term struggles of health workers in El Salvador to resist privatization of public health services and to strengthen services provided in public hospitals and clinics. Then, we analyze the heroic efforts of indigenous communities in Bolivia to protect their water supplies from privatization and takeover by multinational corporations; such "water wars" are becoming more common around the world as corporations seek profits by privatizing increasingly scarce water supplies despite the critical importance of accessible, clean water for a population's health. This chapter concludes with a description of ongoing efforts in Mexico to resist the neoliberal model of privatized, for-profit health services, culminating in the election of a new president who sought a national, public program to provide universal access to care. Social medicine has influenced all these struggles that focus on health, health services, and resources like water that are essential for public health. These efforts reveal a growing, worldwide vision of medicine and public health constructed around principles of justice rather than commodification and profitability.

Transitioning from these examples of struggles around social conditions and health, we present in Chapter 8 a deeper account of Latin American social medicine itself. We start by emphasizing the dangers that some leaders have faced in Latin America simply by practicing social medicine. These dangers have arisen mainly because social medicine, by linking health to underlying social conditions, presents an inherent challenge to those who hold financial and political power in a society. We trace the roots of Latin American social medicine partly to Europe and partly to work in several countries that did not benefit from exposure to European sources. The "golden age of social medicine" in Chile and early efforts in other countries provide examples of work that has inspired later generations of social medicine practitioners and activists. After analyzing the differences between social medicine and public health, we present important work influenced by revolutionary struggles in Cuba, Nicaragua, and Brazil. We also describe the repression that has affected social medicine practitioners, especially during the dictatorships that took power in several countries during the 1960s through the 1980s. To conclude this chapter, we summarize the main theoretical and methodological contributions in Latin America that can serve as models for social medicine throughout the world.

In Chapter 9, we move to the more intimate encounter between patients and health professionals and consider the "micro-politics of health care" as a key focus of social medicine. Our purpose here is to envision how society impinges on the medical encounter. We start by describing the "human experience of access barriers," with information about our patients who have died or suffered major complications because they could not access needed medical care in the United States. Then we consider how the financial and administrative structures of managed care have introduced difficult challenges within the patient–doctor relationship, especially due to distortions in communication and the constraints of the electronic medical record. In this process, health professionals have lost control over the conditions of clinical work, which some have called "proletarianization." Because the social problems that patients experience often enter the conversations of medical encounters, we analyze the constraints that limit professionals' responsiveness and how these limitations could change if health services were organized differently. We conclude the chapter by considering how trauma, especially that generated by militarism, arises as medical and mental health professionals face inherent contradictions in professional roles. In all these variations of encounters, the impact of social conditions on communication becomes a problem whose resolution cannot happen until the social conditions themselves change.

So how to change the social conditions that cause illness, suffering, and early death becomes a key challenge for social medicine, and the last chapter responds to this challenge. We first try to clarify the meaning of praxis, the relationship between theory and practice, which refers in social medicine to activism aimed at changing illness-generating social conditions, guided by a theoretical analysis and understanding of those conditions. To figure out a path toward meaningful change, we distinguish between two types of reform: "reformist reforms," which make limited improvements but do not change underlying conditions based on concentrated wealth and political power, and "non-reformist reforms," which actually do change underlying conditions of wealth and power. Using this distinction, we contrast the ACA and a single-payer national health program ("Improved Medicare for All"), the two main models of health reform considered during recent years in the United States (Trumpcare consisting mainly of attempts to block the construction of an accessible national health program). Despite arguments in favor of unified national health programs that provide a single standard of care for a country's entire population, we recognize a fundamental problem: Recent changes in global capitalism make the construction and preservation of national health programs much more difficult in any country, and the same challenges limit our ability to change illness-generating social conditions in a sustainable way. Most of us find that it is difficult to imagine a viable path from capitalism to postcapitalism (the "TINA" perspective, that is, "There Is No Alternative"). As a result, in social medicine and other worthy endeavors, many of us engage in peculiar efforts to improve our key problems without confronting capitalism, even though we know that capitalism generates and continues to worsen our most important problems. Our praxis in social medicine, and in many arenas of activism, must confront capitalism itself and move beyond it. We present several ways that this confrontation and the transition to healthier, postcapitalist societies are taking place in the United States and other countries. No longer can we afford to defer this struggle for future generations to resolve.

Notes

1 We discuss these sources from Latin American social medicine and collective health in Chapter 8.
2 Chapter 10 provides further information and citations about these and other issues in Obamacare.
3 Please see Chapters 3 and 10 for more information and citations about inequality and costs of care.

Acknowledgments

Thank you!

- Dean Birkenkamp for dreaming up the possibility of this book, for brilliant editing, and for the rare vision of publishing to help build a healthier world
- Rebeca Jasso-Aguilar for comradely collaboration over many years and for encouraging us to use here several key components of our work together
- Mira Lee for profound understanding about the substance, emotional experience, and moral necessity of social medicine
- Compañeros y compañeras de la Medicina Social y Saúde Colectiva en América Latina (comrades of Social Medicine and Collective Health in Latin America) … inspiring role models of courage and praxis under conditions that could not be more challenging … in loving gratitude
- We are deeply grateful and honored that Beatriz Aurora, leading artist of the Zapatista revolution in Mexico, kindly allowed us to use for our cover her painting, "Un Mundo Donde Quepan Muchos Mundos" ("A World Where Many Worlds Fit"). Gabriela Hinojosa provided expert graphic design.

Chapter 1

What Is Social Medicine?

An Outbreak of Fatal Respiratory Disease – Part One

Imagine that you are a health worker, maybe a nurse or a doctor, working in a rural area in the Southwest United States. Consider how you would respond to the following challenge.

You recently started a job with a community health center in Gallup, New Mexico, a town that adjoins the Navajo Nation.[1] During the past two days, you have cared for three Navajo patients, ranging in age from 21 to 60. They all presented with severe cough, high fever, and weakness. The oldest patient developed adult respiratory distress syndrome and required transfer to the medical intensive care unit (ICU) at the University of New Mexico (UNM) Hospital in Albuquerque. The two younger patients presented with less severe respiratory symptoms, and you are treating them with oral antibiotics. However, when they come in again to see you today, their cough has worsened and they are developing symptoms of respiratory distress.

You call UNM Hospital to arrange for them to be admitted. As part of the admission process, you consult with an epidemiologist who is also an infectious disease specialist. She asks you whether the three patients share any characteristics. You reply that all three live in a remote rural area on the Navajo Nation. She replies that no less than six similar patients have entered ICUs at UNM and other local hospitals during the past week, and three of them have died from respiratory failure. Hantavirus is the apparent infection, she says, and has been confirmed by blood tests. She asks that you notify her if you find out any additional, pertinent information.

2 What Is Social Medicine?

> **QUESTIONS TO CONSIDER AND DISCUSS**
>
> In considering these patients, here are some questions to keep in mind:
>
> - How could you determine if an epidemic was developing?
> - If you are, in fact, dealing with an epidemic, what can you do to help control it?
> - Whom could you turn to for help?
> - How does this epidemic reflect larger social factors (sometimes referred to as social determinants)?
> - What relationship does this epidemic have to human rights concerns?

You never have seen a case of hantavirus, although you vaguely remember hearing about it once or twice in medical school. You look it up on the U.S. Centers for Disease Control website.[2] You learn that infected rodents, such as field mice, carry hantavirus. Originally discovered during an epidemic in the Hantan River area in rural Korea, the virus infects humans when they inhale the feces or urine of infected mice or rats. The virus can remain alive in dust and enters the respiratory tract through the nose when people sweep their houses, garages, or barns. There is no known treatment for hantavirus pulmonary syndrome. Among the reported cases in the United States, about 30–40 percent of patients died. While hantavirus infection occasionally affects wealthy people, for instance, those who own ranches, it is overwhelmingly a disease of poverty.

This epidemic of hantavirus actually occurred in 1993 and was the first recognized outbreak of hantavirus in the United States. Sadly, 25 years later people in the Southwest continue to die of the hanta pulmonary syndrome, still mostly in communities affected by poverty and marginalization.

An Outbreak of Fatal Respiratory Disease – Part Two

Now try to imagine yourself as a doctor on December 30, 2019, in Wuhan, a large city in China. Some of your patients have been getting severely ill with a life-threatening pneumonia, requiring hospitalization. You were too young to work in medicine during the epidemic of severe acute respiratory syndrome (SARS) that spread from China to other countries between 2002 and 2004, but you have learned about it in medical school. You know that a coronavirus, called SARS CoV, caused SARS through "zoonotic" spread from bats to civets, the mammals that served as intermediary hosts, and then to humans. SARS had spread throughout east and southeast Asia and also to other countries such as Canada, causing thousands of deaths. You get worried that SARS or a similar infectious epidemic is starting again, so you share this information with medical colleagues who participate in a chat room and ask for feedback. Within days, police authorities accompanied by government public health officials detain you and force you to sign a statement confessing that you were spreading illegal rumors. Eventually COVID-19, caused by a new coronavirus, SARS-CoV-2, spreads rapidly through the population of Wuhan and surrounding areas, and later to nearly the entire world. On February 7, 2020, you die from the same disease at age 33. Later, the Chinese Communist Party exonerates you, apologizes to your family, and names you as a "martyr" of the COVID-19 pandemic.[3]

Dr. Li Wenliang was one among thousands of heroic health workers worldwide who have sacrificed their comfort, health, and lives during the COVID-19 pandemic on behalf of the individual patients and the populations they serve. So far, nurses in particular, but also nursing assistants, workers at nursing homes and other long-term care facilities, non-professional workers at hospitals, and other "essential" but lowly paid workers have suffered severe illness and death due to their exposure to SARS CoV-2. Often these workers' illnesses and deaths have resulted from inadequate personal protective equipment (PPE) and other dangerous work conditions inadequately addressed by employers and governments.[4]

Clinical medicine sometimes can become risky for practitioners, but when practitioners try to address the social dimensions of medical problems, their work and lives can become even riskier. The risks can include dangerous treatment by those who hold economic and political power in societies, because the social medicine perspective (as noted in the Preface) can reveal information that those in power rightfully experience as threatening. In later chapters, especially Chapters 8 and 10, we consider those risks in more depth.

On the other hand, epidemics like COVID-19 show why social medicine, despite its risks, is so important, because epidemics always contain crucial social components. Although some people have referred to the COVID-19 pandemic as an "equalizer," the inequalities in illness and death from COVID-19 actually have followed the same pattern as in other epidemics, and as in many other physical and mental health problems. The worst outcomes have happened in populations that are poor, from minority or indigenous ethnic backgrounds, and suffering from inadequate housing, nutrition, sanitation, discrimination, racism, and other social conditions of marginalization.

Although we previously had decided to begin this book with the hantavirus epidemic that severely impacted the Navajo Nation, COVID-19 has also devastated the same population. Geographically, the Navajo Nation spans the Four Corners area of four U.S. states: New Mexico, Arizona, Utah, and Colorado. As of late April 2020, the rate of COVID-19 per population within the Navajo Nation rose quickly to a level only slightly less than in the so-called "epicenters" of the pandemic in New York and New Jersey. By late May 2020, the infection rate in the Navajo Nation surpassed that of New York state, with 2,680 cases per 100,000 population compared to 1,890 in New York. The Navajo Nation's rate of infection was about ten times higher than the state of Arizona's.

In addition to the Navajo Nation, other indigenous populations have shown much higher risks for infection and mortality. For instance, while Navajo and other Native American communities accounted for about 11 percent of New Mexico's population, they made up 44 percent of the state's cases of confirmed coronavirus. Living conditions in these communities, especially lack of universal access to clean water and soap, made simple precautions like frequent handwashing difficult to implement. Availability of healthy food also remained problematic for these communities, leading to long-standing elevations of key risk factors for COVID-19 mortality such as diabetes, hypertension, and heart disease.

Such conditions emerged from a legacy of colonialism, where colonizers brought with them infectious diseases such as smallpox, cholera, measles, and typhoid, sometimes introduced intentionally into native communities as essentially genocidal practices. The resulting epidemics wiped out a large majority of the indigenous populations of the Americas. These patterns have affected indigenous communities not only in the Americas but also in other countries and continents, including Africa and Asia, where crowded housing, inadequate nutrition, and lack of clean water have fueled the COVID-19 pandemic.[5]

Inequalities in infection rates, illnesses, and mortality during the pandemic also have resulted from dangerous social conditions facing other minority or marginalized populations. African Americans and Latinx communities have suffered much higher rates of infection and death than predicted by their proportion in national or state populations. For instance, as of April 2020 in Illinois, 29 percent of confirmed COVID-19 cases and 41 percent of deaths occurred in people identified as African Americans, even though they comprised only 15 percent of the state's population. Similarly, in Michigan, where 14 percent of the state's population were African Americans, they accounted for 34 percent of confirmed cases and 40 percent of deaths. In the state of Washington, people identified as Latinx comprised 37 percent of confirmed COVID-19 cases, while the state's population included only 13 percent of Latinx people.[6]

The reasons for these higher rates of infection and death are similar to those affecting the Navajo Nation and other indigenous communities: stressful living and working conditions associated with poverty, discrimination, inadequate food and housing, and associated diseases like diabetes, hypertension, and heart disease that increase risk. Members of these minority groups, including undocumented workers, must work to receive survival wages, and they often receive categorization as "essential workers" in meat-packing plants, agriculture, construction, custodial jobs, low-level health work in hospitals and nursing homes, and other jobs that make social distancing extremely difficult.

In social medicine, the visions of "upstream" and "downstream" help us understand causes and effects of important health problems at different levels of analysis.[7] Inequalities of infection and death are "downstream" effects of "upstream" social conditions. These upstream conditions include poverty, discrimination, inadequate access to food and housing, unavailable clean water and sanitation, and similar challenges that play an important role in essentially all major epidemics in the past, present, and future. However, other important upstream causes of epidemics have arisen more recently during the last century through changes that human beings have created in our natural environments and in the industrial production of our food. In Chapter 3, we return to these upstream causes of the COVID-19 pandemic.

Another Outbreak: Typhus in Upper Silesia

Now let us turn back the clock to 1847 and consider the experience of a young German pathologist named Rudolf Virchow. During the winter of 1847–1848, a devastating famine affected the Prussian province of Upper Silesia.[8] There were reports of a typhus epidemic, and the Prussian government appointed Virchow to investigate the suspected outbreak. He visited Upper Silesia from February 20 to March 10, 1848, returning then to Berlin to write his report. He would look back later on these three weeks as being critical for the development of his approach to medicine and what we now consider as social medicine. His scientific mission led to very similar findings concerning social conditions and typhus as those a century and a half later during the hantavirus epidemic in the U.S. Southwest and COVID-19 worldwide.

Typhus causes flu-like symptoms, including fever and headache. Later a rash develops and, after that, inflammation of the brain, often leading to death. At the time of the epidemic in Upper Silesia, the cause of the infection was unknown. Much later, scientists determined that the cause was a bacterium, now called Rickettsia (named after the pathologist Howard Taylor Ricketts, who studied and eventually died from typhus in 1910). Body lice carry the bacteria from one person to another, usually within crowded and unsanitary housing.

Typhus, hantavirus syndromes, and COVID-19 are caused by infections. But if we want to look at the diseases more critically, the three diseases occur in a specific social context. This is what leads us to consider hanta, COVID-19, and typhus largely as "diseases of poverty."

While Virchow discussed the medical aspects of the epidemic in his report, he also undertook a much broader investigation that included factors such as geography, climate, natural resources, the local political structure, and the role of the church. In what was a very novel approach for its time, his medical analysis integrated both social and natural conditions. While the concept of infectious diseases was only just emerging, Virchow put the problem of epidemic typhus into the context of general living conditions, including housing, diet, sanitation, and education. He later wrote:

> This population had no idea that the mental and material impoverishment to which it had been allowed to sink were largely the cause of its hunger and disease, and that the adverse climatic conditions which contributed to the failure of its crops and to the sickness of its bodies, would not have caused such terrible ravages, if it had been free, educated and well-to-do. For there can now no longer be any doubt that such an epidemic dissemination of typhus had only been possible under the wretched conditions of life that poverty and lack of culture had created in Upper Silesia. If these conditions were removed, I am sure that epidemic typhus would not recur.[9]

Virchow went further, putting emphasis on political solutions to the epidemic and famine:

> Medicine has imperceptibly led us into the social field and placed us in a position of confronting directly the great problems of our time. Let it be well understood, it is no longer a question of treating one typhus patient or another by drugs or by the regulation of food, housing and clothing. Our task now consists in the culture of 1½ millions of our fellow citizens who are at the lowest level of moral and physical degradation. With 1½ million people, palliatives will no longer do. If we wish to take remedial action, we must be radical.[10]

In the final pages of his report, Virchow offered a detailed program for developing Upper Silesia that built on the concepts of education, liberty, and prosperity. He advocated economic development through activities such as road building and the promotion of manufacturing.

From Virchow's explicitly political and social approach, we might reconsider the question, "What are the real causes of hanta pulmonary syndrome, COVID-19, and typhus outbreaks?" Surely, these are diseases caused by specific infectious agents. But at the same time, they are also diseases of inadequate housing, poverty, political disenfranchisement, and oppression. It is this central insight, that disease is both a biological phenomenon and a manifestation of specific social conditions, that informs the work of social medicine. The Russian philosopher Georgi Plekhanov captured this combination of biological and social causation in his characteristically sharp style:

> Once the stomach has been supplied with a certain quantity of food, it sets about its work in accordance with the general laws of digestion. But can one, with the help of these laws, reply to the question of why savory and nourishing food descends every day into your stomach, while in mine it is a rare visitor? Do *these* laws explain why some eat so much, while others starve? It would seem that the explanation must be sought in some other sphere, in the working of some other kind of laws.[11]

We will return to Virchow again in Chapter 2.

Other Roots of Social Medicine

Healers probably always have had an intuitive understanding that poverty was associated with ill-health and, conversely, that the wealthy were in general healthier. However, in Europe during the seventeenth and eighteenth centuries, rulers began to pay closer attention to the physical well-being of their subjects. They were interested in maintaining a large standing army to defend their kingdoms and were concerned with controlling the plagues that periodically visited European towns. The Bills of Mortality in London – a record of burials – began in about 1592 as one of the oldest efforts to maintain vital statistics and records of interest to the royalty.[12]

Interest in population health grew in the early 1800s, especially concerning the health consequences of the Industrial Revolution. European cities were filling up with peasants from the countryside – they came attracted by the new industrial jobs to be found in the cities. Little provision was made for the housing and health of the new proletariat, and disease was rampant. This was the terrain on which modern social medicine developed. Social medicine typically (but not always) involved itself in promoting the well-being of the working class and did not limit its view to the treatment of disease – it sought to address the social causes of disease.

The term "social medicine" seems to have been generated independently by Jules Guerin in Paris and Rudolf Virchow in Berlin during the fateful year of European revolutions: 1848.[13] Over time, the field incorporated ideas from many other branches of science, including epidemiology, public health, engineering, and clinical medicine. The ideas of social medicine also traveled far afield from its European roots and have been implanted throughout the world. All of these factors make it difficult to offer one all-inclusive definition of social medicine.

George Rosen, a well-known historian of social medicine, never attempted to write a definition of the term.[14] Rather, he noted that most social medicine initiatives involved the acceptance of three general principles:

- Social and economic conditions profoundly impact health, disease, and the practice of medicine.
- The health of the population is a matter of social concern.
- Society should promote health through both individual and social means.

These principles are rather general, and their implementation depends to a great extent on the social context. For example, social medicine in Latin America today looks very different from contemporary social medicine in the United States. As a result, we see a diversity of initiatives inspired by social medicine ideas, not all of which identify themselves as social medicine. In the rest of this chapter, we explore the principles outlined by George Rosen in greater detail, and throughout this book, we examine not only how social and economic conditions cause disease but also how they shape our understandings about the nature of health, health care, and disease.

Social and Economic Conditions Impacting Health, Illness, and the Practice of Medicine

As noted above, scientists in the early 1800s sought to understand the impact of industrialization on the emerging working class. The growth of manufacturing towns had sparked a vivid debate: Were the new factories good or bad? This debate began on a large scale in England, where a distinct political philosophy known as Manchester Liberalism emerged in the industrial town of Manchester. The leaders of the Manchester School included John Bright, a politician, and Richard Cobden, an industrialist.[15] They argued that free trade and unregulated industry were both economically advantageous and morally justified. The government had no authority to regulate the economy; this would be done by the market.

This policy became known as laissez-faire: The market should be free of government interference. In the United States, laissez-faire economics was largely discredited by the Great Depression, when the government had to step in to rescue the national economy. But in recent decades, attacks on government regulation based on laissez-faire principles have become ever more virulent.

On the other side of this debate in Manchester stood the union movement, supported by progressive physicians like the sanitary reformer Dr. Southwood Smith. They fought for a shortened workday and limitations on the work of women and children. It was also in Manchester that Friedrich Engels, a colleague of Karl Marx, conducted his extensive studies in occupational and environmental health and the impact of capitalist business practices on the health of workers, their families, and their communities.[16] (In Chapter 2, we present more details about Engels's contributions.) Virchow and his colleagues in Germany had similar concerns, although a strong union movement did not develop in Germany until the second half of the nineteenth century.

Virchow theorized that there were "artificial epidemics" during which a generalized illness reflected a particular social imbalance: "Artificial epidemics ... are indicators of defects produced by political and social organization, and therefore affect predominately those classes that do not participate in the advantages of the culture."[17]

Virchow's linkage of social disruption to specific epidemics remains as relevant today as it was in the 1840s. Infectious disease epidemics such as hanta, COVID-19, HIV, and Ebola continue to illustrate the stark inequalities in the impact of infectious agents on populations around the world. Such social determination also shapes the occurrence of noninfectious, chronic diseases such as malnutrition and diabetes.

Virchow's passionate interest in the social causes of diseases and the profound social changes needed to address epidemics was not unusual for his time. But he would develop them further both during and after the revolutionary year of 1848 in his journal *Medical Reform*. His model of the engaged, politically active clinician continues to attract socially minded physicians and other health professionals to the present day. Chapter 2 presents in more depth Virchow's contributions to social medicine.

The Health of the Population as a Matter of Social Concern

Most economically developed societies have accepted the idea that the state has a responsibility for the health and welfare of its citizens. As the world's main economies matured, the ruling classes sought ways to pacify the working class without ceding real power. This process was pioneered by Prussian Chancellor Otto von Bismarck in the latter part of the nineteenth century. Bismarck's strategy began in 1876 with the legal recognition of the (previously) Independent Sickness Funds that workers had created as a form of "self-insurance." Seven years later, the 1883 Health Insurance Law mandated that all industrial workers have health insurance. The costs of this new system were shared by the industrialists (who paid two-thirds) and by the workers (who paid one-third). In 1984, a new law was passed making accident insurance mandatory. Over the next several decades, Germany would develop a national system of social welfare and a robust system of occupational health and safety laws. Some called this "state socialism," but the goal was clearly to defang the working proletariat by providing insurance for health services.[18]

Other European and many Latin American countries created similar systems of social insurance – universal access to health care, old-age pensions, disability insurance, and aid to families – that were based on the Bismarkian model. Often these programs were implemented to placate or to de-radicalize union movements. After World War I, social insurance became an accepted part of a modern society. However, since the Reagan and Thatcher "revolutions" in the 1980s, social insurance has been under attack by a neoliberal ideology that presents government programs as a form of servitude (the so-called nanny state).[19]

The United States, however, has followed a different path, as we will see in Chapter 5. During the Progressive Era (1890s–1920s), the country seemed to be following the European models, particularly Germany's. Theodore Roosevelt made the creation of a German-style welfare state part of his unsuccessful 1912 presidential campaign with the Progressive Party. It was a time when there was an active socialist movement. Support for a mandatory health program that would build on existing union sickness funds led to legislative proposals in both New York and California that aimed to create compulsory health insurance for workers. Both proposals failed, and when the United States entered World War I in 1917, Germany became an enemy to be feared rather than a model to be emulated.

Attempts to develop social insurance programs, however, continued throughout the twentieth century. Major advances were made under the administration of Franklin D. Roosevelt, with the adoption of social security and laws that facilitated union organizing. In his 1941 State of the Union speech (also known as "the four freedoms speech"), Roosevelt spoke of freedom of speech, freedom of worship, freedom from want, and freedom from fear. In the speech, he announced programs creating equality of opportunity for youth, jobs for those who could work, social security for those who needed it, ending special privileges for the few, and the preservation of civil liberties for all.[20] Roosevelt died before realizing his vision.

In the 1960s, health care came back onto the national agenda. It was a time of civil unrest manifested by the civil rights movement and opposition to the war in Vietnam. President Lyndon Johnson brokered a series of laws that would radically change the United States. Among these laws were the Voting Rights Act (which began to address the denial of voting rights for African Americans), the Clean Air Act, the War on Poverty, the Fair Immigration Law, and both Medicare and Medicaid. Medicare provided health care for all citizens over 65 and to persons with disabilities. Medicaid, a joint federal–state program, provided health care to the poor.

Despite fierce opposition from the American Medical Association, Medicare proved very profitable for the medical community. As the proportion of seniors with health care insurance rose from about half in 1965 to nearly all by 1967, doctors' incomes increased. Between 1967 and 1984, Medicare payments rose at an annual rate of nearly 17 percent.[21] Hospitals benefitted not only from the income generated through providing services to the newly insured elderly but also from the direct subsidization provided by Medicare for medical education. Essentially, Medicare assumed the cost of training specialist physicians, thus opening up yet another revenue stream for academic medical centers.

But the massive amounts of money that were now flowing from the federal government did not lead to a comprehensive health care system. Instead, a "medical industrial complex" (MIC) emerged – a network of academic medical centers, often controlling smaller local hospitals and allied with medical industries (such as pharmaceutical and medical equipment companies), insurance companies, and the U.S. government. These power players and their allies in Congress argued that health care was not a human right but instead a commodity to be bought and sold like any other commodity. The goal, harkening back to Manchester Liberalism, was to create a health care market that would operate without interference by the government despite extensive tax-generated government funding.

There were, however, some major problems with the idea of health care as a commodity to be bought and sold in a market governed by laissez-faire principles. First, health care consumers rarely have the necessary information on which to base decisions about which course of action they would prefer. Second, health care consumers rarely pay for services directly; instead, an insurance company or the federal government pays the bills, and patients' contributions are channeled through co-payments, insurance premiums, and taxes. This means that to some extent patients are protected from the full costs of the care they receive. The laws of supply and demand do not operate in health care because consumers are not incentivized to be "prudent, discriminating purchasers."[22] Finally, doctors make most of the decisions in health care through their recommendations to patients, leading to what is called "derived demand."

Despite these concerns, the concept of health care as a commodity has become the dominant ideological model in U.S. politics. Although activists have pushed for extending the Medicare system to the entire population, funds continue to flow from corporations in the MIC into the hands of the lobbyists, who then pass them on to members of Congress. In 2017, four of the top six lobbying groups in Washington were health related: Pharmaceutical Research and Manufacturers of America (PhRMA, $19.9 million in Congressional campaign contributions), Blue Cross/Blue Shield ($17.8 million), the American Medical Association ($17.4 million), and the American Hospital Association ($16.4 million). This money goes mainly to defend the idea of health care as commodity.[23]

The result is that the United States stands alone among economically developed countries in not having a universal health program. By 2007, medical expenses had become the most frequent reason for personal bankruptcy.[24] At the time of this writing, about 30 million people in the United States remain uninsured, and at least twice that number are underinsured[25] – numbers that many consider a national disgrace. In other developed countries, these problems simply do not exist. And the problem is not lack of money; in fact, the United States spends far more on health care than any other developed country. What do we get for all this money? Our health outcomes are not outstanding. For instance, life expectancy in the United States for a girl born in 2016 was 81.1 years and for a boy 76.1 years; these results put the Unites States 27th in rank among the 36 members of the Organization of Economic Cooperation and Development (OECD).[26]

The 2008 Affordable Care Act (ACA, also known as Obamacare) represented a modest attempt to address this situation. This law reduced the number of uninsured Americans but increased the number of underinsured people and conserved the highly inefficient system of private insurance that makes health care so expensive. We consider Obamacare and alternatives to it further in Chapter 10.

Promoting Health through Both Social and Individual Means

The Alma Ata Declaration: primary health care for all. In 1978, the World Health Organization (WHO) convened a meeting in Alma Ata, Kazakhstan, within the Soviet Union. The Alma Ata conference would trace an expansive agenda of public health and "Primary Health Care for All" by the year 2000. Ministers of health came from countries around the world to discuss participation by communities in the solution of their own health problems. The resultant "Declaration of AlmaAta" embodied many of the ideals of the community health movement and also critical social medicine.[27] The declaration reaffirmed WHO's holistic definition of health as "a state of complete physical, mental and social wellbeing, and not merely the absence of disease or infirmity." The declaration signaled that the "existing gross inequality in health" was unacceptable, that people have a right to participate in the organization and implementation of health care, and that primary care should be universally available. Finally, the conference stated:

> A main social target of governments, international organizations and the whole world community in the coming decades should be the attainment by all peoples of the world by the year 2000 of a level of health that will permit them to lead a socially and economically productive life. Primary health care is the key to attaining this target as part of development in the spirit of social justice.[28]

In the rest of this chapter, we will consider some of the experiences that led to and followed from this declaration.

Community-oriented primary care (COPC). COPC emerged as one model for integrating clinical medicine and community health. First developed in South Africa during the 1940s by Doctors Sidney and Emily Kark, this model later contributed to the design of community health centers (CHCs) in the United States and other countries.

The Karks began with the assumption that their patient was not simply the person who walked into their clinic with a problem. They saw their patient as being the entire community. Here is how Dr. Sidney Kark explained his understanding of social medicine:

> The old-time village doctor might well be regarded as a practitioner of social medicine whose major area of practice was within [the community]. It was no doubt his close relationship with the families of the communities among whom he practised that gave meaning to the title 'family doctor'. His action in relation to family and community health was based upon his life experience in the community, the familiarity of daily association giving him an understanding of people's needs.[29]

This definition suggests that for a practitioner of social medicine, clinical activities are informed by a social understanding in a very naturalistic way. It is just part of good doctoring to know the community where you work.

The Karks' model of social medicine was embodied in the cycle shown in Figure 1.1.

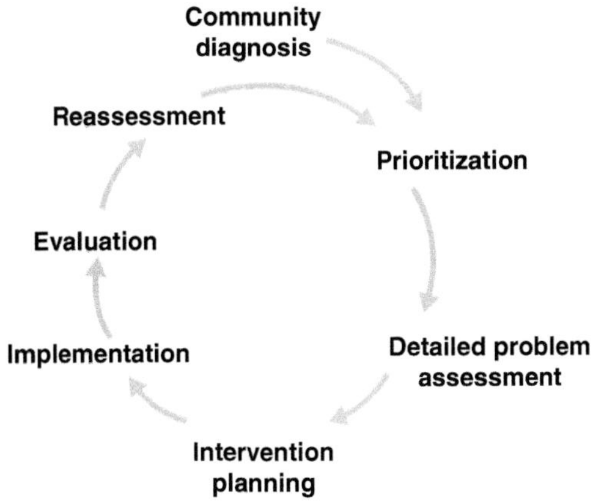

Figure 1.1 Sidney and Emily Kark's model of social medicine in community-oriented primary care.

As shown in Figure 1.1, the first step was to make a diagnosis of the major health care problems in the community. This task was often done by conducting a house-to-house survey. One could then make a diagnosis of the community's most important problems and needs. With participation by members of the community, problems were then prioritized. A detailed assessment of the most important needs was made and was followed by a plan to address these needs. Implementation of community interventions based on the needs assessment then led to a thorough evaluation of the interventions and reassessment of the community's needs; the evaluation and reassessment were key steps for the Karks and people in the communities they served. At this point, the process began anew.[30] Interventions did not necessarily involve medical care. Digging latrines or creating vegetable gardens were concrete means to solve health problems; yet they did not always involve clinical services.

During the early 1960s, Dr. Jack Geiger, who had studied with the Karks, imported the COPC model to the United States. Collaborating with low-income and marginalized communities, Geiger and his colleagues created the first two COPC-style CHCs at Boston's Columbia Point housing project and in Mount Bayou, Mississippi (Figure 1.2).[31] Key to the success of these clinics was the hiring of community organizers who served as a bridge between the communities and the health professionals. The success of these programs provided models and inspiration for the more than 1,400 federally funded CHCs that currently exist in the United States.[32]

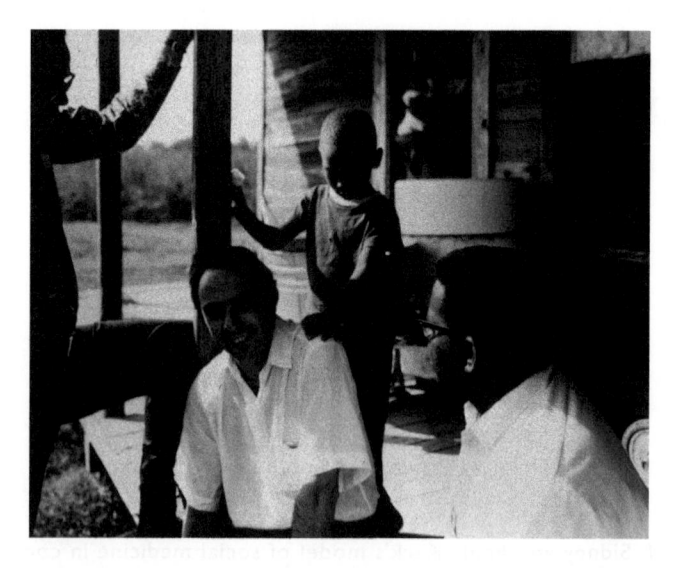

Figure 1.2 Dr. H. Jack Geiger and Dr. John Hatch with people served by an early community health center.

Ninety miles from Miami: the Cuban health system. Cuba, some 90 miles south of the United States, has developed a health care system that has fostered community participation and has served as a model of social medicine for many countries. After the Cuban revolution ended in 1959, many doctors fled the country, and Cuba faced an acute shortage of physicians. In 1960, most of the professors at the country's only medical school, the University of Havana, resigned rather than accept a plan to give students a role in governing the school. Ironically, the decline of the traditional medical establishment allowed the new revolutionary government to undertake a fundamental restructuring of medical education. This shift would serve as a prelude for a reform of the health care system. Young health care professionals now grew up with a new vision of what it meant to address the health of the nation. This vision emphasized preventive care, primary care, and reducing inequalities in access to health services. Similar improvements occurred in Cuba's medical research infrastructure and in the technical quality of its health services. Cuba deliberately located new medical schools outside Havana. This approach allowed local students access to local medical education; the hope was that they eventually would practice in the areas where they were trained. This educational investment produced impressive results, which are reflected in the country's health statistics.

Primary care strongly anchors the Cuban health care system. A physician and a nurse live in a community of approximately 800 people and staff a small office (*consultorio*) where they see patients for half the day. They devote the other half of their workday to home visits. For cases that cannot be treated at the level of the *consultorio*, the country has developed a network of polyclinics located throughout the country, where specialists provide outpatient care. Referral hospitals receive patients with more complex problems. The system has produced excellent health outcomes. According to the World Bank, in 2018 there were 8.4 physicians per 1,000 population in Cuba, compared with 2.6 per 1,000 in the United States. Cuba's infant mortality rate was 4 per 1,000 live births, outperforming the United States with 6 infant deaths per 1,000 live births. The Cuban life expectancy equaled that of the United States (79 years as of 2018), a surprising achievement considering Cuba's much lower level of economic development.[33]

Latin American social medicine (LASM). The Cuban experience is one part of a much larger effort in critical social medicine that continues to evolve in many countries of Latin America. Latin Americans have developed a rich body of theoretical and practical work examining the relationships between health and society.[34] This work emphasizes "praxis": the close relationship between theory and practice. Until recently, due to language barriers, little of the work of LASM has been available in English. This book, in fact, is a small effort to break down some of the linguistic barriers to the exchange of ideas between the global North and global South. Indeed, thousands of practitioners, researchers, and activists from around the world participate in the Latin American Social Medicine Association (Asociación Latinoamericana de Medicina Social, ALAMES) and the Brazilian Association of Collective Health (Associação Brasileira de Saúde Coletiva, ABRASCO).

LASM takes a critical stance toward traditional thinking in medicine and public health. Rather than seeing disease as an isolated state or event, LASM emphasizes the "health–illness dialectic," a concept that expresses the fluid, complex, and ever-changing relationship between the normal and the pathological. This dialectic evolves within a social context that leads to distinct social patterns of diseases and to distinct explanatory models. Debora Tajer, a leading LASM researcher, has described the unique characteristics of LASM in these terms:

- A conceptual framework within the field of public health called *social medicine* or, in Brazil, *collective health* that highlights the economic, political, subjective, and social determinants of the health-disease-care process of human collectivities.
- A political dimension represented by the attempts at political change and social transformation in Latin America, started in the 1950s, that valued the improvement of health status and equitable access to health services as essential pillars of the liberation of the people.
- A view of the concept of subjectivity that is theoretically and practically based on the Marxist tradition that considers the subject as historically conditioned and at the same time a maker of history, and that values political practice as a promoter of solidary subjectivities.[35]

Chapter 8 considers LASM in more depth.

New models of health care in the United States during the 1960s and 1970s. During those years, the dominant medical models drew increasing questions and criticisms. Many came to see medicine as complicit with a large MIC that reinforced existing institutions and power structures. Health served as a vehicle for questioning the system and a way of exploring alternatives. Several creative achievements emerged with close ties to critical social medicine.

The women's movement challenged the control exercised over their bodies by predominately male gynecologists. This challenge emerged in books such as *Our Bodies, Our Selves*, which offered women a chance to understand and care for their own bodies, rather than relying solely on medical professionals.[36] The book took a critical view of capitalism and created a tool that would be open and evolving.

Women began to challenge obstetric practices, and a new generation of midwives promoted alternatives to hospital births. In self-help groups, women learned the anatomy of their bodies as a route to empowerment. Women's clinics initiated more egalitarian ways of providing care – women were encouraged to learn about their bodies and then transmit this knowledge to others.

Beginning in the 1960s, the Black Panther Party developed a thoughtful and ambitious approach to health care. The Panthers created strong community programs grounded in self-defense, health care, and education. Activists in the party carried out mass screening for sickle cell disease, distributed food, initiated programs to feed children, established daycare centers, and set up free clinics and a free ambulance service. These programs achieved a national reach but did not survive, partly due to fierce repression that targeted the group. This repression included the infamous "Cointelpro" campaign run by the Federal Bureau of Investigation with the specific purpose of destroying the party.[37]

The Medical Committee for Human Rights (MCHR), created in 1964, initially provided physicians as witnesses and human shields who were trained as observers of the civil rights marches and other protests in the southern United States. By the end of the decade, MCHR was providing medical services for large demonstrations against the Vietnam War and also for draft resisters and military service members who opposed the war. Although MCHR disbanded during the 1970s, when the next wave of large protests began with the Seattle uprising against globalization in 1999, a national network of street medics provided similar medical services. MCHR was the most prominent but not the only medical civil rights group; many other health professionals with a perspective of critical social medicine worked against war and for civil rights.[38]

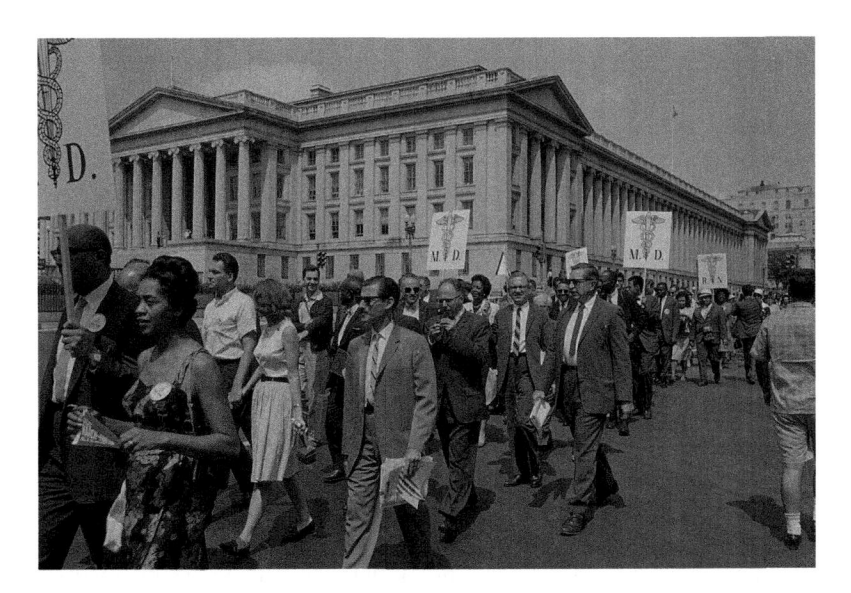

Figure 1.3 Demonstration in Washington, DC, organized by the Medical Committee for Human Rights.

The neoliberal retreat from Alma Ata. The 1978 Alma Ata meeting was both the pinnacle of the community health movement and the beginning of its decline. When Margaret Thatcher (1979) and Ronald Reagan (1980) won elections in the United Kingdom and the United States, respectively, the world began a turn to the right. The union movement came under sharp attack, as did the institutions of the welfare state. Neoliberalism, a policy that favored "free market" economic activities with reduced regulation by governments as well as cutbacks and privatization of public services, became the dominant economic policy throughout the world.

This change exerted an enormous impact on health care systems. Many government systems – modeled on Bismarck's reforms in Germany – had been universal, comprehensive, and cost free at the point where services were delivered. Such systems now were considered too expensive, particularly for poor countries. In 1979, Walsh and Warren published an article advocating "selective primary health care," a strategy that limited health care to a set of supposedly cost-effective interventions rather than comprehensive care.[39] This model advanced in less wealthy countries of Latin America and other regions, where having health insurance increasingly meant coverage with a limited panel of services. Sometimes this policy led to contradictory situations in which, for example, screening for cervical cancer was covered, while treatment for cervical cancer was not.

Limitation of clinical services accompanied disease-specific initiatives, such as the under-financed Global Fund to Fight AIDS, Tuberculosis and Malaria. Such "vertical" programs address only one problem. "Horizontal" programs, such as comprehensive primary care, address many problems at the same time. Funding agencies, including international financial institutions and large foundations, favored vertical programs because they were thought to provide better data on outcomes and were simpler to organize. But for recipient countries, vertical programs with external funding often disrupted other initiatives that received less funding but might have achieved more profound effects on health outcomes. Vertical programs generally led to a recipient country's loss of autonomy in creating and maintaining comprehensive horizontal programs.

The period between 1990 and 2010 also saw a boom of health initiatives funded by wealthy donors such as the Bill and Melinda Gates Foundation. The Gates Foundation currently is estimated to be the second largest donor to WHO – preceded by the U.S. government and followed by the United Kingdom. The 2006 gift of $30 billion to the Gates Foundation by Warren Buffett prompted Gates to remark: "It was the biggest gift anyone's ever given for anything."[40] In comparison, WHO's total budget is only about $4.5 billion.[41] Gates and Buffett have made arrangements so that after their deaths their money does not go to national governments as taxes. Instead, ultra-rich individuals spend huge sums of money on their pet interests without any social accountability and with substantial tax benefits. This form of "philanthrocapitalism" has become yet another element of the retreat from the universalism of Alma Ata.[42]

Why Is Critical Social Medicine Relevant Now?

For those of us working in critical social medicine, the fundamental flaw of neoliberal health care reforms, including the ACA and some of its potential replacements, is that health care is seen as a commodity and not as a right. The market orientation puts health care under pressure to produce profits, and this pressure goes counter to providing good, inexpensive, and universal health care. Market-oriented health care has not achieved any notable success in improving quality and reducing costs.

Market reforms have not provided universal, affordable, high-quality health care, nor are they likely to do so. Efforts to create a universal system, including Obamacare, have not been successful in the United States despite a hundred years of advocacy. As we discuss in Chapter 10, this failure contrasts starkly with the achievement of universal systems in all other economically developed countries. Virchow argued that "physicians surely are the natural advocates of the poor and the social problem largely falls within their scope."[43] Many contemporary physicians and other health workers have taken up this stance as part of their professional identities. Critical social medicine can guide the struggle toward a universal system in the United States, as it continues to do in other countries. The struggle toward a universal health care system must accompany a struggle to change the broader social conditions that foster illness and early death.

Notes

1 The Spanish conquistadors used the term "Navajo" to refer to the geographical location where the Diné people lived. In the Navajo Nation, people usually prefer the term Diné to refer to themselves. Diné also refers to their language. Because the term Navajo has been used legally in the United States and is more widely known, we reluctantly decided to use that term rather than the preferred Diné in this book.
2 Centers for Disease Control and Prevention, "Hantavirus," January 31, 2019, www.cdc.gov/hantavirus/index.html.
3 Chris Buckley, "Chinese Doctor, Silenced after Warning of Outbreak, Dies from Coronavirus," *New York Times*, February 7, 2020, https://www.nytimes.com/2020/02/06/world/asia/chinese-doctor-Li-Wenliang-coronavirus.html; Elliot Hannon, "Rare Public Anger in China After Silenced Doctor Who Warned of Coronavirus Dies of the Virus," *Slate*, February 7, 2020, https://slate.com/news-and-politics/2020/02/china-doctor-li-dies-coronavirus-whistleblower-public-anger-dissent.html; Andrew Green,

"Li Wenliang," *Lancet*, February 29, 2020, https://www.thelancet.com/journals/lancet/article/PIIS0140-6736(20)30382-2/fulltext. For comprehensive information supportive of the Chinese government's response, see Tricontinental: Institute for Social Research, "Coronashock No. 1: China and Coronashock," April 2020, https://www.thetricontinental.org/wp-content/uploads/2020/04/20200427_CoronaShock_1_EN_Web.pdf.

4 Peter Kenny, "90,000 Healthcare Workers Infected with COVID-19: ICN," Anadolu Agency, May 6, 2020, https://www.aa.com.tr/en/europe/90-000-healthcare-workers-infected-with-covid-19-icn/1831765#; Sarah Marsh, "Doctors, Nurses, Porters, Volunteers: the UK Health Workers Who Have Died from COVID-19," *The Guardian*, May 22, 2020, https://www.theguardian.com/world/2020/apr/16/doctors-nurses-porters-volunteers-the-uk-health-workers-who-have-died-from-covid-19; National Nurses United, "Honor Fallen Nurses," May 2020, https://honorfallennurses.org/nurses-weve-lost/.

5 For recent journalism on the impact of COVID-19 in Indian Country: Simon Romero, "How New Mexico, One of the Poorest States, Averted a Steep Death Toll," *New York Times*, April 24, 2020, https://www.nytimes.com/2020/04/24/us/coronavirus-new-mexico.html; Delilah Friedler, "Navajo Nation Is Behind Only New York and New Jersey in Rates of COVID-19 Infection," *Mother Jones*, May 5, 2020, https://www.motherjones.com/politics/2020/05/navajo-nation-covid-outbreak-deaths/; Kalen Goodluck, "Every Corner of the Navajo Nation Has Been Hit By COVID-19," *Mother Jones*, May 21, 2020, https://www.motherjones.com/politics/2020/05/every-corner-of-the-navajo-nation-has-been-hit-by-covid-19/; Nina Lakhani, "Why Native Americans Took COVID-19 Seriously: 'It's Our Reality,'" *The Guardian*, May 26, 2020, https://www.theguardian.com/us-news/2020/may/26/native-americans-coronavirus-impact. For an in-depth historical analysis of biological warfare directed against indigenous communities in what are now the United States of America: Elizabeth A. Fenn, "Biological Warfare in Eighteenth-Century North America: Beyond Jeffery Amherst," *Journal of American History* 86, no. 4 (March 2000): 1552–80. Published by Oxford University Press on behalf of Organization of American Historians, https://www.jstor.org/stable/2567577. For more on genocidal practices toward indigenous communities: Roxanne Dunbar-Ortiz, *An Indigenous Peoples' History of the United States* (Boston, MA: Beacon Press, 2014); Roxanne Dunbar-Ortiz and Dina Gilio-Whitaker, "The United States Did Not Have a Policy of Genocide," in *"All the Real Indians Died Off" and 20 Other Myths About Native Americans* (Boston, MA: Beacon Press, 2016); Gerald Horne, *The Apocalypse of Settler Colonialism: The Roots of Slavery, White Supremacy, and Capitalism in Seventeenth-Century North America and the Caribbean* (New York: Monthly Review Press, 2017).

6 Elizabeth Cooney, "'We're Flying Blind': African Americans May Be Bearing the Brunt of Covid-19, But Access to Data is Limited," *StatNews*, April 6, 2020, https://www.statnews.com/2020/04/06/flying-blind-african-americans-disparities-covid-19-data-limited/. See also "Coronavirus Disease 2019 (COVID-19): Racial and Ethnic Minority Groups," Centers for Disease Control and Prevention (CDC), April 22, 2020, https://www.cdc.gov/coronavirus/2019-ncov/need-extra-precautions/racial-ethnic-minorities.html; Clyde W. Yancy, "COVID-19 and African Americans," *JAMA* 323, no. 19 (May 19, 2020): 1891–92, https://jamanetwork.com/journals/jama/fullarticle/2764789; Washington State Department of Health, "2019 Novel Coronavirus Outbreak (COVID-19)," May 24, 2020, https://www.doh.wa.gov/Emergencies/Coronavirus.

7 For details on the upstream-downstream vision, see Howard Waitzkin, "John D. Stoeckle and the Upstream Vision of Social Determinants in Public Health," *American Journal of Public Health* 106, no. 2 (February 2016): 234–36.
8 Most of this territory today belongs to Poland.
9 Rudolf Virchow, *Collected Essays on Public Health and Epidemiology*, volume 1, edited by L. J. Rather (Boston, MA: Science History Publications, 1985), pp. 204–319.
10 Virchow, *Collected Essays on Public Health and Epidemiology*. Also cited in: Rudolf Virchow, "Report on the Typhus Epidemic in Upper Silesia," *American Journal of Public Health* 96, no. 12 (December 2006): 2102–05.
11 Georgi Plekhanov, *The Development of the Monist View of History* (New York: International Publishers, 1947), p. 188.
12 Kristin Heitman, "Of Counts and Causes: The Emergence of the London Bills of Mortality," *The Collation: Research and Exploration at the Folger*, http://collation.folger.edu/2018/03/counts-causes-london-bills-mortality/.
13 Juan César García, "Juan César García Entrevista a Juan César García," *Medicina Social* 2 (2007): 153–59, www.medicinasocial.info/index.php/medicinasocial/article/viewFile/132/269.
14 George Rosen, "What Is Social Medicine? A Genetic Analysis of the Concept," *Bulletin of the History of Medicine* 21 (1947): 674–733.
15 Norman Davies, *Europe: A History* (New York: Oxford University Press, 1996), pp. 803 ff.
16 Friedrich Engels, *The Condition of the Working Class in England in 1844* (Moscow: Progress Publishers, 1973 [1845]).
17 Cited in George Rosen, *From Medical Police to Social Medicine* (New York: Science History Publications, 1974).
18 Adam Gaffney, *To Heal Humankind: The Right to Health in History* (New York: Routledge, 2017), chapter 4; Lorraine Boissoneault, "Bismarck Tried to End Socialism's Grip—By Offering Government Healthcare," *Smithsonian Magazine*, July 14, 2017, https://www.smithsonianmag.com/history/bismarck-tried-end-socialisms-grip-offering-government-healthcare-180964064/.
19 Gaffney, *To Heal Humankind*, chapters 5 and 7.
20 Franklin D. Roosevelt, "1941 State of the Union Address: 'The Four Freedoms,'" January 6, 1941. http://voicesofdemocracy.umd.edu/fdr-the-four-freedoms-speech-text/.
21 Margaret H. Davis and Sally T. Burner, "Three Decades of Medicare: What the Numbers Tell Us," *Health Affairs* 14, no. 4 (1995): 231–43.
22 Arnold S. Relman, "The New Medical-Industrial Complex," *New England Journal of Medicine* 303, no. 17 (1980): 963–70. Although most sources cite Relman as the source of the term "medical industrial complex," it actually originated from the Health Policy Advisory Center. For more on the MIC: Robb Burlage and Matthew Anderson, "The Transformation of the Medical Industrial Complex: Financialization, the Corporate Sector, and Monopoly Capital," in Howard Waitzkin and the Working Group on Health beyond Capitalism, *Health Care under the Knife: Moving beyond Capitalism for Our Health* (New York: Monthly Review Press, 2018).
23 OpenSecrets.org: Center for Responsive Politics, "Top Spenders," www.opensecrets.org/lobby/top.php?indexType=s&showYear=2017, accessed August 27, 2018.
24 David U. Himmelstein, Elizabeth Warren, Deborah Thorne, and Steffie Woolhandler, "Medical Bankruptcy in the United States, 2007: Results of a National Study," *American Journal of Medicine* 122 (2009): 741–46.
25 Robin A. Cohen, Emily P. Zammitti, and Michael E. Martinez, "Health Insurance Coverage: Early Release of Estimates from the National Health

Interview Survey, 2017, National Center for Health Statistics, 2018, www.cdc.gov/nchs/data/nhis/earlyrelease/insur201805.pdf, accessed July 7, 2018.
26 OECD Data, "Life Expectancy at Birth," https://data.oecd.org/healthstat/life-expectancy-at-birth.htm.
27 World Health Organization, "Declaration of Alma-Ata: International Conference on Primary Health Care," Alma-Ata, USSR, September 6–12, 1978, www.who.int/publications/almaata_declaration_ en.pdf; Fran Baum, "Health for All Now! Reviving the Spirit of Alma Ata in the Twenty-First Century: An Introduction to the Alma Ata Declaration," *Social Medicine* 2, no. 1 (2007): 34–41.
28 World Health Organization, "Declaration of Alma-Ata."
29 Sidney Kark and Guy W. Steuart, eds., *A Practice of Social Medicine: A South African Team's Experiences in Different African Communities* (Edinburgh and London: E&S Livingstone Ltd., 1962), pp. 3–4.
30 Jane Westberg, "An Interview of Jaime Gofin, a Promoter of COPC," *Education for Health* 19, no. 2 (July 2006): 256–63, https://pdfs.semanticscholar.org/9e8f/85cb0d0c1866beeefafb7e3d75f440e6c0cb.pdf.
31 *Out in the Rural* is a film that captures the COPC vision in Mississippi, https://vimeo.com//118063052.
32 Tory Waldron, "How Many Federally Qualified Health Centers Are There?" The Definitive Blog, July 1, 2019, https://blog.definitivehc.com/how-many-fqhcs-are-there; "About Community Health Centers," National Association of Community Health Centers, *Community Health Center Chartbook, 2020*, https://www.nachc.org/wp-content/uploads/2020/01/Chartbook-2020-Final.pdf.
33 World Bank, "Physicians Per 1000 People," https://data.worldbank.org/indicator/SH.MED.PHYS.ZS; "Mortality Rate, Infant (Per 1,000 Live Births)," https://data.worldbank.org/indicator/SP.DYN.IMRT.IN; "Life Expectancy at Birth, Total (Years)," https://data.worldbank.org/indicator/SP.DYN.LE00.IN.
34 For references, please see Chapter 8.
35 Debora Tajer, "Latin American Social Medicine: Roots, Development during the 1990s, and Current Challenges," *American Journal of Public Health* 93, no. 12 (2003): 2023–27.
36 Our Bodies, Ourselves, "History," www.ourbodiesourselves.org/our-story/history/.
37 Alondra Nelson, *Body and Soul: The Black Panther Party and the Fight against Medical Discrimination* (Minneapolis: University of Minnesota Press, 2011).
38 John Dittmer, *The Good Doctors: The Medical Committee for Human Rights and the Struggle for Social Justice in Health Care* (Jackson: University Press of Mississippi, 2017).
39 Julia A. Walsh and Kenneth S. Warren, "Selective Primary Health Care, an Interim Strategy for Disease Control in Developing Countries," *New England Journal of Medicine* 301 (1979): 967–74.
40 Ben Paynter, "Warren Buffet Gave Bill Gates $30 Billion: Here's How It's Paying Off," *Business Breaking News*, last updated February 14, 2017, www.fastcompany.com/3068134/warren-buffet-gave-bill-gates-30-billion-heres-how-its-paying-off.
41 World Health Organization, "Programme Budget 2018–2019," http://open.who.int/2018-19/budget-and-financing/summary.
42 Anne-Emanuelle Birn and Judith Richter, "U.S. Philanthrocapitalism and the Global Health Agenda: The Rockefeller and Gates Foundations, Past and

Present," in Howard Waitzkin and the Working Group on Health beyond Capitalism, *Health Care under the Knife: Moving beyond Capitalism for Our Health* (New York: Monthly Review Press, 2018).
43 Virchow, *Collected Essays on Public Health and Epidemiology*, vol. 1, p. 4.

Chapter 2

One and Half Centuries of Forgetting and Remembering the Social Origins of Illness

> And as a doctor I suffered from two very difficult diseases. I was only beginning to make my way as a surgeon when I came down with a bad case of tuberculosis.... My second "sickness"...well, that wasn't so simple.... I came to understand that tuberculosis was not merely a disease of the body but a social crime.... I have learned what must be done to cure this second sickness.
> – Norman Bethune, M.D., surgeon to the liberation forces of China, 1939[1]

Norman Bethune, a Canadian surgeon, provided an early inspiration for social medicine, both internationally and in the United States. In his work with poor and marginalized patients in Detroit, Bethune became infected by tuberculosis.[2] Bethune saw clearly, as do most people who dedicate their work to social medicine, that social conditions often lie behind medical disorders. Without addressing these illness-generating social conditions, health professionals frequently find that the impact of their work remains limited, unfulfilling, and not fully effective. Bethune analyzed tuberculosis first as an infection of the body but secondly as a disease of society. He argued that the cure of tuberculosis in China and many other countries of the world required fundamental changes in the social conditions that generate illness. Bethune's understanding of the "second sickness" became a focus of subsequent work in social medicine and the title of a book written to clarify collective action toward change.[3]

The conditions of society that generate illness and mortality have become largely forgotten and rediscovered with each new generation. Now, when social conditions create environmental catastrophes, risk of nuclear war, and other dangers that threaten the survival of humanity and other life forms, it is not surprising that such problems again would start to receive attention. There is a long history of research and analysis about the relationships among political economic systems, the social determination of health, and the health of populations.[4] This work has remained largely overlooked, despite its importance now. During our current period of history, as such problems have become ever more critical, it is important to look back and to learn.

How This Viewpoint Emerged

There are many modern-day heroes who have taken up social medicine as their cause[5]; yet, they are not the first to point out the social determination of health. Three people – Friedrich Engels, Rudolf Virchow, and Salvador Allende – made major contributions to understanding the social origins of illness under capitalism and empire. Although other writers also have examined this topic,[6] the works of Engels, Virchow, and Allende are important in several respects. All three writers emphasized political economic systems as causes of illness-generating social conditions. Engels and Virchow provided analyses of the impact of political economic conditions on health that essentially created the perspective of social medicine. Both men were active during the tumultuous years of the 1840s and both took decisive – though divergent – personal actions to correct the conditions they described through political economic change. Allende's key work appeared

TUBERCULOSIS VERSUS COVID-19

Because social conditions have affected sickness and death from tuberculosis and COVID-19 so profoundly, the question arises: How do these two diseases compare in their impacts on human populations? We won't know the answer for a while, but the available data so far indicate that tuberculosis has greater adverse impacts than COVID-19. In the first five months of 2020, about 6 million cases of COVID-19 were diagnosed, and about 367,000 deaths attributed to COVID-19 occurred worldwide (Johns Hopkins COVID-19 Dashboard, https://coronavirus.jhu.edu/map.html). Most researchers in the field believe that these figures are underestimates due to incomplete testing.

During 2017, about 10 million new cases of tuberculosis were diagnosed worldwide, with 1.6 million deaths (World Health Organization, Global Health Observatory, https://www.who.int/gho/tb/epidemic/cases_deaths/en/). Tuberculosis is an ongoing epidemic, in which roughly the same or more new cases and deaths happen each year. The COVID-19 pandemic may extend beyond one year, but that scenario is not very likely. If tuberculosis leads to about the same magnitude of illness and death every year as COVID-19 does in a single year, why does COVID-19 generate so much more attention and fear? What do you think?

(Continued)

> Hint: Tuberculosis threatens poorer countries of the global South much more than richer countries of the global North. COVID-19 threatens richer countries of the global North also, even though its overall impact also will become more devastating in poorer countries of the global South. We will talk more about more how social medicine analyzes such differences between the global South and global North, including the challenges of infectious diseases like tuberculosis and COVID-19, as the book proceeds.

during a later historical period, the 1930s, and in a different geopolitical context. While Engels and Virchow documented the impact of early capitalism, largely before the expansion of empire, Allende focused on empire and the underdevelopment of health in countries affected by empire. Although little known in North America and Western Europe, Allende's studies in social medicine have influenced efforts to achieve political economic changes that improve health conditions in Latin America and elsewhere in the "global South."[7]

While Engels, Virchow, and Allende all connected health, capitalism, and empire, they also diverged in major ways, especially regarding the structures of oppression that cause disease, the social contradictions that inhibit change, and directions of reform that would foster health rather than illness. A look at their work clarifies issues that today gain even more urgency. This work has influenced a new generation of practitioners, researchers, teachers, and activists, who also focus in large part on political economic systems as social determinants of health and illness.

Before considering these pioneers' work, we want to explain briefly why we are using the term "social origins" in this chapter and "social determination" versus "social determinants" in the next two chapters. During the last 20 years or so, the term "social determinants of health" has become more widely used in studies about the associations between social conditions and health. Because research on social determinants usually refers to associations between social characteristics of individuals and their health experiences, the deeper mechanisms by which social conditions cause illness and early death often remain unclear. For that reason, scientists and activists have criticized the term "social determinants" and have preferred the term "social determination," which refers to the deeper processes by which social conditions cause unfavorable health outcomes. We explain these distinctions further in the next two chapters. In this chapter, we are using the terms "social origins" or "social causes," which during the last two centuries usually have referred to the deeper mechanisms by which social conditions affect health.

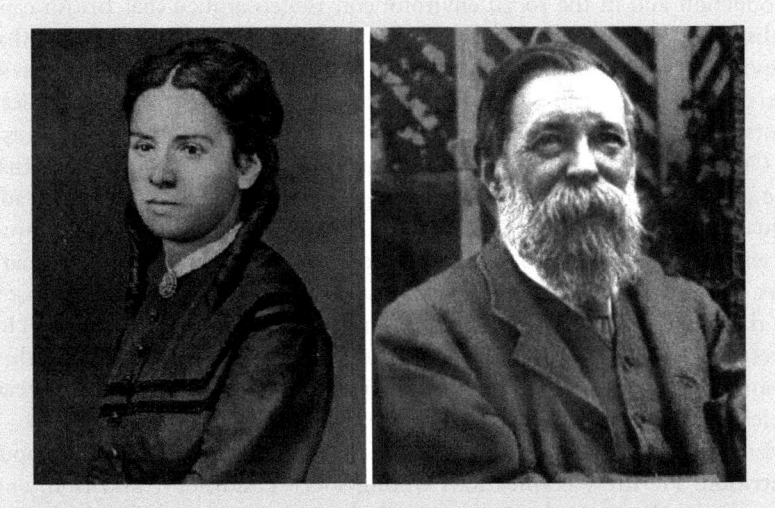

Figure 2.1 Friedrich Engels, who initiated some of the first studies from the perspective of social medicine while he was collaborating with Karl Marx.

MARY BURNS AND FRIEDRICH ENGELS

Mary Burns was a working-class, Irish woman whom Engels met early during his stay in Manchester. During their 20-year relationship until Burns' premature death at age 41, she introduced him to the realities of workers' lives in the squalid homes and factories of a large industrial city during capitalism's early history. In private, Engels acknowledged Burns's impact on his perceptions and thinking – but not enough to cite her or to share co-authorship in his book that presented one of the first detailed accounts analyzing the "condition of the working class," which became an early classic in social medicine. (Figure 2.1 probably shows Mary Burns, but it may show her sister, Lizzie, with whom Engels lived after Mary's death.)

Friedrich Engels

Engels worked as a middle-level manager at a textile mill in Manchester, England, between 1842 and 1844. His father was co-owner of the mill. Engels benefited from the perks of his managerial role. Despite this success, however, he immersed himself in English working-class life, partly due to the influence of his partner, Mary Burns. His experiences and observations went into his first book, *The Condition of the Working Class in England in 1844*.[8] For Engels, the roots of illness lay in the organization of economic production and in the social environment. Engels argued that British capitalism forced working-class people to work and live in circumstances that inevitably caused sickness and that those who controlled the capitalist system were well aware of this fact. The contradiction between profit and safety worsened health problems and stood in the way of necessary improvements.

Considering the effects of environmental toxins, Engels argued that the poorly planned housing in working-class districts did not permit adequate ventilation of toxic substances. For example, carbon-containing gases from burning fossil fuels gathered and lingered within living quarters. There were no proper disposal systems for human and animal waste, so these materials were left in courtyards, apartments, or the street. The overcrowding and insufficient ventilation contributed to a high mortality from tuberculosis – an airborne infection – in London and other industrial cities. Typhus, carried by lice, also spread due to inadequate sanitation.

Engels went beyond living conditions, however, and also wrote about nutrition. He drew connections among social conditions, nutrition, and disease, emphasizing the expense and chronic shortages of food supplies for urban workers and their families. Lack of proper storage facilities at markets led to contamination and spoilage. As a result, children were often malnourished. Engels was able to describe the skeletal deformities of rickets as a nutritional problem long before the medical finding that vitamin D deficiency was the cause.[9]

He viewed alcoholism as the result of social forces that fostered excessive drinking, for example, a response to the miseries of working-class life: "The working man... must have something to make work worth his trouble, to make the next day bearable.... They who have degraded the working man to a mere object have the responsibility to bear."[10] Therefore, the treatment for alcoholism involved basic changes in those social conditions rather than treatment programs that focused on the individual. Limited medical interventions, from this viewpoint, would never yield the improvements most needed.

Engels also analyzed structures of oppression within the social organization of medicine. He emphasized the maldistribution of appropriately trained medical personnel and the lack of access due to lack of resources. According to Engels, the working class coped with the "impossibility of employing skilled physicians" when they fell sick.[11] Some infirmaries would offer charitable services, but this only met a fraction of people's needs. Engels also criticized the then burgeoning pharmaceutical market. Apothecaries would provide "remedies" for childhood illness containing a variety of ingredients, including opiates. Engels argued that the high rate of infant mortality in working-class districts could be explained partly by the lack of medical care, but also partly by the promotion of inappropriate medications.

To back up his claim, Engels then took on an epidemiological investigation of mortality rates and social class, using demographic statistics collected by public health officials. His data suggested that mortality rates were inversely related to social class, not only for entire cities but also within specific geographic districts of cities. For example, he noted that in Manchester, childhood mortality was substantially greater among working-class children than among children of higher classes. In addition, Engels commented on the cumulative effects of class and urbanism on childhood mortality. He cited data that demonstrated higher death rates from epidemics of infectious diseases like smallpox, measles, scarlet fever, and whooping cough among working-class children. For Engels, crowding, poor housing, inadequate sanitation, and pollution – the standard features of urban life – combined with low social class were responsible for causing disease and early mortality.

In describing particular types of industrial work, Engels provided early accounts of occupational diseases that did not receive intensive study until well into the twentieth century. Among others, Engels identified several orthopedic disorders as caused by the physical demands of industrialism. He discussed curvature of the spine, deformities of the lower extremities, flat feet, varicose veins, and leg ulcers as manifestations of work demands that required long periods of time in an upright posture. The insight that chronic musculoskeletal disorders could result from unchanging posture or small, repetitive motions seems simple enough today. Yet, this source of illness – quite different from a specific accident or exposure to toxic substance – only entered occupational medicine as a serious topic of concern toward the end of the twentieth century.[12] Again, Engels was ahead of his time in developing a social medicine approach to diseases caused by work.

Engels focused in particular on occupational lung disease. His description of textile workers' pulmonary pathology predated the medical diagnosis of byssinosis, or brown lung:

> In many rooms of the cotton and flax-spanning mills, the air is filled with fibrous dust, which produces chest affections, especially among workers in the carding and combing-rooms... The most common effects of this breathing of dust are [blood spitting], hard, noisy breathing, pains in the chest, coughs, sleeplessness, in short, all the symptoms of asthma.[13]

Engels also offered a parallel description of "grinders' asthma," a respiratory disease caused by inhaling metal dust particles in the manufacture of knife blades and forks. The pathologic effects of cotton and metal dusts on the lung were similar; Engels noted the similarities of symptoms experienced by those two diverse groups of workers. He also analyzed the ravages of pulmonary disease among coal miners. Engels proposed that the unventilated coal dust caused both acute and chronic pulmonary inflammation that frequently progressed to death. He noted that "black spittle" – the syndrome now called coal worker's pneumoconiosis, or black lung – was associated with gastrointestinal, cardiac, and reproductive complications. By pointing out that this lung disease was preventable, Engels illustrated the contradiction between profit and safety as a political economic determinant of disease in capitalist industry: "The profit-greed of mine owners which prevents the use of ventilators is therefore responsible for the fact that this working-man's disease exists at all."[14] After more than a century and a half, the same structural contradiction impedes the prevention of black lung. In Appalachian coal mines, unprecedented numbers of workers continue to suffer from this fatal disease.[15]

Engels interspersed his remarks about disease with many other perceptions of class oppression. His argument implied that the solution to these health problems required basic political economic change; limited medical interventions would never yield the improvements that were most needed. Although Engels's early work on medical issues has been lost to many later researchers and activists, his analysis exerted a major influence on one of the founders of social medicine, Rudolf Virchow.

Rudolf Virchow

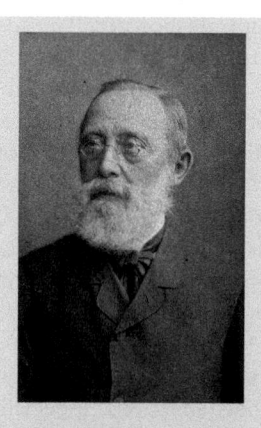

Figure 2.2 Rudolf Virchow, "father of cellular pathology" and "father of social medicine," during the late 1800s when he was working as a professor in Berlin and serving as an elected representative in Germany's parliament (Reichstag).

As we mentioned in Chapter 1, Virchow was a prominent nineteenth-century German pathologist, who used his background in medicine to offer a unified explanation of the physical and social forces that cause human disease and suffering. Throughout his career, he made important medical discoveries. He was among the first to recognize leukemia as a unique illness, to describe the mechanisms of pulmonary thromboembolism (later known as "Virchow's triad" of hypercoagulability, hemodynamic stasis or turbulence, and injury or dysfunction of the endothelial cells within blood vessels), and to coin the well-known phrase "every cell stems from another cell."[16] His best-known work, *Cellular Pathology*, presented the first comprehensive exposition of the cell as the basic unit of physiologic and pathologic processes (Figure 2.2).[17]

YOUNG VIRCHOW WRITES TO HIS PARENTS ABOUT THE TYPHUS EPIDEMIC

Until their deaths, Virchow maintained an extensive correspondence with his parents, which serves as a remarkably

Virchow emphasized the concrete historical and material circumstances in which disease appeared, the contradictory political economic forces that impeded prevention, and researchers' role in advocating reform.[18] In this multifaceted approach, Virchow claimed that the most important causes of illness were the material conditions of people's everyday lives. Therefore, even the most effective health care system could be unsuccessful in treating the pathophysiological disturbances of the individual.

By studying epidemics of typhus, tuberculosis, and cholera, Virchow developed a theory that political economic structures fostered the spread of illness. He argued that defects of society allowed such outbreaks to occur. The specific disease entities – such as typhus, scurvy, tuberculosis, leprosy, cholera, and some mental disorders – he called "artificial diseases."[19] According to his analysis, inadequate social conditions increased the population's susceptibility to climate, infectious agents, and other specific causal factors – the perfect combination to create a devastating epidemic. For the prevention and eradication of such rampant diseases, social change was, therefore, just as important as medical intervention: "The improvement of medicine would eventually prolong honest record of family life and parental reaction to a precocious son.

In late 1847, a typhus epidemic broke out in Upper Silesia, a chronically impoverished area of East Prussia with a large Polish-speaking minority. By the beginning of 1848, thousands were dying, and famine complicated the problems. Virchow convinced his superiors to support a pathologically oriented investigation that would lead to recommendations about stopping the epidemic and preventing recurrences. He departed for a brief but intensive field trip to Upper Silesia. Within days of his arrival, the horrors of the epidemic produced a profound emotional impact.

Although he revealed some of these feelings in his formal reports, he reserved most of them for his correspondence with his parents (Rudolf Virchow, Briefe an Seine Eltern [Letters to His Parents] (Leipzig, Germany: Engelmann, 1907, pp. 125–27). In these letters, Virchow gave a passionate account of suffering. He described the available diet in detail, expressed indignation about the continuing hunger, and began to draw a connection between hunger and disease: "It is rather certain that hunger and typhus are not produced apart from each other but that the latter has spread so extensively only through hunger." Inadequate housing conditions also predisposed to transmission of the disease. He complained to his father that the epidemic's persistence was the fault of public officials, who did not take aggressive action to correct the social conditions that fostered illness. He also blamed the local medical profession for not attending to the poor properly, because of "love of money" and reluctance "to put bills aside." Only a "public health service" (Die Öffentliche Gesundheitspflege), in which doctors and medical facilities would function under state control, could hope to deal with such problems effectively.

human life, but improvement of social conditions could achieve this result even more rapidly and successfully."[20]

The social contradictions that Virchow emphasized most strongly were those of class structure. He described the deplorable conditions that the working class endured and linked disease patterns to these deprivations. For example, he noted that morbidity and mortality rates – especially infant mortality rates – were much higher in working-class districts of cities than in the more affluent areas. As documentation, Virchow cited the statistics in Engels's book on the condition of the working class in England, as well as data he himself gathered from German cities. He described inadequate housing, poor nutrition, and threadbare clothing, all the while criticizing the apathy of government officials for ignoring such basic causes of illness. While the list of disease-causing social conditions was long, Virchow became particularly outraged in his discussion of epidemics like the cholera outbreak in Berlin. Again, Virchow believed these diseases were caused not by a defect in human immunology, but by a problem in human society:

> Is it not clear that our struggle is a social one, that our job is not to write instructions to upset the consumers of melons and salmon, of cakes and ice cream, in short, the comfortable bourgeoisie, but is to create institutions to protect the poor, who have no soft bread, no good meat, no warm clothing, and no bed, and who through their work cannot subsist on rice soup and camomile tea...? May the rich remember during the winter, when they sit in front of their hot stoves and give Christmas apples to their little ones, that the shiphands who brought the coal and the applies died from cholera. It is so sad that thousands always must die in misery, so that a few hundred may live well.[21]

For Virchow, the deprivation of working-class life created a susceptibility to disease. When infectious organisms, climate changes, famine, or other causal factors also came into play, disease would then spread rapidly through the community.

Because he clarified the social origins of illness, Virchow advocated a broad scope for public health and the medical scientist. He attacked structures of oppression within medicine, particularly the hospital policies that required payment from the poor rather than assuming their care as a matter of social responsibility. Virchow envisioned the creation of a "public health service," an integrated system of publicly owned and operated health care facilities, staffed by health workers employed by the state. Such a system would define health care as a constitutional right of citizenship.[22]

Virchow's concept of public health also focused on prevention of disease as well as the state's responsibility to ensure material security for its citizens. Virchow believed that epidemics could be prevented by straightforward changes in social policy. For example, Virchow noted that some recent epidemics had been preceded by poor potato harvests. These poor harvests resulted in malnutrition, making the impoverished susceptible to disease. Virchow argued that the government officials should have prevented malnutrition by distributing foodstuffs from other parts of the country. The half-hearted attempt at health care that followed as a result of the epidemic was too little, too late. As Virchow explained: "Our politics were those of prophylaxis; our opponents preferred those of palliation."[23]

Prevention of disease was in fact a political economic problem and not just a medical one. Beyond the necessities, such as food and adequate clothing, Virchow also believed that the governmental structures of the state should provide work for its "able-bodied" citizens. By the state's assuring conditions of economic production that guaranteed employment, workers could obtain their own economic security necessary for good health. Likewise, the physically disabled should also enjoy the right of financial support and security supplied by the state.[24]

Virchow lived during a time of great medical accomplishments, to many of which he contributed. Indeed, his name is recognizable to any current medical student. In many respects, however, Virchow worked ahead of his time. His theories on the social origins of illness pointed out the enormity of the medical task. He knew that it was necessary to study social conditions as part of medical and clinical research, and he argued that health professionals had an obligation to engage in political action. On the other hand, the era of microbiology – of reducing the focus rather than expanding it – had just begun. During the twenty-first century, we are returning to Virchow's connections among medicine, social medicine, and politics, with a perspective that medicine arguably is a "...social science, and politics is nothing more than medicine in larger scale."[25] His contributions set a standard for our current attempts to understand and to challenge the social, political, and economic conditions that generate illness and suffering.

Salvador Allende

Although better known for his political than for his medical career, Salvador Allende, like Virchow, was a physician and pathologist. His efforts became one of the most important influences on social medicine, especially in Latin America. Allende acknowledged his intellectual debts to Engels, Virchow, and others who analyzed the social roots of illness in nineteenth-century Europe. Allende learned about social medicine partly due to the influence of a professor of pathology previously at the University of Chile, Max Westenhöfer, who had studied with Virchow in Germany (more on this connection through Westenhöfer appears in Chapter 8). Throughout his working life, Allende implemented a political economic model of medical problems in the context of empire and economic underdevelopment. His model emphasized the specific characteristics of society that could be transformed (Figure 2.3).

Writing during 1939 as minister of health for a popular-front government, Allende presented his analysis of the relationships among political economy, disease, and suffering in his book, *The Chilean Medico-Social Reality* (*La Realidad Médico-Social Chilena*).[26] This work recognized that the health problems of the Chilean people derived largely from the country's political and economic conditions. It also implied that social change was the only potentially therapeutic approach to many health problems. After

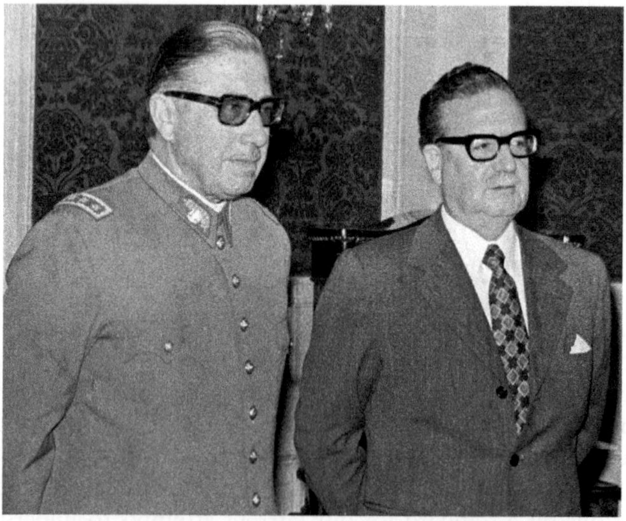

Figure 2.3 Doctor Salvador Allende as President of Chile and General Augusto Pinochet shortly before Pinochet led the military coup on September 11, 1973, that resulted in Allende's death by suicide.

Allende introduced these connections, he presented some geographic and demographic "antecedents" to contextualize specific health problems. Sharing a similar focus with Engels and Virchow, he focused on the living conditions "of the working classes."

In his account of working-class life, Allende emphasized capitalist imperialism, particularly the multinational corporations that extracted profit from Chilean natural resources and inexpensive labor. He claimed that to improve health, a popular-front government must change the nature of empire:

> For the capitalist enterprise it is of no concern that there is a population of workers who live in deplorable conditions, who risk being consumed by diseases or who vegetate in obscurity... [Without] economic advancement... it is impossible to accomplish anything serious from the viewpoints of hygiene or medicine... because it is impossible to give health and knowledge to a people who are malnourished, who wear rags, and who work at a level of unmerciful exploitation.[27]

Allende's analytic tone and statistical tabulation thinly veiled his outrage at the contradictions of class structure and the underdevelopment that empire fostered.

Allende focused first on wages, which he viewed as a primary determinant of workers' health. Many of his political economic observations anticipated future problems, such as wage differentials for men and women, the impact of inflation, and the inadequacy of laws claiming to ensure subsistence-level income. He linked his exposition of wages directly to the problem of nutrition and presented comparative data on food availability, earning power, and economic development. The production of milk and other needed foodstuffs was less efficient than in more developed countries, and Chilean workers' inferior earning power also made food less accessible. Reviewing the minimum requirement to ensure adequate nutrition, he found that the majority of Chilean workers could not obtain the elements of this diet on a regular basis. The Chilean people, Allende argued, did not have access to the food needed for efficient work. Inadequate nutrition also contributed to high infant mortality, skeletal deformities, and tuberculosis and other infectious diseases.

With the same focus on concrete, material conditions, Allende then turned to clothing, housing, and sanitation facilities. He found that working people in Chile were inadequately clothed, largely because wages were low and the greatest proportion of income went for food and housing. The effects of insufficient clothing, Allende observed, were apparent in the rates of upper respiratory infections, pneumonia, and tuberculosis that were higher than in any economically developed country.

In his analysis of housing problems, Allende focused on population density, which largely reflected the geography of economic production.

He noted that Chile had one of the highest rates of inhabitants per residential structure in the world. As a result of this overcrowding, infectious diseases spread easily. Again, he cited comparative data that showed a correlation between population density and overall mortality. In a style similar to that of Engels and Virchow, Allende presented a concrete description of housing conditions, including details about insufficient beds, inadequate construction materials, and deficiencies in apartment buildings. He reviewed private initiatives in construction, found them unsatisfactory, and outlined the need for major public sector investments in new housing. Allende then presented data on drinking water and sewage systems for all provinces of Chile, noting that vast areas of the country lacked these rudimentary facilities, linked to a shortage of suitable housing.

Allende's study of the material conditions affecting the working class laid the groundwork for his analysis of concrete medical problems. When he discussed specific diseases, he looked for their sources in the social and material environment. The medical problems that he considered included maternal and infant mortality, tuberculosis and other infectious diseases, sexually transmitted diseases, emotional disturbances, and occupational illnesses. He observed that maternal and infant mortality rates generally were far lower in developed than in less developed countries. After reviewing the major causes of death, he concluded that malnutrition and poor sanitation, both rooted in the political economy of underdevelopment, were major explanations for this excess mortality.

Allende designated tuberculosis as a "social disease" because its incidence differed so greatly among social classes. Writing before the antibiotic era, Allende reached conclusions similar to those of modern epidemiology — that the major decline in tuberculosis followed economic advances rather than therapeutic medical interventions. From statistics of the first three decades of the twentieth century, he noted that tuberculosis had decreased consistently in the economically developed countries of Western Europe and the United States. On the other hand, in economically less developed countries like Chile, little progress against the disease had occurred. Within the context of underdevelopment, tuberculosis exerted its most severe impact on the poor.

Regarding other infectious diseases, Allende turned to typhus, the same disease that shaped Virchow's views about the relationships between illness and the political economic system. Allende began his analysis with a straightforward statement: "Some [infectious diseases], like typhus, are an index of the state of pauperization of the masses."[28] Like Virchow in Upper Silesia, Allende found a disproportionate incidence of typhus in the Chilean working class. He then showed that bacillary and amebic dysentery as well as typhoid fever occurred because of inadequate drinking water and sanitation facilities in residential areas densely populated by working-class families. Similar problems fostered other infections, such as diphtheria, whooping cough, scarlet fever, measles, and trachoma.

In his discussion of sexually transmitted diseases, Allende emphasized political economic conditions that favored the spread of syphilis and gonorrhea. He discussed deprivations of working-class life that encouraged prostitution. Citing the prevalence of prostitution in the capital city of Santiago and other cities, as well as recruitment of women from poor families, he argued that social programs to eliminate prostitution through expansion of employment opportunities must precede significant improvements in sexually transmitted diseases. Allende also gave one of the first analyses of illegal abortion. He noted that a large proportion of deaths in gynecological hospitals, about 30 percent, derived from abortions and their complications. Pointing out the high incidence of abortion complications among working-class women, he attributed this problem to economic deprivations of class structure. After a statistical account of the complications, Allende allowed his outrage to surface:

> There are hundreds of working mothers who, because of anxiety about the inadequacy of their wages, induce abortion in order to prevent a new child from shrinking their already insignificant resources. Hundreds of working mothers lose their lives, impelled by the anxieties of economic reality.[29]

Drug addiction was another topic that troubled Allende deeply. In *La Realidad*, Allende analyzed the social and psychological problems that motivated people to use addictive drugs. Allende's political economic analysis of the cause of alcohol intoxication showed similarity to that of Engels:

> We see that one's wages, appreciably less than subsistence, are not enough to supply needed clothing, that one must inhabit inadequate housing... [and that] one's food is not sufficient to produce the minimum of necessary caloric energy... The worker reaches the conclusion that going to the tavern and intoxicating oneself is the apparent solution to all these problems. In the tavern one finds a lighted and heated place, and friends for distraction, making one forget the misery at home. In short, for the Chilean worker... alcohol is not a stimulant but an anesthetic.[30]

Rooted in social misery generated by conditions of capitalist production, alcoholism exerted a profound effect on health, an impact that Allende documented for a variety of illnesses, including gastrointestinal diseases, cirrhosis, delirium tremens, sexual dysfunction, birth defects, and tuberculosis. He also traced some of the subtler societal outcomes of alcoholism, offering an early analysis of alcohol's impact on accidental deaths.

Allende analyzed monopoly capital and international expansion by pharmaceutical industry, criticizing issues such as brand-name medications and pharmaceutical advertising. In perhaps the earliest discussion of its type, Allende compared the prices of brand-name drugs with their generic equivalents:

> Thus, for example, we find for a drug with important action on infectious diseases, sulfanilamide, these different names and prices: Prontosil $26.95, Gombardol $20.60, Aseptil $18.00, Intersil $13.00, Acetilina $6.65. All these products, which in the eye of the public appear with different names, correspond, in reality, to the same medication which is sold in a similar container and which contains 20 tablets of 0.50 grams of sulfanilamide.[31]

Beyond the issue of drug names, Allende also anticipated a later theme by criticizing pharmaceutical advertising: "Another problem in relation to the pharmaceutical specialties is... the excessive and charlatan propaganda attributing qualities and curative powers which are far from their real ones."[32] Throughout his career, he maintained his concern with exploitation by multinational drug companies. As president, he helped develop a national generic drug formulary and proposed nationalization of the pharmaceutical industry that remained dominated by North American firms.

Allende concluded by proposing the policy position and plan for political action of the Ministry of Health within the popular-front government. In considering reform and its dilemmas, he refused to discuss specific health problems in isolation from macro-level political economic issues. He introduced his policy proposals with a chapter titled "Considerations Regarding Human Capital." Analyzing the detrimental economic impact of ill-health among workers, he argued that a healthy population was a worthy goal both in its own right and also for the sake of national development. The country's productivity suffered because of workers' illness and early death; yet, improving the health of workers was impossible without fundamental changes in society. These changes would include "an equitable distribution of the product of labor," state regulation of "production, distribution, and price of articles of food and clothing," a national housing program, and special attention to occupational health problems. The links between medicine and the broader political economy were inescapable: "All this means that the solution of the medico-social problems of the country would require precisely the solution of the economic problems that affect the proletarian classes."[33]

He then proposed specific reforms that he viewed as preconditions for an effective health system. These reforms called for profound changes in the existing structures of power, finance, and economic production. First, he suggested modifications of wages, which if enacted would have led to a major redistribution of wealth. Regarding nutrition, he developed a plan to improve milk supplies, fishing, and refrigeration and suggested land reform provisions to enhance agricultural productivity. Allende proposed a concerted national effort in publicly supported construction as well as rent control in the private sector.

Allende did not emphasize programs of research or treatment for specific diseases. Instead, he assumed that the greatest advances toward lowering morbidity and mortality would follow fundamental societal change. This orientation also pervaded his proposed "medico-social program." In this program, he suggested innovations including reorganization of the Ministry of Health, planning activities, control of pharmaceutical production and prices, occupational safety and health policies, measures supporting preventative medicine, and sanitation programs. Since the major social origins of illness included low wages, malnutrition, and poor housing, the first responsibility of the public health system was to improve these conditions, some of which derived from the actions of multinational corporations. Allende's vision implied that medical intervention without basic political economic change would remain ineffectual and, in a deep sense, misguided.

Capitalism, Empire, Illness, and Early Death

Engels, Virchow, and Allende developed divergent, though complementary, views about the social etiology of illness, which later generations have tended to forget and then rediscover. Their work conceptualized unnecessary illness and premature death as inherent outcomes of capitalist production and the expansion of empire. The divergences, however, reflected certain differences in theoretical orientation. For Engels, economic production was primary. Even in his early work, Engels emphasized the organization and process of production as a potential cause of morbidity and mortality. Disease and early death, in his view, developed directly from exposure to dusts, chemicals, time pressures, demands about body position, visual demands, and related difficulties that workers faced in their jobs. Environmental pollution, bad housing, alcoholism, and malnutrition also contributed to the poor health of the working class, but these factors mainly reflected or exacerbated the structural contradictions of production itself.

While he shared Engels's view that the working class suffered disproportionately, Virchow focused on inequalities in the distribution and consumption of social resources. In Virchow's analysis, important sources of illness and early death included poverty, unemployment, malnutrition, cultural and educational deficits, political disenfranchisement, linguistic difficulties, inadequate medical facilities and personnel, and similar deficiencies that affected the working class. He believed that public officials could prevent epidemics by distributing food more efficiently. Disease and mortality, he argued, would improve if a "public health service" made medical care more available. Virchow did criticize profiteering by businessmen and the high fees of the private medical profession, but he did not emphasize the illness-generating conditions of production itself. Instead, he viewed unequal access to society's products as the principal problem of social medicine.

Allende also concerned himself with the impact of class structure but focused on the context of empire and underdevelopment. The deprivations that the working class experienced in countries like Chile reflected the exploitation of less developed countries by advanced capitalist nations. Allende attributed low wages, malnutrition, poor housing, and related problems directly to the extraction of wealth by international imperialism. He recognized that production itself could produce illness, but, unlike Engels, devoted less attention to occupational illness per se. He did document distributional inequalities of goods and services that, as in Virchow's analysis, ravaged the working class. On the other hand, the most crucial political economic determinant of illness and death, in Allende's view, was the contradiction of development and empire. Economic advancement of the society as a whole was the major precondition for meaningful improvements in medical care and individual health.

The contributions of Engels, Virchow, and Allende shared the framework of social causation. These writings conveyed a vision of multiple social structures and processes impinging on the individual. Disease was not the straightforward outcome of an infectious agent or pathophysiological disturbance. Instead, a variety of problems – including malnutrition, economic insecurity, occupational risks, bad housing, and lack of political power – created an underlying predisposition to disease and death. Although these writers differed in the specific factors they emphasized, they each saw illness as deeply embedded in the complexities of social reality. To the extent that social contradictions affected individual disease, therapeutic intervention that limited itself to the individual level proved both naïve and futile. Social etiology implied social change as therapy, and the latter linked medical practice to political practice.

Another crucial divergence concerned policy, reform, and political strategy. Engels, Virchow, and Allende differed in their views of the strategies needed for change. They also held varying visions of the society in which these policies would take effect. Although their explanations of the social origins of illness complemented one another, the question of how to change illness-generating conditions evoked different strategic analyses.

Already present in his early work, Engels's strategy involved revolution, not reform. His documentation of the occupational and environmental conditions that caused illness and early death did not aim toward limited reform of these problems. Instead, he intended his data to serve, at least in part, as propaganda. The purpose was to provide a focus for political organizing among the working class. Notably, Engels did not advocate specific changes in the conditions he described. While he detailed the defects of housing, sanitation, occupational safety, maldistribution of medical personnel, and promotion of drugs, he did not explicitly seek reform in any of these areas. The alternatives he occasionally suggested, such as cursory outlines of a public health service, were always speculation about how a more effective system might appear in a postrevolutionary society. The many deprivations of working-class life required fundamental change in the entire social order, rather than limited improvements in parts of society. The companion piece of *The Condition of the Working Class in England* was clearly *The Communist Manifesto*,[34] with its aim to address problems such as unnecessary illness and early death through broad social revolution. From this perspective, reformism in health care made as little sense as any other piecemeal tinkering with capitalist society.

Taking a different approach to social change, Virchow favored policies of reform. Although he participated in the agitation of the late 1840s and doubted that the ruling circles would permit needed changes in response to peaceful challenges alone, he ultimately opted for reform rather than revolution. While the conditions he witnessed in the Upper Silesian typhus epidemic were horrifying, he believed that a series of reforms could correct the problems. The reforms he advocated transcended medicine to include rationalized food distribution, modifications in the educational system, political enfranchisement, and other changes at the level of social structure. He also adopted a broad view of the systematic reforms that were necessary in health care. An adequate health system, for example, demanded a public health service. In this service, health care professionals would work as employees of the state and would act to correct maldistribution across class, geographical, and ethnic lines. As an overall political goal, Virchow favored a constitutional democracy that would reduce the power of the monarchy and nobility. He supported principles of socialism, particularly those that involved public ownership and rational organization of health and welfare facilities. However, Virchow argued against communism, which he saw as a naïve view that a just society was feasible without a strong state apparatus. Virchow firmly believed that limited reforms within a capitalist society were both appropriate and desirable, and he was optimistic that they would be effective.

Allende's conceptualization of political strategy was more complex than those of Engels or Virchow. In *La Realidad*, he unambiguously stated that the health problems of the working class were inherent in the contradictions of class structure, underdevelopment, and the oppressive international relations of empire. Without basic modification of these structural problems, he argued, limited medical reform would prove futile. In Allende's view, revolutionary social change was necessary to achieve needed improvements in health services and outcomes. Throughout his life, Allende believed that progressive forces could achieve a socialist transformation of society through a sequence of peaceful actions within the framework of constitutional democracy. He and his co-workers based this position on a reading of prior socialist strategists, examples of other revolutions, and a detailed analysis of Chile's concrete historical and material reality.

From this viewpoint, the most important health-related reforms transcended medicine. Allende called for improvements in housing, nutrition, employment, and other concrete manifestations of class oppression. Such reforms were preconditions for reduced morbidity and mortality; without them, changes in health services could not succeed. On the other hand, structural reforms in the social organization of medicine, including a public health service and a nationalized pharmaceutical and equipment industry, were desirable goals along the path to a socialist society. Allende did not accurately anticipate the violence of national and international groups about to be dispossessed on the peaceful road to socialism. This grim result left the balance between reform and revolutionary alternatives incompletely resolved in strategies for change.

The social pathologies that distressed Engels, Virchow, and Allende continue to create suffering and early death. Public health generally has adopted the medical model of etiology. In this model, social conditions may increase susceptibility or exacerbate disease, but they are not primary causes like microbial agents or disturbances of normal physiology. Partly because research rarely has clarified causes of illness within political economic systems, political strategy – both within and outside medicine – seldom has addressed the social roots of disease.

Inequalities of class, exploitation of workers, and conditions of capitalist production in the context of empire remain with us now as previously. The links between political economic conditions and disease become ever more urgent, as economic instability, unreliable food supplies, depletion of petroleum, nuclear and toxic chemical wastes, global warming, and related problems threaten the survival of humanity and other life forms. In future chapters, we will discuss more recent perspectives on the social determination of health, based on work in social medicine. As Engels, Virchow, and Allende argued and as more recent studies in social medicine have confirmed, efforts to improve the health of populations without addressing the social origins of illness ultimately will fail. Strategies that do address these social origins reveal the scope of reconstruction that is necessary for meaningful solutions, which we consider in the last part of the book.

Notes

1 Norman Bethune, "Wounds," in Joshua S. Horn, ed., *Away with All Pests...: An English Surgeon in People's China, 1954–1969* (New York: Monthly Review Press, 1939 [1969]).
2 Disclosure: One of the authors, Howard, became infected by tuberculosis while taking care of a family at La Clínica de la Raza, a community health center in Oakland, California, and similarly began to address the "second sickness" in social medicine.
3 Howard Waitzkin, *The Second Sickness: Contradictions of Capitalist Health Care*, 2nd ed. (Lanham, MD: Rowman & Littlefield, 2000).
4 Due to the varying usages of the term "political economy," a brief definition may help. In this book, political economy refers to the conditions under which economic production is organized. This definition follows the usage of the term in Marxian and neo-Marxian studies, as well as previous work by Adam Smith and David Ricardo. In this sense, "political economic systems" refer to the different organizational frameworks for organizing economic production, such as capitalism and socialism. From this point of view, class structure, particularly the distinction between those who do own or control the means of production (capitalists) and those who do not (workers), is a crucial focus of political economy. Waitzkin, *The Second Sickness*, Chapter 1.
5 The Social Medicine Portal reports many of these efforts around the world: www.socialmedicine.org. See also the Social Medicine Consortium, www.socialmedicineconsortium.org.
6 George Rosen, "What Is Social Medicine?" *Bulletin of the History of Medicine* 21 (1947): 674–733; George Rosen, *A History of Public Health* (New York: MD Publications, 1958), pp. 192–293; René Sand, *The Advance to Social Medicine* (London: Staples Press, 1952), pp. 295–343, 507–89; Henry E. Sigerist, *Civilization and Disease* (Ithaca, NY: Cornell University Press, 1944), pp. 6–64.
7 For the distinction between global South and global North, we like many others feel deeply indebted to the work of Samir Amin, who has illuminated the historical and contemporary importance of the exploited peripheries in the South and exploiting centers in the North. For instance, in this book we are trying to extend Amin's recently expressed vision: "In the countries of the South, most people are victims of the system, whereas in the North, the majority are its beneficiaries.... The possible, but difficult, conjunction between the struggles of peoples in the South with those of peoples in the North is the only way to overcome the limitations of both." See Samir Amin, "Revolution from North to South," *Monthly Review* 69, no. 3 (July–August 2017): 113–27.
8 Friedrich Engels, *The Condition of the Working Class in England in 1844* (Moscow: Progress Publishers, 1973 [1845]). For background on Engels's situation when writing this book, see W.O. Henderson, *The Life of Friedrich Engels* (London: Frank Cass, 1976), vol. 1, pp. 43–78. Regarding the influence of Mary Burns and for other details about Engels: Mike Dash, "How Friedrich Engels' Radical Lover Helped Him Father Socialism," *Smithsonian.com*, Smithsonian Institution, August 1, 2013, www.smithsonianmag.com/history/how-friedrich-engels-radical-lover-helped-him-father-socialism-21415560; Howard Waitzkin, "The Social Origins of Illness: A Neglected History," *International Journal of Health Services* 11, no. 1 (November 1, 1981): 77–103.
9 George Wolf, "The Discovery of Vitamin D: The Contribution of Adolf Windaus," *Journal of Nutrition* 134, no. 6 (June 1, 2004): 1299–302.
10 Engels, *Condition*, pp. 141–42.

11 Ibid., pp. 142–43.
12 Ibid., pp. 190–93.
13 Ibid., p. 200.
14 Ibid., pp. 279–84.
15 David J. Blackley, James B. Crum, Cara N. Halldin, Eileen Storey, and A. Scott Laney, "Resurgence of Progressive Massive Fibrosis in Coal Miners—Eastern Kentucky, 2016," *Morbidity and Mortality Weekly Report* 65, no. 49 (December 16, 2016): 1385–89, www.cdc.gov/mmwr/volumes/65/wr/mm6549a1.htm; Howard Berkes, "Advancing Black Lung Cases Surge in Appalachia," *NPR*, December 15, 2016, www.npr.org/documents/2016/dec/blacklungreport121516.pdf.
16 Myron Schultz, "Rudolf Virchow (1821–1902)," *Emerging Infectious Diseases* (Centers for Disease Control and Prevention) 14, no. 9 (September 2008), www.nc.cdc.gov/eid/article/14/9/08-6672_article.
17 Rudolf Virchow, *Cellular Pathology* (London: John Churchill and Co., 1860), https://archive.org/details/in.ernet.dli.2015.221222.
18 Rudolf Virchow, *Disease, Life, and Man*, translated by L. J. Rather (Stanford, CA: Stanford University Press, 1958), pp. 27–29. Unless otherwise noted, Howard Waitzkin prepared the translations from German and Spanish for this chapter.
19 Erwin H. Ackerknecht, *Rudolf Virchow: Doctor, Statesman, Anthropologist* (Madison: University of Wisconsin Press, 1953), p. 52.
20 Rudolf Virchow, *Gesammelte Abhandlungen aus dem Gebiet der Öffentlichen Medicin und der Seuchenlehre* (Berlin: Hirschwald, 1879), vol. 1, pp. 121–22; Ackerknecht, *Rudolf Virchow*, pp. 125–29.
21 Rudolf Virchow, *Werk und Wirkung* (Berlin: Rütten & Loenig, 1957), p. 110.
22 Virchow, *Werk und Wirkung*, p. 55; Ackerknecht, *Rudolf Virchow*, pp. 131–38.
23 Virchow, *Werk und Wirkung*, pp. 127, 108.
24 Ibid., p. 106.
25 Ibid., p. 117; Virchow, *Disease, Life, and Man*, p. 106.
26 Salvador Allende, *La Realidad Medico-Social Chilena* (Santiago: Ministerio de Salubridad, Previsión y Asistencia Social, 1939).
27 Ibid., pp. 6, 8.
28 Ibid., p. 105.
29 Ibid., p. 86.
30 Ibid., p. 119.
31 Ibid., pp. 189–90.
32 Ibid, p. 191.
33 Ibid., p. 198.
34 Karl Marx and Frederick Engels, *Manifesto of the Communist Party* (New York: International Publishers, 1983).

Chapter 3

The Social Determination of Illness, Part I

Health and Social Contradictions

T.B., a 30-year-old worker in the pesticide division of a chemical company in California, and his co-workers began to wonder why they and their wives were not having children. After several years, they contacted a local medical clinic, where sperm examinations revealed sterility or decreased fertility. Later studies showed similar findings among pesticide workers in other states. Eventually, the problem was traced to dibromo-chloropropane (DBCP), a soil fumigant used to kill worms that feed on crop roots. Laboratory experiments showed that DBCP caused testicular damage in rats. Then reports of testicular cancer in pesticide workers exposed to DBCP began to appear. In an investigation, the California Department of Health found hazardous DBCP levels in more than forty municipal water wells, as the chemical had leached down to groundwater. Health officials estimated that about 200,000 people had been drinking water contaminated by DBCP. Although the Department of Health issued a ban on DBCP, chemical and agricultural corporations resisted the ban through legal actions and used similar compounds instead.[1]

★ ★ ★

R.L. was a 32-year-old Spanish-speaking mother of five who moved from rural Mexico to Oakland, California, where she began to work as a part-time housekeeper. She knew no English, held no legal documents regarding residency in the United States, and had no insurance. She became pregnant again. During the last month of her pregnancy, she went to the emergency rooms of two private hospitals because she felt that labor might have begun. Emergency room staff refused to see her because she did not have insurance; as an undocumented immigrant, she was not eligible for public support through Medicaid. She then went to the emergency room of a county hospital three times in one week; the interns who examined her found high blood pressure but did not test for fetal distress and did not refer her to a prenatal program. Twelve hours after her last visit, she delivered a stillborn infant at home. Three months later, the county hospital threatened to send her bill to a collection agency for nonpayment.

★ ★ ★

G.M. was a 74-year-old Italian American man who was admitted to a medical center in Boston because of rectal bleeding. As part of his evaluation on admission, an electrocardiogram showed that he was having a heart attack, though he had no chest pain or other symptoms. He was taken to the intensive care unit (ICU), where studies of cardiac enzymes confirmed that a heart attack had, indeed, occurred. The doctor who had followed him at a neighborhood health center reported that several months earlier the patient had presented to him with chest pain and a pattern of electrocardiogram changes consistent with a heart attack. On the previous occasion, at the patient's request, the doctor had chosen not to admit the patient to a hospital but instead had followed him at home, where he recuperated uneventfully. During the current admission, he had no further symptoms or cardiac instability, although he became very distressed when he could not sleep due to the constant lights and noises in the ICU. He was transferred from the ICU to the ward after four days and discharged after eight days. A plan was made to evaluate the source of his rectal bleeding about six weeks after discharge.

★ ★ ★

The health care systems of the United States and some other economically developed countries reveal many troubling deficiencies, as shown in these case summaries. For example, occupational and environmental hazards threaten survival in ways that are difficult to predict. Essential health care services remain inaccessible to the poor and to minority populations. Technologically oriented medicine continues to increase the cost and stress of care. In this and later chapters of the book, we present data and citations that provide more information.

For now, we ask: How can such problems exist in wealthy and powerful nations? These issues have not been ignored: They have received wide attention in research, media coverage, politics, and legislatures. Yet, despite the best attempts, a true and lasting solution has remained elusive. This may be because each separate problem is its own object of analysis, debate, and very limited reform. Meanwhile, the fundamental social conditions that are responsible for a variety of health-related issues escape serious study. The cases of a man suffering infertility from pesticide exposure, a woman whose infant dies needlessly, and a man who endures expensive and unnecessary medical procedures may seem isolated from one another, but the social conditions that their cases reflect are not isolated problems. It is important to seek out the underlying realities that provide a more unified explanation and would lead to a more coherent strategy for change.

Social Contradictions – Effects on Health

Major problems in medicine and public health are also problems of society: The health system is so intimately tied to broader social conditions that attempts to study one without the other can be misleading. Difficulties in health and medical care emerge from social contradictions and rarely can be separated from those contradictions. These relationships are not only important for clearer understanding; they also suggest directions for change. From this view, health reforms that do not address the relationships among health, the health care system, and broader social structures are doomed to fail.

The strength of social medicine comes from its ability to analyze the relationships that link the health care system with the political, economic, and social conditions of a society. Without attention to these connections, the health care system falsely takes on the appearance of an autonomous, free-floating entity whose defects purportedly can be corrected by limited reforms in the medical sphere. Karl Marx and Friedrich Engels – the originators of Marxist theory and methodology – analyzed the political, economic, and social conditions of society. (In the previous chapter, we already have considered Engels's classic study, *The Condition of the Working Class in England in 1844*, that helped initiate the field of social medicine.) Their dialectic approach, the principal analytic tool of Marxism, involves several key features.

First, social reality contains structural contradictions. Contradictions are defined as antagonistic or opposing characteristics that arise among social groups, within organizations and institutions, across nations, and in the realm of ideas. Contradictions in social systems are more than simply problems or difficulties: They are destructive tendencies that emerge from and are intertwined with a system's creative capacities. If a specific feature is necessary for a system's accomplishments, a contradictory feature is that one undermines these accomplishments. However, both sides of a contradiction are integrally related to each other. A central purpose of the dialectic approach is to clarify the "unity of opposites": the social contradictions that are at once creative and destructive.

Certain social contradictions illustrate this theoretical approach. For example, a primary structural contradiction in capitalist societies is that of social class. Within capitalism, from this perspective, the capitalist class owns or controls the means of economic production, which consist of the nonhuman inputs of production such as factories, machines, tools, and natural resources (raw materials used to make products). Because capitalists own the means of production and workers do not, a fundamental conflict arises between the capitalist class and the working class. The accumulation of wealth by the capitalist class depends on the productivity of workers, who in return seek their own prosperity. In historical periods of higher wages, fringe benefits, and relatively easier working conditions, this contradiction of class may be less obvious. Yet, the potentially antagonistic relationship between classes is inherent in a system that aims toward amassing wealth by the few, largely through the work of the many. The state's conflicting roles also contribute to the problem: Inconsistent public policies provide limited social welfare to citizens while protecting the ability of private enterprise to accumulate great wealth.

An additional contradiction of capitalist society is that the private accumulation of wealth tends to occur more in specific geographic areas than in others; as a result, wealthy regions contrast with areas of stark poverty. Natural resources tend to flow from the countryside to cities, and from poor nations to wealthy ones. This contradiction between development and underdevelopment manifests itself in regional inequalities within a nation and in international inequalities among nations. However, social policies that aim to redistribute wealth on a geographic basis are weak or lacking.

In the realm of ideas, discrepant ideologies justify and legitimize contradictions of society. For instance, the notion of "equality" masks the continuing inequalities of class structure. However, these contradictions do not disappear in socialist societies: There is a tendency toward the reemergence of class structure based on expertise and bureaucratic authority rather than the ownership of economic production. Although we are emphasizing here the social contradictions that lead to health problems in capitalist societies, social medicine also tries to analyze the contradictions that have created challenges for health in socialist and so-called mixed capitalist–socialist societies.

Social Determinants versus Social Determination

The social determination of health involves the concrete ways in which social contradictions impinge on groups and, ultimately, on individuals in a society to cause illness and early death. Historically, people working in social medicine, like Engels and Virchow, used terms like "social origins" or "social causes"; Allende referred to "socio-medical reality." Others influenced by social medicine, especially John D. Stoeckle and John B. McKinlay, formulated the "upstream" vision in public health, which focused on sources of illness and early death in the social and physical environment, that is, at a broader level of analysis "upstream" from the individual.[2] During recent years, the term "social determination" mostly has replaced the previously used terms. The processes by which social contradictions affect groups and individuals involve several levels of analysis, including the society as a totality; communities, neighborhoods, workplaces, schools, families, and other social institutions; and psychological and biological processes within the individual. Through these sometimes complex processes, social origins become "embodied," with illness and early death as the results.[3]

Social determination generally has replaced the earlier terms mainly because it contrasts with the now frequently used term, "social determinants." What are called "social determinants of health" (SDOH) keep getting forgotten and rediscovered in each succeeding generation. This recurrent amnesia might be called "1 1/2 centuries of forgetting and remembering the social origins of illness."[4] As we described in the last chapter, this history goes back at least to Engels and Virchow during the 1840s and has reemerged roughly every 30 years since then, including some particularly important work in Latin America during the 1930s (e.g., by Allende) and again from the 1960s to the present time. The current rapidly expanding literature on the SDOH, while sometimes admirable and usually well meaning, rarely mentions this earlier work.

One example among many of this apparent amnesia is the World Health Organization's (WHO) influential report, published in 2008 from the Commission on the Social Determinants of Health[5] (Table 3.1 presents a summary). This report stimulated much of the continuing epidemic of new studies on the SDOH, again replicating the findings of prior generations. Some of the leadership for the WHO report were well aware of the earlier intellectual and scientific history, even though they chose not to cite that literature. As a result, most of the current literature on the SDOH, both research findings and educational efforts, comes across as though this field and its discoveries are new, while they actually address relationships between social oppression and health that prior generations have illuminated earlier.

A reason for this amnesia, unintentional or not, involves the theoretical approach and implications for policy in current approaches to the SDOH. The current popularity of the SDOH, and one main reason that the SDOH in such areas as inequality and racism worsen with each succeeding year (as we will see in the next chapter), is that the theoretical approach does not emphasize forces of oppression and sources of social conflict within our societies. Work on the SDOH usually does not threaten those responsible for the SDOH, even when the work concerns such critical problems as the deepening inequality of wealth and the injurious social structures of racism. Although the WHO report does refer to power and concentrated wealth, it nowhere refers to capitalism or the possibility that capitalism might need to change if the SDOH are to be addressed. The data in the WHO report involve almost exclusively correlations between individual characteristics (especially income) and adverse health outcomes. But the report does not clarify causal relationships or processes of change under real-world conditions. So the assumption in the WHO report, as in most subsequent research and educational efforts, is that scientific data will lead

Table 3.1 WHO's Report on the Social Determinants of Health

Summary of Findings

- The poor health of the poor, the social gradient in health within countries, and the marked health inequities between countries are caused by:
  - the unequal distribution of power, income, goods, and services, globally and nationally;
  - the consequent unfairness in the immediate, visible circumstances of peoples lives:
    - their access to health care, schools, and education, their conditions of work and leisure, their homes, communities, towns, or cities
    - their chances of leading a flourishing life.

Summary of Recommendations

- Together, the structural determinants and conditions of daily life constitute the social determinants of health and are responsible for a major part of health inequities between and within countries.
  - Three principles of action are recommended:
    - Improve the conditions of daily life – the circumstances in which people are born, grow, live, work, and age.
    - Tackle the inequitable distribution of power, money, and resources – the structural drivers of those conditions of daily life – globally, nationally, and locally.
    - Measure the problem, evaluate action, expand the knowledge base, develop a workforce that is trained in the social determinants of health, and raise public awareness about the social determinants of health.

to enlightened policies decided by those who govern our societies and control our societies' financial resources.

History shows, however, that the relationship between knowledge and power is rarely, if ever, straightforward.[6] Those who hold power and control wealth seldom rely on knowledge about social problems in taking action and in implementing policies that relate to those problems, unless social movements force them to do so. In our current period of history, political and economic leaders in the United States and some other countries not only disregard findings about the SDOH but also implement policies that continue to worsen the SDOH, such as:

- tax cuts for the rich that increase economic inequality, which is the most important social determinant of health;
- lax regulations affecting the environment and climate, which lead to more illness-generating pollution, occupational diseases, dangerous extreme weather, and even epidemics like COVID-19;

- laws that encourage increasing incarceration, with adverse effects on health and mortality through police brutality and unsanitary conditions in prisons, also contributing to epidemics like COVID-19;
- structural racism, by which non-enforcement of laws and regulations that prohibit discrimination leads to chronic stress and worse outcomes among racial/ethnic minorities for such diseases as hypertension, heart disease, stroke, cancers, and COVID-19;
- militarism, which affects health through food insecurity, housing insecurity, migration to escape war, and reduced government spending for health and public health due to the financial costs of war – all in addition to the direct health effects of war through combat and "collateral damage" to civilian populations; and
- inadequate funding and services for maternal and infant care and for birth control, which result in higher rates of infant and childhood mortality, maternal mortality, and infectious diseases like measles and polio that respond to immunizations.

In this and later chapters and in our references, we provide more details about how these policies have worsened the SDOH, as well as explanations about the political and economic motivations for the policies. Meanwhile, political leaders show little hesitancy in funding unthreatening research and education on the SDOH. These activities focusing on the SDOH create a symbolic image of concern even though key policies continue to worsen the SDOH, to the benefit of those at the top in hierarchies of power and finance.

Many constructive critiques of current work on the SDOH have appeared during the decade since the WHO report appeared. Several organizations have criticized the SDOH approach, including the International Federation of Medical Student Associations, the international People's Health Movement, the Latin American Association of Social Medicine (ALAMES), and the Center for Brazilian Studies on Health (CEBES). Critical analyses also have appeared in scientific articles.[7] Scholars and activists with ALAMES have produced especially helpful analyses that distinguish between "social determinants" (the orientation of the WHO report as well as research, educational efforts, and policy initiatives from this framework) and "social determination" (the orientation of social medicine). These leaders show that these terms reflect important ethical and political differences that focus on contrasting ideas about causality, risk, concepts of health and illness, and causes of inequity (referring to unfair distribution of resources) and inequalities (referring to unfair differences in health outcomes).

In Table 3.2, we summarize some of the main differences between social determinants and social determination,[8] and we discuss these differences further in Chapter 8, where we talk about the differences between

Table 3.2 Differences between Social Determinants and Social Determination

Social Determinants	Social Determination
Society as sum of individuals Health–illness as dichotomous states Change achieves equilibrium; functionalist perspective Variables at individual level of analysis, viewed as risk factors: income, education, job, social cohesion	Society as a totality Health–illness as a dialectic process Change results from social contradictions that lead to mass movements and social conflicts. Hierarchies of determination, production, and reproduction at a societal level
Social position generates different exposures and vulnerabilities.	Power relations, accumulation of capital, and discrimination (classism, racism, sexism) create inequality, exploitation, and chronic stress, which lead to illness and early death.
Reforms achieved through "political will" can change SDOH as risk factors. Such changes can occur within the global capitalist system. Example: Individual-level poverty is associated with increasing obesity and diabetes. Interventions focus on changing the eating and exercise habits of poor people.	Meaningful, lasting improvements in social determination will happen only through societal transformation, including moving beyond the characteristics of global capitalism that generate illness, early death, and fundamental threats to the future of humanity and other forms of life on planet earth. Example: Obesity and diabetes increase when low-income communities lose their ability to grow and to consume healthy foods through collaborative activities that involve physical labor and mutual aid. Unhealthy foods containing high sugar content are promoted by the capitalist food industry, and healthy foods are more expensive or unavailable due to "food deserts" linked to corporate decisions about profitable investments. Interventions focus on self-sufficiency in collaborative food production, distribution, and consumption at the community level, which reduce profiteering and food insecurity.

public health and social medicine. Those who study the SDOH usually assume that society is the sum of the individuals in the society's population. Disease in individuals is either present or absent. Changes in disease patterns result from persuasion based on research "evidence"; policy makers facilitate helpful programs based on their rational assessment of research findings. The individuals in a population show differing "demographic" characteristics, called "variables," which include income, education, occupation, gender, racial–ethnic background, and age. Such variables comprise differing "risk factors" for disease and mortality. As a result, social position involves different exposures and vulnerabilities, and public health interventions target individual risks and behaviors. To improve inequities in access to resources and inequalities in health outcomes, "political will" can lead to reforms that reduce the harmful impacts of social determinants. These reforms can occur within the current global capitalist political economic system. For instance, obesity and diabetes linked to poverty will improve through interventions that change individuals' behaviors in reducing dietary sugar and increasing exercise.

The perspective of social determination leads to different data, interpretations, and recommendations for change. Social determination views society as a totality, rather than as a sum of individuals, and the overall characteristics of a society require analysis in studying the impacts of social conditions on health. Instead of health or illness as dichotomous categories, social determination considers health–illness as a dialectic process. A dialectic vision requires a multilevel analysis of how social conditions, such as economic production, reproduction, marginalization, and political oppression, affect a dynamic process of health–illness among different groups within a population, such as workers versus capitalists, poor versus rich, women versus men, and ethnic–racial minorities versus non-minorities. Rather than processes of persuasion and assessment of evidence, changes in policies and in societies emerge from social contradictions and the social movements and conflicts that arise from those contradictions. Hierarchies of determination, production, and reproduction at the societal level impact health–illness, as opposed to individual-level variables that measure risk. Such hierarchies involve power relations, accumulation of capital, and discrimination (classism, racism, sexism) that create inequality, exploitation, and chronic stress, and these conditions lead to illness and early death. Lasting improvements emerge through societal transformation, for instance, transforming the structural characteristics of capitalism that generate illness, early death, environmental degradation, war, and multiple injurious effects on humanity, other forms of life, and the earth. Considering the example of obesity and diabetes, social determination focuses on the capitalist food industry that promotes unhealthy food and that restricts access to healthy food; organizing to increase food self-sufficiency through collaborative food production, distribution, and consumption at the community level aims to overcome dependency on industrial agriculture.

From here on, we apply the perspectives of social determination to devastating health problems. In the sections that follow, we consider occupational and environmental illnesses that show how social determination works in real-world situations. These examples provide gripping examples of social contradictions that stand in the way of healthy workplaces and a healthy environment. In the next chapter, we analyze three "variables" that studies of the SDOH usually identify as important: social class, race, and gender. But we use the approach of social determination to move beyond the associations between variables and adverse health outcomes. Specifically, we try to clarify the mechanisms by which discrimination and oppression lead to the effects of classism, racism, and sexism in health.

Plastic Workers' Liver Cancer

Social contradictions manifest themselves in many health conditions that social medicine aims to clarify. One disturbing example of such a contradiction regarding occupational health has arisen in the plastics industry. Vinyl chloride is an industrially produced colorless gas used to make polyvinyl chloride, commonly known as PVC, which in turn is used to make a variety of plastic products. In the early 2000s, researchers began to identify an increased risk of liver cancer in plastic-manufacturing employees. This issue gained worldwide attention due to the poor prognosis of the particular type of cancer, hepatic angiosarcoma. Continued research also suggests that exposure to vinyl chloride can cause other types of cancer as well. However, despite the apparently strong evidence that vinyl chloride causes cancer of the liver and other organs, the plastics industry resisted attempts to reduce occupational exposure.[9]

The production of plastic has involved several steps. During one step, the cleaning stage, workers have crawled into reactors where PVC is formed; within these reactors the concentration of vinyl chloride has exceeded 1,000 parts per million (ppm). However, in a study with rodents, researchers found that liver damage could occur with exposure to as little as 50 ppm. Although the minimum toxic level for humans is unknown, professionals working in occupational safety and health recommended that companies should ensure exposure levels of 1 ppm or less. The plastic industry generally refused to comply, stating that this recommendation would raise the cost of production by about 50 percent. As a compromise, the U.S. Occupational Safety and Health Administration set a standard that allowed exposure levels up to 25 ppm. The plastic industry still did not agree with the concession and challenged exposure regulation through court appeals. This action delayed the implementation of new regulations, and employees continued to be exposed to dangerously high levels of the chemical.

While the impact of increased production cost on profit is the industry's main concern, this issue also affects organized labor. The implementation of safer standards is costly and time consuming, and it is likely that some plants producing PVC would close, either permanently or temporarily. If plants were closed until safe production procedures or substitutes for PVC were developed, many workers would lose their jobs for extended periods of time.

This is labor's classic dilemma in occupational disease. Workers frequently face a choice between job safety and continued employment. Workmen's compensation laws provide financial benefits only after a worker has suffered injury or disability from the work process; there are no adequate provisions for financial assistance during changes in the production process that would prevent the development of occupational diseases. Workers' desire for a safe workplace is, thus, an ambivalent desire, as the threat of unemployment is present in any struggle to reduce occupational hazards. Historically, organized labor has favored safety legislation and tighter regulations, but when workers confront job loss, they often have accepted compromises that they recognize are inadequate.

As the dangers of vinyl chloride have become clearer, plastic workers' unions have supported the recommendation of 1 ppm, but political and economic realities have restrained the unions' activism. In general, unions have not opposed the compromise regulation of 25 ppm, since they receive no assurance of alternative employment during the industry's transition to safer standards. Profitability imposes a structural impediment on the industry's willingness to modify production in order to ensure a safe workplace. To keep their jobs, workers are left with no choice but to accept a risk of cancer.

Asbestos Workers' Lung Disease and Cancer

Asbestos is another one of the many compounds that can cause occupational disease. Industries that have exposed workers to asbestos include manufacturers of insulation (pipes, heatproof screens, etc.), construction, shipyards, and textile makers. The disease "asbestosis" occurs in the following way: Industrial dusts containing asbestos settle in the small airways of the lungs, form dust deposits, and cause inflammation. This inflammation leads to scarring, or fibrosis, in the cell layers between airways and small blood vessels. As a result of fibrosis, it becomes more and more difficult for oxygen to move from the lungs into the bloodstream.

Workers in many industries develop similar chronic lung diseases from exposure to other types of dust: aluminosis ("bauxite lung") from aluminum in smelting, explosives, paints, and fireworks manufacturing; baritosis from barium sulfate in mining; beryllium disease from beryllium in aircraft manufacturing, metallurgy, and rocket fuels; kaolinosis from hydrated aluminum silicates in china making; platinum asthma from platinum salts in electronics and chemical industries; siderosis from iron oxides in welding and iron ore; silicosis from silica in mining, pottery, sandblasting, foundries, quarries, and masonry; stannosis from tin oxide in smelting; and talcosis from hydrated magnesium silicates in the rubber industry.

Although many of these diseases produce chronic disability and early death from lung pathology alone, asbestos has the added danger of cancer. Since 1935 the medical literature has contained reports of lung cancer associated with asbestosis. The industry's response followed a pattern of denial and suppression of information: For many years, major asbestos companies in the United States and Canada publicly claimed that evidence of cancer caused by asbestos was not convincing enough to reduce exposure levels. Several companies also gave financial support to researchers whose published studies showed no relation between asbestos and cancer. Retrospectively, all these studies used inadequate methods. For example, industry-sponsored research studied young people who worked in asbestos production for short periods of time; this research generally ignored the latent period between exposure and development of disease.

During the 1960s, for the first time, several investigators who were not receiving industry support were able to study workers who had longer periods of occupational exposure to asbestos. These definitive studies showed a clear-cut association between asbestos exposure and a specific cancer called "mesothelioma," an otherwise rare cancer growing from the lining of the chest or abdominal cavity.[10] Sixty years after the initial reports of asbestosis, and 50 years after the observed association between asbestos and cancer, it has been only during the past four decades that there have been serious attempts to reduce workers' exposure to safe levels.

As in other occupational health problems, the industry's profits have stood in the way of change. The prospect of unemployment also has inhibited unions of asbestos workers from taking a strong stand on working conditions. Many asbestos workers have lost their jobs during production cutbacks resulting from environmental protection regulations. This discouraging outcome, however, is not inevitable. Some positive changes can happen when workers take control of their factories, as can be seen in the example of the Vermont Asbestos Company (VAC), although even those improvements can deteriorate due to the continuing contradiction between profit and safety.

For many years, the GAF Corporation of New York – a multinational corporation controlling numerous industrial subsidiaries – owned and operated an asbestos mine in northern Vermont. The mine served as the main employer for two local towns. In 1974, the U.S. Environmental Protection Agency and the Vermont Occupational Safety and Health Administration asked the mine to install dust-control devices and procedures to lower asbestos exposures to appropriate levels. The estimated cost of these changes was about $1 million. Rather than spend the money, GAF decided to close the mine.

Facing massive unemployment, workers at the mine began to consider an alternative: owning and running the mine themselves. At first, the price of $5 million seemed impossible. With outside technical support, however, workers obtained the necessary loans, bought the mine, and began operating it themselves. Workers and their families purchased shares in the company. Productivity increased, and soon VAC had repaid its loans. In one and a half years, the mine was making a profit. As a result, the board (composed jointly of manual and managerial workers, all whom held shares in the company) decided to invest in a new plant, located in an area of high unemployment, that would make construction material from asbestos waste products. VAC also installed dust-control devices that brought asbestos levels close to recommended standards.

Despite these early successes with worker ownership and management, the contradiction between profit and safety did not disappear when "profit" returned to workers. At first, since VAC's revenues no longer went to an external corporation, they were hardly profits in the traditional sense. Monetary rewards meant little if workers faced disability, cancer, and early death. The importance of safety in the workplace became a higher priority when workers owned the workplace.

The initial accomplishments of VAC and similar cooperative ventures in worker ownership do not, of course, imply that such a strategy will solve all occupational health problems under capitalism. Worker ownership within the overall framework of capitalism faces basic structural limitations. In the case of VAC, one investor gradually bought out the interests of workers and assumed dominant control of the company, which took on the name Vermont Asbestos Group (VAG). Later, the profitability of asbestos production declined rapidly after its health hazards became more widely known. The mine eventually closed in 1993, leaving a huge environmental clean-up problem that has persisted until the present day. Experiments in worker ownership clarify the contradiction of profit versus safety, and the improvements that become possible when profit is no longer an impediment to change in the production process. But the temporary time course of such improvements also shows the fragility of these attempts in the context of an overall economic system founded on profitability rather than health.[11]

Farmworkers' Back

The contradiction between profit and safety arises not only in industry but also in agriculture. Chronic back injury, for example, is one of the most common occupational diseases that farmworkers have endured in the United States. This disease has occurred mostly in agricultural work that has depended almost entirely on manual labor.

Although contradictions like the one between profit and safety manifest themselves at the level of social structures, they also have direct effects on the lives of individuals. Therefore, it is again useful to consider these effects more concretely. The following case history concerns a patient followed by one of the authors (Howard) at a clinic of the United Farm Workers Union in California.

> J.C. was a 32-year-old Chicano father of five. He began working as a farm laborer at age 14. He generally worked ten to twelve hours a day, in stoop labor with an arched back, on such crops as lettuce. For about ten years he used the "short hoe" required of many farmworkers in Western states. At age 28, while bending at work, he suddenly felt a sharp pain in his back with radiation down his left leg. Physical exam at that time showed tenderness over the L4–L5 intervertebral space of the back, decreased reflexes and sensation of the left leg, weakness of the muscles in the left foot and ankle, and positive straight-leg raising test (a test for impingement of a nerve root). X-rays showed advanced degenerative arthritis of the entire lower spine and a slipped disc at the L4–L5 level. Severe pain on bending persisted despite back surgery. The patient knew no English, could not find a job outside farm labor, and was forced to apply for permanent disability benefits.

The short hoe has a small wooden handle about one foot in length. To use the short hoe, a person must work in a stooped posture, bent forward at the waist, so that the hoe can reach the ground. The short hoe has no intrinsic advantage over the long-handled hoe, which a farmworker can use in an erect posture. The only reason to prefer the short hoe is supervision: If the foreman sees that all workers in a crew are bent over, he can be assured that everybody is working. Using long-handled hoes, workers can stand with their backs straight. Therefore, with a small number of supervisors, it can be hard to make sure that large numbers of workers are actually working.

Farmworker's back is a preventable disease. It occurs in an industrialized agricultural sector of the economy that is highly oriented toward profit. That profit historically has come with the short hoe's human toll of crippling back disease for thousands of farmworkers; the main injuries are slipped discs and degenerative arthritis of the spine. These problems have occurred in young workers doing stoop labor, and their physical effects are irreversible. Since migrant workers most often lack educational opportunities and frequently know little English, farmworkers' back usually means permanent economic disability.

There is nothing new about this disease. Medical specialists have testified about the short hoe's devastating effects for several decades. Yet, for many years farm owners, especially the agribusiness corporations that have gained control of many agricultural enterprises, refused to stop the short hoe's use. Farm owners generally gave no reason for this policy, except that long-handled hoes would require higher costs of supervision. A few companies also argued that the wood for longer handles increased costs; when analyzed, however, the costs of longer handles were minimal. It was the profit motive and the nature of agricultural production that led directly to this disease-generating labor practice.

Until the mid-1960s, farmworkers were largely unorganized. Additional workers needing employment, which Engels first called the "reserve army of the unemployed" in *The Condition of the Working Class in England in 1844*,[12] were available to replace those crippled by farmworkers' back or objecting to the conditions of work. Individual farmworkers were powerless and had no alternative to the disabling effects of the short hoe, because resistance meant loss of work.

The United Farm Workers (UFW) organization has organized farmworkers throughout the West, Southwest, and Southeast. Like other unions, the UFW has fought for basic improvements in wages and benefits. Beyond these economic gains, however, the union has focused on the conditions of work. The UFW organized and launched publicity campaigns concerning the short hoe, dangerous insecticides and chemicals, and other occupational health issues.

In response to this pressure, the California legislature ultimately passed a law banning the short hoe. Agribusiness corporations then obtained a series of court injunctions against the new law. These rulings accepted the companies' claim that conversion to the long-handled hoe would lead to excess costs. Other courts later reversed these injunctions. But even after legislation, some California farmworkers (as well as workers in other states without such laws) continued to use and suffer from the short hoe. In addition, because growers still require stoop labor for activities such as weeding organic vegetables by hand, the musculoskeletal problems of farmworkers persist.

Meanwhile, activists have hardly scratched the surface of occupational health problems in agriculture such as pesticides, herbicides, and toxic chemicals. Progress occurs, albeit slowly. In the fall of 2015, the UFW won a long-fought battle for pesticide worker protection. The new act would enforce pesticide application requirements, create whistleblower protections for complaints, and provide access to records for employees. At that time, Arturo S. Rodriguez, president of the UFW of America, said: "Is it ever too late to do the right thing? It's been a long time coming, but it has come today."[13] Under the Trump administration, which prioritized elimination of even the limited occupational health protections achieved in prior years, these advances again began to deteriorate. The contradiction between profit and safety, therefore, persists in agriculture as it does in industry.[14]

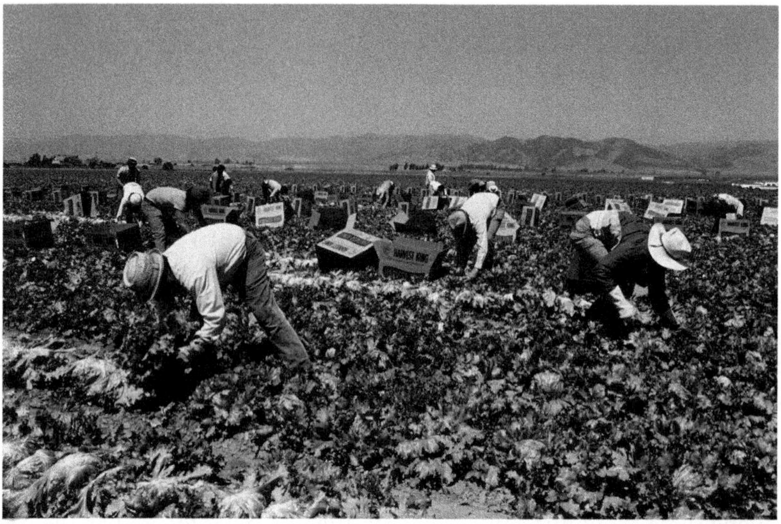

Figure 3.1 Farmworkers weeding organic lettuce by hand without a hoe. An online photo shows the similarity of work positions before and after the short hoe was banned.

Brain Disease from Mercury Poisoning

It is also important to understand how this contradiction extends beyond the workplace to affect entire communities and larger populations. In 1907, a chemical company built a factory in Minamata, Japan. Minamata is a small seacoast community whose economy for centuries had been based on fishing. Over the years, the factory grew and became part of a large petrochemical conglomerate, the Chisso Corporation. Because the factory dumped its waste products into Minamata Bay, fish began to die or to avoid the area. In 1925, Chisso started to give payments to local fisherman who complained.

In 1932, Chisso began to produce acetylaldehyde, a chemical used in the manufacturing of drugs, perfumes, plastics, and many other products. Organic mercury, which is highly toxic to humans and other animals, is a catalyst for acetaldehyde production. Beginning in 1952, cats in Minamata began to die after developing convulsions, bizarre behavior, and paralysis. Between 1956 and 1957, 52 children and adults started to show similar neurologic disorders; 21 people died. Outside investigators reported that the cause of the disease was probably heavy metal poisoning carried to humans and cats that ate the fish from Minamata Bay.

In 1959, a scientist working for Chisso fed material from an acetaldehyde waste pipe to a cat in his laboratory. Soon after the cat showed the typical signs of what is now called "Minamata Disease." This scientist reported this finding to Chisso management. The management suppressed the finding and ordered the scientist not to conduct more experiments concerning Minamata Disease. The scientist remained silent, but the results of his experiment would eventually come to light during trials that took place in the late 1960s. Prior to the trials, the company publicly announced there was no scientific proof that Minamata Disease was related to Chisso manufacturing processes. The company installed a "purification device" in 1959. But Chisso continued to dump waste products containing mercury into Minamata Bay until 1968, when it switched to catalysts that were technically more effective than mercury.

During the 1960s and 1970s, over 3,000 patients brought legal suit against Chisso for financial compensation and medical expenses. Residents also held demonstrations, sit-ins, and other protests at the Minamata plant. Company guards, together with unionized workers at the plant, physically attacked the protestors several times; there were many injuries, some serious. Despite the company's resistance, in 1973 the Central Pollution Board decided that Chisso would pay medically verified patients $68,000 for "heavy" cases and $60,000 for "lighter" cases. Many of the patients were children with congenital Minamata Disease, whose mothers had eaten mercury-containing fish during pregnancy. Meanwhile, the provincial government announced that fish outside Minamata Bay, marked by buoys, were safe to eat. This decision ignored the seemingly obvious fact that fish throughout the Shiranui Sea, of which Minamata Bay is a part, can swim past buoys. Researchers in Japan estimated that as many as 10,000 people, previously eating fish from Shiranui Sea, eventually fell ill with Minamata Disease.

The structure of capitalist production is responsible for such tragedies of environmental poisoning. For more than a decade, Chisso management suppressed evidence of the company's responsibility for Minamata Disease; management recognized the financial burden it would face if it accepted responsibility. Indemnity payments would drastically affect profits. There were no mechanisms by which Japanese society as a whole could compensate the victims or pay their medical expenses. Moreover, in this situation, workers at Chisso had structural interests that overlapped with management's. By reducing profitability, major payments to Minamata victims or a less efficient production process without mercury catalysts would ultimately threaten workers' jobs. During the protests and suits, these economic realities led unionized workers at Chisso to side with their managers against their injured neighbors. If profit were not the guiding motivation of industry, and if society guaranteed people's material subsistence, prevention and protection from industrial poisoning would not encounter such fundamental resistance.[15]

The implications of Minamata Disease go far beyond Japan and mercury. During the 1960s, a paper company in northern Ontario, Canada, dumped mercury-containing wastes into the English and Wabigoon Rivers. This region of Canada is fairly isolated: The people who live there are mainly indigenous communities and the operators of tourist camps. Several citizens, concerned about the mercury problem, obtained tests that showed toxic levels in the river fish. Government officials investigated the situation. The paper company reduced, but did not eliminate, the mercury in its waste discharges. Although it is estimated that the river fish will contain toxic mercury levels for about 70 years, the government did not stop the company's mercury dumps, nor did the government ban fishing, apparently responding to pressures from the tourist industry that caters to visiting sports fishermen. Inaction persisted despite the fact that several people in the region developed classic symptoms of Minamata Disease and showed high mercury levels in tests of blood and hair. Mercury poisoning is still a major problem for the indigenous communities in Canada.[16]

Outbreaks of mercury and other heavy metal poisoning occur periodically in many parts of the United States and in other countries as well. In the early phases of the Minamata epidemic, investigators found that Chisso was pouring into the sea more than 50 chemicals that can cause disease in humans. Later research showed that thallium, manganese, and selenium – all present in high concentrations in Chisso's effluents – were not the cause of symptoms; mercury was.[17] Other industries have discharged these elements and related compounds, including lead, hydrocarbons, asbestos, and radioactive spills. Environmental poisons have caused temporary epidemics of acute illness; their chronic effects, especially in the development of cancer, are only recently receiving more attention. The social, economic, and political issues involved in many geographic areas, and related to specific poisons, resemble those of Minamata. While the structure of capitalist production remains what it is, one can expect more of the same devastation that people of Minamata have faced. The contradiction between profit and safety persists as a major source of illness, suffering, and death.

Leukemia and Lymphoma among Electronic Workers

It is difficult to believe that such occupational and environmental health atrocities, stemming from the contradiction between profit and safety, could occur at this point in history. However, these challenges continue to affect those who are vulnerable. In 2012, researchers in South Korea reported a cluster of leukemia and non-Hodgkin lymphoma among workers in the electronics industry. These researchers have pursued their work against obstacles erected by the Samsung Group and the government of South Korea. Because most of us use cellphones, computers, video displays, and other electronic products, our actions as consumers become intertwined with the health problems of workers who make the products we use.

In February 2012, the Korean government's Occupational Safety and Health Research Institute announced their findings from a three-year investigation that identified several known cancer-causing agents being used in the electronics production process. These carcinogens were commonly employed especially in the production and handling of semiconductors, which are essential components of many electronic products. The carcinogens included chemicals like benzene, formaldehyde, and arsenic, as well as ionized radiation. Benzene is a product derived from coal and petroleum; it is employed in the manufacture of items such as plastics, detergents, and pesticides. Studies suggest that there may be an association between occupational exposure to benzene and the development of lymphoid and myeloid leukemia.[18]

Samsung has refused to allow independent researchers to obtain essential information concerning their industrial processes. Previously Samsung has come under fire for concerns about public health, labor rights, the environment, and fair trade. For example, Samsung prohibits union organizing and has fired employees for attempting to do so. Community members and their supporters have criticized and resisted Samsung for participation, through its construction subsidiary, in the destruction of environmentally and culturally sensitive habitat on the South Korean island of Jeju, linked to the construction of a new naval base. Jeju's economy is largely dependent on fishing and agriculture; construction of a naval base will exert major effects on the fragile ecosystem.

In this context, Samsung's occupational health policies appear consistent with the corporation's overall approach to profitability as the driving force of policy making. Although researchers and activists have called attention to the clusters of leukemia and other cancers among Samsung's electronic workers, the corporation has not cooperated meaningfully in attempts to resolve the scientific questions involved or in acknowledging its responsibility to compensate workers.

Even if Samsung eventually does succumb to pressure and begins to collaborate in a forthright way to investigate the impact of toxic exposures on its workers, methods to establish causality are not straightforward. In particular, the usual epidemiological methods to assess the impact of exposures on disease outcomes contain some inherent limitations. For example, a case-control study follows all workers who are exposed to a certain chemical or carcinogen and identifies those who developed disease and those who did not. To do this, however, a large number of people are needed to reach statistical significance. Due to this methodological challenge of proving causality with small numbers of cases, clusters of cancer like those that have appeared among Samsung workers may not receive the urgent attention and action that they deserve.

To address the impediments to occupational safety and health that Samsung has created, actions that go beyond research are urgently needed. Those who care about the health of electronics workers – and workers in general – need to consider ways to exert pressures on Samsung and to publicize these concerns in ways that motivate Samsung to address fully workers' health issues. Economic leverage could encourage Samsung's honest and open disclosure of information on workers' exposures, improved protection of workers from toxic exposures in the production process, respect for workers' right to unionize, and facilitation of independent research on the cancer-causing effects of semiconductor production. These efforts, like many in social medicine pertaining to occupational and environmental health, cry out for urgent attention. At the time of this writing, two small children became motherless after the 32nd death from cancer among workers at a single Samsung semiconductor manufacturing plant, and 118 deaths, among more than 250 victims, have occurred overall at Samsung electronics manufacturing facilities.[19]

Upstream Causes of COVID-19 and Other Epidemics to Follow[20]

Through dangerous and sometimes heroic efforts, people working in social medicine and clinical medicine around the world have struggled to lessen the many downstream effects of COVID-19, which we described in Chapter 1. In particular, we referred to the devastating impacts that the pandemic has exerted on indigenous, black, Latinx, incarcerated, migrant, and other minority and marginalized populations. We drew a linkage between these downstream effects and upstream causes rooted in poverty, discrimination, insecure access to food and housing, unavailable clean water, and sanitation; such challenges play an important role in essentially all major epidemics.

Other upstream causes of the COVID-19 pandemic are linked to the social contradictions that we have been considering. Again, these contradictions derive from the characteristics of the global capitalist political-economic system, especially the contradiction between profit and safety. Clarity about such upstream causes rarely emerges in discussions of the pandemic, even in the scientific and public health communities, and hardly ever in pronouncements of the public health institutions on which many of us rely: the World Health Organization (WHO), U.S. Centers for Disease Control and Prevention (CDC), U.S. National Institute of Allergy and Infectious Diseases (NIAID), Pan American Health Organization (PAHO), Gates Foundation, and so forth.

Identifying the upstream causes of epidemics has been a central goal of epidemiology since the 1840s. At that time, the pathologist Rudolf Virchow, as we describe in Chapters 1 and 2, did his path-breaking investigation of the upstream social conditions – poverty, inequality, food insecurity, inadequate housing, and social marginalization – that led to a devastating typhus epidemic in Upper Silesia, as well as epidemics of tuberculosis and cholera elsewhere.[21] Due to the COVID-19 pandemic's magnitude, one would expect that the upstream causes would be crystal clear for all to see, so we could address them directly, but amazingly this is not the case.

Many people attribute the origins of the pandemic to the strange and retro marketing practices of some individuals and groups in Wuhan, China, who were selling wild animals in the market from which the virus spread, eventually worldwide. But such marketing practices involving wild animals have been going on for a long time, probably hundreds of years or more. Why did a pandemic arise in 2019 and not earlier?

Upstream Causes in Agriculture

Although the source of COVID-19 remains uncertain at the time of this writing (spring 2020), most evidence suggests this pandemic and every other important emerging viral epidemic in the recent past and predictably into the future come from the same upstream causes: capitalist industrial agriculture, destruction of natural habitat, and production of meat. For several decades, the intensity and worldwide scale of capitalist industrial practices in agriculture have increased rapidly. Pioneering microbiological and epidemiological studies have clarified these upstream causes of emerging epidemics, whose effects we now are confronting every day.[22] In addition to viral epidemics, these and similar agricultural practices also deepen the parallel crises of multi-drug-resistant bacterial infections (through overuse of antibiotics in industrial meat and fish production), climate change (by destruction of rainforest habitats and long-distance transportation of food that requires burning of petroleum), plastic pollution (by agricultural packaging methods), and other severe environmental problems.[23]

LABORATORY ACCIDENT AS AN ALTERNATIVE EXPLANATION FOR COVID-19

An alternative but less likely explanation for the source of COVID-19 focuses on the unintentional release of the virus from a laboratory in China. This explanation also involves "upstream" conditions, including the laboratory-based development of dangerous viruses as part of "biodefense" procedures and vaccine production, with participation by multinational pharmaceutical corporations, military organizations, government agencies including those of China and the United States, non-governmental organizations focusing on ecology, and foundations that favor drugs and vaccines as solutions for public health challenges. While we do not review the evidence here, we do agree that the possibility of unintentional release from a laboratory warrants detailed investigation and attention. For more information, please see note 23.

Natural forest habitat previously provided ecological control for microbes such as SARS-CoV-2 and their hosts such as bats. Because humans entered these forests infrequently and because human communities remained small and mostly isolated, infections rarely spread from forest animals to humans; when they did spread, they usually did not affect larger population centers in different regions. Clearing habitat for industrial agriculture emerged as a central characteristic of China's economy as it "liberalized" after Mao Zedong into a bastion of the capitalist world system.[24] Similar "zoonotic" sources of transmission from wild animals in destroyed habitats have happened in China with the previous coronavirus in severe acute respiratory syndrome (SARS); Ebola in Africa; Zika in Africa, Latin America, and elsewhere; and arguably HIV in Africa.[25]

Another practice stemming from the capitalist model of agriculture involves the industrial production of meat. Especially for pigs and chickens but also other species, reproduction of offspring, growth to adulthood, slaughter, and packaging increasingly occur under factory conditions that receive little regulatory oversight and control. Worldwide, a small number of large multinational corporations dominate factory farming. In enormous factory farms, animals live their entire lives in small cages, contaminated by feces and urine, which slowly drain into large pits and pools that may leak into the surrounding environment. As with the other diseases considered in this chapter, corporations trying to maximize their profits usually do not choose to improve health and safety conditions through costly changes in sanitation. Because of these conditions, viruses spread and mutate to more virulent organisms in unsanitary factory conditions, leading to epidemics of swine flu, avian flu, and a variety of emerging influenza viruses.[26]

Deemphasis on Agriculture in Public Health

Even though sources of information like CDC and WHO remain widely recommended, do they provide a complete picture? Some well-motivated people work for these agencies, and helpful information is available. But mistakes get made, as have occurred multiple times during the COVID-19 pandemic, and more importantly these sources rarely address the upstream causes of epidemics. Many have commented about the devastating funding cutbacks and de-prioritization that have crippled these organizations' capacity to protect public health. As just one example, the annual program budget of WHO for the whole world is smaller by about half than the operating budget of a large medical center in the United States (WHO: $4.34 billion; New York Presbyterian Hospital: about $8 billion).[27]

Into the financial crisis of international health organizations have stepped the World Bank, International Monetary Fund, Gates Foundation, and other agencies of "philanthrocapitalism," whose financial priorities and ideologies dominate the policies and practices of WHO and its affiliated organizations worldwide.[28] This is one reason that the global People's Health Movement produces "WHO Watch" and "Global Health Watch" to monitor WHO critically and offer alternatives that WHO and its affiliates do not pursue because of their financial dependency on international financial institutions and philanthrocapitalism.[29] Partly due to such financial support, international and national health organizations almost always promote reductionist initiatives that focus on so-called magic bullets such as vaccines and antiviral medications, as well as behavioral change at the level of individuals, rather than upstream causes.

Financial conflicts of interest can also distort the organizations' policies. For instance, the Gates Foundation has invested in and promoted genetically modified crops through such corporations as Monsanto/Bayer. Farmlands for such crops produce mainly animal feeds, required for increased meat production, which causes further loss of forest habitat.[30] In addition, Gates' investments emphasize new medications and vaccines produced by pharmaceutical corporations and other companies that profit from intellectual property, which in the realm of computer software creates most of Gates' wealth. Similarly, CDC and its employees regularly attract criticism based on revelations about conflicts of interest at both the organizational level (especially regarding grants and other financial support that a foundation connected to CDC receives from the pharmaceutical industry) and individual level (employees' and committee members' investments in and gifts from the industry).[31]

Agricultural Corporations

So WHO, CDC, Gates, and their affiliates have obscured the upstream causes of emerging viral epidemics not only in COVID-19 but also in all other recent epidemics. An especially disheartening example was the swine flu epidemic of 2009, which began within 1 mile of Smithfield Foods' notorious industrial pig farm operation in a rural area of Veracruz state in Mexico. Smithfield had outsourced this operation from the United States partly due to occupational and environmental cleanup requirements. Although public health authorities and investigators in Mexico and other countries reported this epidemiological association between swine flu and capitalist industrial agriculture (one of the authors, Howard, was involved), CDC, WHO, Gates, and all other international health organizations pursued reductionist strategies like a vaccine, rather than confront radical change in the meat-processing industry.[32]

During the COVID-19 pandemic, Smithfield's practices became even more startling. Less than a decade after the swine flu epidemic, a Hong Kong-based investment corporation, WH Group Ltd, had acquired Smithfield Foods. In 2018, an ongoing epidemic of African swine fever, a coronavirus that was causing the deaths or intentional killing (to prevent further spread of disease) of millions of pigs in Europe and Asia. Because a reduced global supply of pork would lead to major increases in prices and profitability for the corporation, Smithfield executives based at U.S. headquarters in Smithfield, Virginia, welcomed the African swine flu epidemic.[33] When COVID-19 struck, Smithfield executives reassured U.S. consumers that, despite ownership in Hong Kong, the corporation did not import pork from China but instead exported U.S. pork to China, where prices were higher.[34] The Smithfield pork-processing plant in Sioux Falls, South Dakota, became one of the largest COVID-19 hotspots in the United States. Rapid spread of the infection to workers because of similar unsanitary working conditions affected other corporations' meat-processing plants as well.[35]

The role of capitalist industrial agriculture through loss of habitat and meat production occasionally does surface in the mainstream media. Such media attention, while limited, happened occasionally during the COVID-19 pandemic, although the term "capitalist" did not enter the discussion.[36] But the impacts of such corporations on emerging epidemics rarely appear in communications or policies of international health organizations or the Gates Foundation.

The leaders of these agencies are fully aware that emerging viral epidemics come from capitalist industrial agriculture. They showed this awareness in "Event 201" on October 18, 2019, ironically about two months before the COVID-19 epidemic began in Wuhan.[37] In this "tabletop exercise," coordinated by the Johns Hopkins Center for Health Security, Gates Foundation, and World Economic Forum, a novel coronavirus pandemic begins at pig farms in Brazil and spreads rapidly around the world, resulting in 65 million deaths and catastrophic effects on the global economy, political stability, and international security. After the COVID-19 epidemic actually began, the sponsors of Event 201 emphasized that they did not predict the timing of COVID-19 and that the projected death toll did not necessarily apply. But they did not say anything about an initiative to eradicate the practices of capitalist industrial agriculture that led to the hypothetical scenario of Event 201, to the current global COVID-19 pandemic, and to the inevitable future pandemics that will occur on a similar scale or even worse if these current upstream causes do not change.

Better Ways to Produce Food

Is there an alternative to capitalist industrial agriculture? Yes. Around the world, often against resistance from corporations and governments, farmers are returning to peasant agricultural practices. A whole body of research has shown that peasant agriculture is not only safer than capitalist agriculture but actually is more efficient and productive as well.[38] Millions of people worldwide already are making this transition, often because they/we see no other choice. Especially in the context of economic collapse, capitalist agriculture – with its tendency to overproduce and even destroy surplus food while hunger and food insecurity worsen – is ill suited to feed the world's peoples.

Changing the upstream causes of epidemics like COVID-19 and others yet to come becomes a key scientific and practical priority for medicine and public health, considering the future of humanity and other inhabitants of the planet. If that transformation doesn't happen, we can expect even more devastating pandemics, stemming from the same upstream causes.

The Narrative of Economic Collapse

The official narrative of COVID-19 states that the pandemic caused the global capitalist economy to collapse, or at least to enter a deep recession and possibly great depression, but is that correct?

A more accurate interpretation is that the pandemic triggered a collapse that was going to happen anyway. For many years, the global capitalist economy has been crisis ridden, unstable, and "bubbly... subject to blowups."[39] During August 2019, months before the COVID-19 pandemic began, the interest yield on a ten-year U.S. Treasury bond fell below that of a two-year bond. This inversion, indicating a marked decline in investors' confidence in long-term earnings, has preceded every recession since the 1950s. These and other economic trends led the editors of the journal *Monthly Review* to predict: "There is now little doubt that the world economy is on the verge of a recession after a long sluggish recovery from the Great Financial Crisis of 2007–09.... In this instance, however, there lurks a bigger fear, the possibility of a financial Armageddon on the level of the Great Financial Crisis of 2008—or worse."[40]

The COVID-19 narrative assigns blame for the economic crash to a virus, taking attention away from the structural contradictions and instabilities that would have led to a crash in any case, as predicted for many months before the pandemic began. The global capitalist economy has switched to the expansion of finance capital and away from production of useful goods and services. Financialization now creates "fictitious capital" such as packages of risk, derivatives, and futures. These fictional financial instruments involve gambles on the future valuation of an imaginary reality that does not correspond to any concrete economic good, service, or property. Global markets in financial instruments therefore become a more elite version of gambling that traditionally takes place in poker games, casinos, and racetracks.

Creation of fictitious capital and accumulation of capital through gambling create a vulnerability to burst financial bubbles and crashes like that of 2008. That particular crash derived from the collapse of collateralized loan obligations (CLOs). CLOs refer to financial instruments that bundled housing loans for investment in global financial markets. As the COVID-19 pandemic worsened, large investors spurred the rapid decline in prices of stocks and fictional financial instruments, as they rapidly sold off holdings that had become overvalued. Blaming a virus for the crash mystified the economic contradictions actually responsible for the abrupt end of the latest capitalist bubble.[41]

The false narrative of viral infection as the cause of economic collapse also justified public health policies with little or no scientific basis. Such influential but mostly non-evidence-based public health policies include lockdowns, travel bans, closed schools and factories, and forced quarantines of large populations rather than individuals and clustered groups who harbor the infection.[42] For instance, multiple research studies of school closures during this pandemic and prior epidemics show that risks for mortality due to loss of health workers who can't access alternative childcare balance or outweigh benefits from reduced contagion through children.[43]

The advantages that arise from these drastic measures happen mainly in countries that didn't prepare adequately for the pandemic, didn't respond quickly enough with more focused measures to test and isolate people infected with the virus, and have health care systems either organized by capitalist principles or suffering cutbacks and privatization in recent years due to capitalist economic ideologies such as austerity. Unprepared countries, especially the United States, did not even try to implement the procedures that we learn in Epidemiology 101:

- quickly identify individuals and groups at high risk, especially those who have traveled from specific geographical areas where an epidemic already has spread;
- test those individuals and groups to find out if they have the infection;
- strictly quarantine those individuals and groups who are waiting for test results and/or test positive;
- make sure that those in quarantine have enough food, toilet paper, money, and other necessities of life so that they don't try to escape from the quarantine;
- make sure that those who test positive receive free or very cheap medical treatment and surveillance, with a clearly established end point to determine when they are ready to leave quarantine;
- convey honest and transparent information to the general population about specific geographical locations with prevalent infection so people can get tested if they have been there and can avoid the areas if they have not been there;
- provide financial support for anybody who suffers economic hardship during an epidemic, especially if a person becomes unemployed but

also if there are other sources of vulnerability such as poverty, disability, ethnic/racial minority status, young or old age, recent migration, and chronic illnesses;
- initiate economic policies that preserve people's jobs during an epidemic by paying employers to continue wages and benefits while people can't work, rather than allowing large numbers of people to be laid off and face the insecurity of uncertain future employment.[44]

Health professionals and politicians who advocate more general, population-based interventions like lockdowns either didn't take Epidemiology 101 and therefore don't have a clue how to respond to epidemics, or they did take Epidemiology 101 and understand that their political-economic system doesn't provide a public health infrastructure that permits the above procedures, either early enough during an epidemic or at all – for instance, in the United States, which has lacked a viable public health infrastructure for decades, at least since the drastic cutbacks achieved as part of neoliberal policies starting in the 1980s.

Countries that did prepare, did test and isolate infected people, and have health care systems organized around universal access to services and a well-financed and organized approach to public health have done much better in controlling the pandemic.[45] Complete lockdowns have not occurred in these countries. Such harsh measures, with their devastating economic effects leading to massive unemployment, lost income and retirement accounts, and worsening food and housing insecurity, may seem reasonable for countries whose leaders didn't act decisively at an early stage. But we shouldn't delude ourselves about the scientific evidence for these measures' effectiveness, or about the viral pandemic itself as the cause of the overall economic collapse.

Although the health benefits of such policies remain dubious, the benefits for protecting what remains of global capitalism are substantial. As in 2008, a massive injection of tax-generated, public-sector funding to private corporations creates a kind of socialism for the rich. This process includes a version of disaster capitalism, in which corporations receive public subsidies to protect the capitalist economy.[46] Authoritarian tactics applied by some governments purportedly to contain the pandemic and to protect the economy pave the way to anti-democratic rule, militarism, and fascism. This path becomes especially dangerous when police and military forces get involved in repressive tactics justified by public health and humanitarian rationales. These harsh policies, purportedly implemented to protect the public's health, also exert their most adverse effects on poor, minority, incarcerated, immigrant, and otherwise marginalized populations, who already suffer from the worsening economic inequality that global, financialized capitalism has fostered.[47]

Levels of Analysis in Social Medicine

The problems considered so far show how social contradictions impinge on individuals and groups, especially those who live and work in jobs and environments that make them vulnerable. In particular, the fundamental contradiction between profit and safety in capitalist societies increases the likelihood of illness and early death, within specific industries and communities more than others. This contradiction has generated the upstream causation of many problems considered by social medicine, including COVID-19. However, social medicine also moves the level of analysis higher, to illness-generating characteristics of whole societies. The next chapter shows how social determination happens in this larger context.

Notes

1 Occupational Safety and Health Administration, Department of Labor, "1,2-Dibromo-3-Chloropropane (DBCP)," 2012, www.gpo.gov/fdsys/pkg/CFR-2012-title29-vol6/html/CFR-2012-title29-vol6.htm; D. Shemi, Z. Marx, J. Kaplanski, G. Potashnik, and U. A. Sod-Moriah, "Testicular Damage Development in Rats Injected with Dibromochloropropane (DBCP)/Entwicklung eines Hodenschadens bei der Ratte durch Dibromchlorpropan," *Andrologia* 20, no. 4 (1988): 331–37; David B. Cohen, *Ground Water Contamination by Toxic Substances: A California Assessment*, ACS Symposium Series, Washington, DC: American Chemical Society, 1986; "Groundwater Information Sheet, Dibromochloropropane (DBCP)," State Water Resources Control Board, Division of Water Quality, July 2016, www.waterboards.ca.gov/water_issues/programs/gama/docs/coc_dbcb_infosheet_jz0610.pdf.
2 Howard Waitzkin, "John D. Stoeckle and the Upstream Vision of Social Determinants in Public Health," *American Journal of Public Health* 106, no. 2 (2016): 234–36; John B. McKinlay, "A Case for Refocusing Upstream – The Political Economy of Sickness," in: J.D. Enelow and J.B. Henderson, eds., *Applying Behavioral Science to Cardiovascular Risk* (Dallas, TX: American Heart Association, 1975).
3 See Chapter 2 for more on Engels, Virchow, and Allende. About the concept of embodiment, see Nancy Krieger, "Living and Dying at the Crossroads: Racism, Embodiment, and Why Theory Is Essential for a Public Health of Consequence," *American Journal of Public Health* 106, no. 5 (2016): 832–33; "Public Health, Embodied History, and Social Justice: Looking Forward," *International Journal of Health Services* 45, no. 4 (2015): 587–600; *Epidemiology and the People's Health: Theory and Context* (New York: Oxford University Press, 2013), especially Chapter 7.
4 Howard Waitzkin, "One and a Half Centuries of Forgetting and Rediscovering: Virchow's Lasting Contributions to Social Medicine," *Social Medicine* 1 (2006): 5–10; *Medicine and Public Health at the End of Empire* (Boulder, CO: Paradigm Publishers, 2011), Chapter 2.
5 Commission on Social Determinants of Health, *Closing the Gap in a Generation: Health Equity through Action on the Social Determinants of Health* (Geneva: World Health Organization, 2008), www.who.int/social_determinants/final_report/en/.

6 Howard Waitzkin and F. Allan Hubbell, "Truth's Search for Power: Critical Applications to Community Oriented Primary Care and Small Area Analysis," *Medical Care Review* 49 (1992): 161–89.
7 Anne-Emanuelle Birn, "Making it Politic(al): Closing the Gap in a Generation: Health Equity through Action on the Social Determinants of Health," *Social Medicine* 4, no. 3 (2009): 166–82; Vicente Navarro, "What We Mean by Social Determinants of Health," *International Journal of Health Services* 39, no. 3 (2009): 423–41.
8 Carolina Morales-Borrero, Elis Borde, Juan C. Eslava-Castañeda, and Sonia C. Concha-Sánchez, "¿Determinación Social o Determinantes Sociales? Diferencias Conceptuales e Implicaciones Praxiológicas," *Revista de Salud Pública* (Colombia) 15, no. 6 (2013): 797–808; Elis Borde and Mario Hernández, "Revisiting the Social Determinants of Health Agenda from the Global South," *Global Public Health* (2018), doi:10.1080/17441692.2018.1551913; Jaime Breilh, "La Determinación Social de la Salud Como Herramienta de Transformación hacia una Nueva Salud Pública (Salud Colectiva)," *Revista de la Facultad Nacional de Salud Pública* 31, Supplement 1 (2013): 13–27; Catalina Eibenschutz, Silvia Tamez, and Rafael González, eds.,¿*Determinación Social o Determinantes Sociales de la Salud?* (México: Universidad Autónoma Metropolitana, 2011).
9 The following references also apply to the paragraphs that follow about vinyl chloride: Occupational Safety and Health Administration, Department of Labor, "Vinyl Chloride," 2018, https://www.osha.gov/laws-regs/regulations/standardnumber/1910/1910.1017; Eileen McGurty, *Transforming Environmentalism: Warren County, PCBs, and the Origins of Environmental Justice* (New Brunswick, NJ: Rutgers UP, 2007), pp. 26–28; Laszlo Makk, John L. Creech, and Joseph G. Whelan, Jr., "Liver Damage and Angiosarcoma in Vinyl Chloride Workers: A Systematic Detection Program, *JAMA* 230, no. 1 (1974): 64–68; C. Bossetti, C. La Vecchiia, L. Lipworth, and J.K. McLaughlin, "Occupational Exposure to Vinyl Chloride and Cancer Risk: A Review of the Epidemiologic Literature," *European Journal of Cancer Prevention* 12, no. 5 (2003): 427–30; "Groups Head to Court to Seek Protection from PVC Plant Pollution," *Earthjustice*, October 22, 2008; http://earthjustice.org/news/press/2008/groups-head-to-court-to-seek-protection-from-pvc-plant-pollution.
10 Irving J. Selikoff, Jacob Churg, and E. Cuyler Hammond, "Asbestosis Exposure and Neoplasia," *JAMA* 188, no. 1 (1964): 22–26. Regarding suppression of scientific information about the dangers of asbestos: Gerald Markowitz and David Rosner, 'Unleashed on an Unsuspecting World': The Asbestos Information Association and Its Role in Perpetuating a National Epidemic," *American Journal of Public Health* 106 (2016): 834–40.
11 For comments about the early history of asbestos workers' ownership in a mainly positive light: Howard Waitzkin, "Asbestos Workers' Lung Disease and Cancer," in *The Second Sickness: Contradictions of Capitalist Health Care* (New York: Free Press, 1983). The analysis here updates the story with problems that developed later. For more on this history, see: Kayla Collier, "30 Million Tons of Asbestos Leftovers," *Stowe (Vermont) News & Citizen*, August 18, 2017, www.stowetoday.com/news_and_citizen/news/local_news/million-tons-of-asbestos-leftovers/article_f4f10bae-8366-11e7-8fb7-e363f8bc6585.html; State of Vermont, Department of Labor, "R. P., Estate of R. P., H. P. v. Vermont Asbestos Group," January 23, 2007, http://labor.vermont.gov/wordpress/wp-content/uploads/X-01358Pion.pdf.

12 Friedrich Engels, *The Condition of the Working Class in England in 1844* (Moscow: Progress Publishers, 1973 [1845]).
13 Farm Workers Win Long-fought Battle for Pesticide Worker Protections under New EPA Rules," United Farm Workers, September 28, 2015, http://ufw.org/Farm-workers-win-long-fought-battle-for-pesticide-worker-protections-under-new-EPA-rules. For more on the UFW's accomplishments, including those in health, see Inga Kim, "UFW Successes through the Years," April 3, 2017, https://ufw.org/ufw-successes-years/. For a balanced account that does not focus on health issues: Frank Bardacke, *Trampling Out the Vintage: César Chávez and the Two Souls of the United Farm Workers* (London and New York: Verso, 2011).
14 For other important work on the health problems of migrant farmworkers, see: Sarah Bronwen Horton, *They Leave Their Kidneys in the Fields: Illness, Injury, and Illegality among U.S. Farmworkers* (Oakland: University of California Press, 2016); Seth Holmes, *Fresh Fruit, Broken Bodies: Migrant Farmworkers in the United States* (Oakland: University of California Press, 2013).
15 For a gripping pictorial description and analysis of what happened in Minamata, see W. Eugene Smith and Aileen M. Smith, *Minamata* (New York: Holt, Rinehart and Winston, 1975), especially pp. 140–43.
16 Susan Goldberg, "The Town Where Mercury Still Rises," *New York Times*, April 19, 2017, www.nytimes.com/2017/04/19/opinion/the-town-where-mercury-still-rises.html.
17 Smith and Smith, *Minamata*.
18 Fatemeh Saberi Hosnijeh, Yvette Christopher, Petra Peeters, et al., "Occupation and Risk of Lymphoid and Myeloid Leukaemia in the European Prospective Investigation into Cancer and Nutrition (EPIC)," *Occupational & Environmental Medicine* 70, no. 7 (2013): 464–70.
19 Elizabeth Grossman, "Toxics in the 'Clean Rooms': Are Samsung Workers at Risk?" *Yale Environment 360*, June 9, 2011, http://e360.yale.edu/features/toxics_in_the_clean_rooms_are_samsung_workers_at_risk; Barbara Kyle, "Samsung Apologizes To Semiconductor Workers Who Contracted Cancer, Promises Compensation," Electronics Take Back Coalition, May 27, 2014, www.electronicstakeback.com/2014/05/27/samsung-apologizes-to-semiconductor-workers-who-contracted-cancer-promises-compensation; Youkyung Lee, "Samsung Workers Are Falling Sick And Dying; Company Mum Due To 'Trade Secrets,'" *Huffington Post*, August 10, 2016, www.huffingtonpost.ca/2016/08/10/samsung-workers-sick-dying_n_11424158.html; "Samsung's Recent Moves Highlight Inability To Clean Its House of Malfeasance, Supporters for the Health and Rights of People in the Semiconductor Industry (SHARPS), February 25, 2020, https://stopsamsung.wordpress.com; "Another Samsung Victim Dies As SHARPS Reaches New Momentum," Supporters for the Health and Rights of People in the Semiconductor Industry (SHARPS), October 6, 2017, https://stopsamsung.wordpress.com. For more on the challenges of research and advocacy: Inah Kim, Hyun J. Kim, Sin Y. Lim, and Jungok Kongyoo, "Leukemia and Non-Hodgkin Lymphoma in Semiconductor Industry Workers in Korea," *International Journal of Occupational and Environmental Health* 18, no. 2 (2012): 147–53; K. Lee, S.-G. Kim, and D. Kim, "Potential Risk Factors for Haematological Cancers in Semiconductor Workers," *Occupational Medicine* 65, no. 7 (2015): 585–89; Mira Lee and Howard Waitzkin, "A Heroic Struggle to Understand the Risk of Cancers among Workers in the Electronics Industry: The Case of Samsung," *International Journal of Occupational and Environmental Health* 18, no. 2 (2012): 89–91.

20 Howard Waitzkin dedicates this section to the memory of John D. Stoeckle – teacher, colleague, friend, comrade – who developed the upstream focus in medicine and public health and who died in April 2020 from COVID-19. (See Howard Waitzkin, "John D. Stoeckle and the Upstream Vision of Social Determinants in Public Health," *American Journal of Public Health* 106, no. 2 (2016): 234–36.) May his efforts live on as we cope with this pandemic and its aftermath, and as we struggle to prevent those coming in the future if we don't address their upstream causes.

21 Howard Waitzkin, *Medicine and Public Health at End of Empire* (Boulder, CO: Paradigm, 2011), Chapter 2; "One and a Half Centuries of Forgetting and Rediscovering: Virchow's Lasting Contributions to Social Medicine," *Social Medicine* 1 (2006): 5–10, https://www.academia.dk/MedHist/Biblioteket/pdf/virchow_intro.pdf.

22 Rodrick Wallace, Luis Fernando Chaves, Luke Bergmann, et al., *Clear-Cutting Disease Control: Capital-Led Deforestation, Public Health Austerity, and Vector-Borne Infection* (New York: Springer, 2018); Carles Muntaner and Robert Wallace, "Confronting the Social and Environmental Determinants of Health," in Howard Waitzkin, coordinator, *Health Care Under the Knife: Moving Beyond Capitalism for Our Health* (New York: Monthly Review Press, 2018): pp. 224–38; Robert G. Wallace and Rodrick Wallace, eds., *Neoliberal Ebola: Modeling Disease Emergence from Finance to Forest and Farm* (New York: Springer, 2016); Rob Wallace, *Big Farms Make Big Flu: Dispatches on Infectious Disease, Agribusiness, and the Nature of Science* (New York: Monthly Review Press, 2016); Rob Wallace, Alex Liebman, Luis Fernando Chaves and Rodrick Wallace, "COVID-19 and Circuits of Capital," *Monthly Review* 72, no. 12 (May 2020), https://monthlyreview.org/2020/04/01/covid-19-and-circuits-of-capital/; David W. Redding, Peter M. Atkinson, Andrew A. Cunningham, et al., "Impacts of Environmental and Socio-economic Factors on Emergence and Epidemic Potential of Ebola in Africa," *Nature Communications* 10 (2019): 4531, doi:10.1038/s41467-019-12499-6; Aneta Afelt, Roger Frutos, and Christian Devaux, "Bats, Coronaviruses, and Deforestation: Toward the Emergence of Novel Infectious Diseases?" *Frontier in Microbiology* 9 (April 2020): 1–5, https://www.frontiersin.org/articles/10.3389/fmicb.2018.00702/full; Mike Davis, *The Monster Enters: COVID-19, Avian Flu and the Plagues of Capitalism* (New York: OR Books, 2020).

23 For information about the possible release of COVID-19 from a laboratory, see: Rob Wallace, "Midvinter-19: On the Origins of SARS-CoV-2," *Patrion*, May 6, 2020, https://www.patreon.com/posts/midvinter-19-36797182; Sam Husseini, "Did This Virus Come from a Lab? Maybe Not – But It Exposes the Threat of a Biowarfare Arms Race," Salon.com, https://www.salon.com/2020/04/24/did-this-virus-come-from-a-lab-maybe-not--but-it-exposes-the-threat-of-a-biowarfare-arms-race/; Jonathan Latham and Allison Wilson, "The Case Is Building That COVID-19 Had a Lab Origin," *Independent Science News for Food and Agriculture*, June 2, 2020, https://www.independentsciencenews.org/health/the-case-is-building-that-covid-19-had-a-lab-origin/.

24 Chuǎng, "Social Contagion," 2020, http://chuangcn.org/2020/02/social-contagion/; Wallace, Liebman, Chaves, and Wallace, "COVID-19 and Circuits of Capital."

25 World Health Organization, "Ebola Virus Disease," February 10, 2020, https://www.who.int/news-room/fact-sheets/detail/ebola-virus-disease; Mary Kay Kindhauser, Tomas Allen, Veronika Frank, Ravi Shankar Santhana, and Christopher Dye, "Zika: the Origin and Spread of a Mosquito-borne

Virus," *Bulletin of the World Health Organization* 94 (2016): 675–86C; Nuno R. Faria, Andrew Rambaut, Marc A. Suchard, et al., "The Early Spread and Epidemic Ignition of HIV-1 in Human Populations," *Science* 346 (2014): 56–61, DOI: 10.1126/science.1256739.

26 Muntaner and Wallace, "Confronting the Social and Environmental Determinants of Health"; Wallace and Wallace, eds., *Neoliberal Ebola*; Wallace, *Big Farms Make Big Flu*; Wallace, Liebman, Chaves, and Wallace, "COVID-19 and Circuits of Capital."

27 World Health Organization, "Programme Budget 2018-2019," May 2017, p. 5, https://www.who.int/about/finances-accountability/budget/PB2018-2019_en_web.pdf?ua=1; *Forbes*, December 11, 2018, https://www.forbes.com/companies/new-york-presbyterian-hospital/#4f9f3f6551e2.

28 Anne-Emanuelle Birn and Judith Richter, "U.S. Philanthrocapitalism and the Global Health Agenda: the Rockefeller and Gates Foundations, Past and Present," in Howard Waitzkin, coordinator, *Health Care Under the Knife: Moving Beyond Capitalism for Our Health* (New York: Monthly Review Press, 2018), pp. 155–74.

29 People's Health Movement, "Global Health Watch," "WHO Watch," https://phmovement.org.

30 "Tanzania Orders Destruction of Monsanto/Gates Foundation GMO Trials," *Sustainable Pulse*, November 24, 2018, https://sustainablepulse.com/2018/11/24/tanzania-orders-destruction-of-monsanto-gates-foundation-gmo-trials/#.XrDf5i-cbAw; Silvia Ribeiro, "Two Hundred Million against Monsanto," Etc Group, June 9, 2013, https://www.etcgroup.org/content/two-hundred-million-against-monsanto; The Oakland Institute, "The Unholy Alliance: Five Western Donors Shape a Pro-Corporate Agenda for African Agriculture," 2016, https://www.oaklandinstitute.org/sites/oaklandinstitute.org/files/unholy_alliance_web.pdf.

31 Judith Garber, "CDC 'Disclaimers' Hide Financial Conflicts of Interest," Lown Institute, November 6, 2019, https://lowninstitute.org/cdc-disclaimers-hide-financial-conflicts-of-interest/.

32 Smithfield continued to deny that the swine flu epidemic originated from the pig farm in Veracruz, but a later international study provided conclusive evidence that this industrial meat-processing plant was the source: Ignacio Mena, Martha I. Nelson, Francisco Quezada-Monroy, et al. "Origins of the 2009 H1N1 Influenza Pandemic in Swine in Mexico," *eLife* 5 (2016): e16777, DOI: 10.7554/eLife.16777, https://www.ncbi.nlm.nih.gov/pmc/articles/PMC4957980/.

33 Lydia Mulvany and Isis Almeida, "Smithfield CEO Looks Ahead to 2019: Ken Sullivan Sees Spread of African Swine Fever and Trade Deals as Positive for the Hog Market," *National Hog Farmer*, December 21, 2018, https://www.nationalhogfarmer.com/marketing/smithfield-ceo-looks-ahead-2019. An early report on the issues reported here appeared in Robert Kennedy, Jr., "Smithfield Foods: the Truth behind Its Pigs and Factories," *The Ecologist*, December 1, 2003, https://theecologist.org/2003/dec/01/smithfield-foods-truth-behind-its-pigs-and-factories.

34 "Read Our COVID-19 Statement," Smithfield Marketplace, April 18, 2020, https://www.smithfieldmarketplace.com/covid-19_statement.

35 Dawn Geske, "Meatpacker Smithfield Foods Becomes Largest COVID-19 Hotspot in US with 518 Employees Testing Positive," *International Business Times*, April 16, 2020, https://www.ibtimes.com/meatpacker-smithfield-foods-becomes-largest-covid-19-hotspot-us-518-employees-testing-2960006.

36 Nick Paton Walsh and Vasco Cotovio, "Bats Are Not to Blame for Coronavirus. Humans Are," CNN Health, March 20, 2020, https://edition.cnn.com/2020/03/19/health/coronavirus-human-actions-intl/index.html.
37 Johns Hopkins Center for Health Security, "The Event 201 Scenario," October 18, 2019, http://centerforhealthsecurity.org/event201/scenario.html.
38 Jan Douwe van der Ploeg, *The New Peasantries: Rural Development in Times of Globalization* (London: Routledge, 2018); "Peasant-Driven Agricultural Growth and Food Sovereignty," Food Sovereignty: A Critical Dialogue, International Conference, September 14–15, 2013, https://www.tni.org/files/download/8_van_der_ploeg_2013.pdf. For an orientation to peasant agriculture and educational materials from throughout the world, see La Via Campesina/ International Peasant's Movement, https://viacampesina.org/en/; Food First, https://foodfirst.org/; Eric Holt-Giménez, *A Foodie's Guide to Capitalism* (New York: Monthly Review Press, 2017).
39 Craig Allan Medlen, *Free Cash, Capital Accumulation and Inequality* (New York: Routlege, 2018), p. 14.
40 "Notes from the Editors," *Monthly Review* 71, no. 5 (October 2019): inside cover, https://monthlyreview.org/2019/10/01/mr-071-05-2019-09_0/.
41 Eric Toussaint, "The Capitalist Pandemic, Coronavirus and the Economic Crisis," Committee for the Abolition of Illegitimate Debt, March 19, 2020, http://www.cadtm.org/The-Capitalist-Pandemic-Coronavirus-and-the-Economic-Crisis; "No, the Coronavirus is Not Responsible for the Fall of Stock Prices," Committee for the Abolition of Illegitimate Debt, March 5, 2020, http://www.cadtm.org/No-the-coronavirus-is-not-responsible-for-the-fall-of-stock-prices; Howard Waitzkin, "Revolution Now: Teachings from the Global South for Revolutionaries in the Global North," *Monthly Review* 10, no. 2 (June 2017): 18–36, https://monthlyreview.org/2017/11/01/revolution-now/.
42 Matthew Kavanagh, "Transparency and Testing Work Better Than Coercion in Coronavirus Battle," *Foreign Policy*, March 16, 2020, https://foreignpolicy.com/2020/03/16/coronavirus-what-works-transparency-testing-coercion/; John P.A. Ioannidis, "A Fiasco in the Making? As the Coronavirus Pandemic Takes Hold, We Are Making Decisions without Reliable Data," *StatReports*, March 17, 2020, https://www.statnews.com/2020/03/17/a-fiasco-in-the-making-as-the-coronavirus-pandemic-takes-hold-we-are-making-decisions-without-reliable-data/.
43 Russell M. Viner, Simon J. Russell, Helen Croker, et al., "School Closure and Management Practices During Coronavirus Outbreaks Including COVID-19: A Rapid Systematic Review," *Lancet Child and Adolescent Health*, April 6, 2020, https://www.thelancet.com/pdfs/journals/lanchi/PIIS2352-4642(20)30095-X.pdf; Simon Cauchemez, Neil M. Ferguson, Claude Wachtel, et al., "Closure of Schools During an Influenza Pandemic," *Lancet Infectious Disease* 9 (2009): 473–81, https://www.ncbi.nlm.nih.gov/pmc/articles/PMC7106429/.
44 Emmanuel Saez and Gabriel Zucman, "Jobs Aren't Being Destroyed This Fast Elsewhere. Why Is That?" *New York Times*, March 30, 2020, https://www.nytimes.com/2020/03/30/opinion/coronavirus-economy-saez-zucman.html.
45 Comparisons of countries' success in controlling the COVID-19 will occupy researchers' attention for quite some time. Preliminary comparisons of countries' differing approaches to the COVID-19 pandemic appear in Howard Waitzkin and Colleagues, *COVID-19: Moving the Narrative, and the Struggle, Upstream* (Ottawa, Canada: Daraja Press, 2020, in press).

46 Marie Solis and Naomi Klein, "Coronavirus Is the Perfect Disaster for 'Disaster Capitalism,'" *Vice*, March 16, 2020, https://www.vice.com/en_in/article/5dmqyk/naomi-klein-interview-on-coronavirus-and-disaster-capitalism-shock-doctrine.

47 Amy Kapczynski and Gregg Gonsalves, "Alone Against the Virus: Class and Inequality," *Boston Review*, March 13, 2020, http://bostonreview.net/class-inequality-science-nature/amy-kapczynski-gregg-gonsalves-alone-against-virus; Nomi Prins, "The Global Economy Catches the Coronavirus," TomDispatch.com, March 12, 2020, http://www.tomdispatch.com/post/176674/tomgram%3A_nomi_prins%2C_the_global_economy_catches_the_coronavirus/#more. For more on the impending global crisis of food insecurity caused by lockdowns as a claimed public health policy, see: Vijay Prasad, "Hunger Gnaws at the Edges of the World," Tricontinental: Institute for Social Research, May 14, 2020, https://mailchi.mp/thetricontinental.org/hunger-gnaws-at-the-edges-of-the-world-the-twentieth-newsletter-2020?e=7aac4cc929; Michael Pollan, "The Sickness in Our Food Supply," *The New York Review of Books*, June 11, 2020, https://www.nybooks.com/articles/2020/06/11/covid-19-sickness-food-supply/.

Chapter 4

The Social Determination of Illness, Part 2

Inequality, Class, Race, Ethnicity, and Gender

Improving Research on Worsening Social Determination

Throughout the world, research on the social determinants of health (SDOH) has flourished. As we already pointed out in the last chapter, this helpful work rarely acknowledges its roots in the classic studies of Engels and Virchow, or its similarities with the efforts of Allende and current researchers in Latin America. Nevertheless, recent investigations have advanced knowledge about the social conditions that shape illness and early death. The findings of these studies again lead to humility about the impact of improved access to medical services. Instead, the conclusions from this field suggest that in addition to improved access, basic changes in social conditions will be needed if the goal is to improve the health outcomes of populations.

In this chapter, we examine three key dimensions of the SDOH that have received wide attention: social class, race, and gender. Inequality creates harmful effects in each of these areas. However, rather than just describing the associations between these dimensions and adverse health outcomes, we use the analytic framework of social determination. So instead of referring simply to social class, race, and gender, we analyze classism, racism, and sexism, to show that these social conditions exert concrete effects on health within a larger social context. This context includes discrimination, oppression, violence, police brutality, militarism, marginalization, despair, drug and other abuse, suicide, and unhealthy social processes linked to our overall political economic system. Looking at these "determinants" through the lens of social determination reveals that meaningful solutions are not likely to emerge from rational efforts using research data to convince the rich and powerful that changes are needed. In other words, social determination requires more profound actions to change the societal structures that generate illness and early death.

Social Class and Classism

In the United States and around the world, social class remains arguably the most important cause in determining a population's health outcomes. Social class also intersects with race and racism, as well as gender and sexism, in determining health, and we will consider these intersections later. Research continues to show that the poor suffer much worse overall mortality than the wealthy. This is not a new finding: The living conditions of the poor historically were powerful predictors of who would die of infectious diseases, occupational illnesses, environmental health problems, and more. When the standard of living rose, the death rates from measles, tuberculosis, and polio fell. Interestingly, the decline in the death rate for some of the most feared infectious diseases occurred before the implementation of antibiotics and vaccines. Better health due to rising levels of income and improved standards of living played a more important role than advances in medical care and technology.[1]

In addition to overall poverty, research comparing states, counties, and metropolitan areas in the United States, as well as research comparing countries, has found that geographic units with the highest measures of income inequality manifest the most unfavorable life expectancy and health outcomes. Areas with the highest income inequality are also the least likely to invest in public education and a comprehensive health infrastructure, which also impact population health. Although social determination, as we are discussing it, is not their main focus, researchers such as Marmot, Wilkinson, and colleagues have clarified some mechanisms by which the SDOH exert their adverse effects: The perception of one's economic position as unfavorable becomes a major psychosocial stressor that mediates the effects of social inequality at the individual level. Meanwhile, epidemiologists have developed more sophisticated methods that attempt to trace the multilevel psychosocial processes by which social conditions, such as income inequality, exert their effects on individuals' health.[2]

The injurious effects of social class operate through a cluster of deprivations and oppressions that affect people who occupy the lower end of social class hierarchies. We and others view these unhealthy deprivations and oppressions as "classism." In the United States, alarming trends show deteriorating health and mental health conditions for the white population, and these changes mostly reflect deteriorating socioeconomic conditions. During the past decade, the white population has experienced worsening life expectancy, mainly among people in mid-life and in rural areas. Death rates from drug overdoses, suicide, poisonings, and alcohol-related liver disease have been increasing rapidly. These trends have occurred to a much greater extent in rural than in urban areas. Researchers have attributed these changes to a massive increase in "despair" about declining economic opportunities and day-to-day financial stress. In the 2016 presidential election, voters in counties with higher levels of inequality, worsening health outcomes, increasing suicide rates, and higher use of prescription opiates voted more for Donald Trump. These worsening trends of adverse health and mental health effects of inequality, poverty, and economic insecurity have been impacting disproportionately the white population, although this population still shows more favorable outcomes compared with minority groups.[3] Figures 4.1 through 4.6 present data and explanations based on recent research that conveys these worrisome trends in more detail.

It is now important to take a step back and discuss the meanings and implications of social class. Why are there different classes? What is inequality? To help answer these questions, we briefly discuss two theoretical approaches to understanding socioeconomic position and health.

Karl Marx argued that in order to understand the concept of a social class, one must understand the economic structure of society. In this theory, social class refers to a group's relationship to the means of production. Those who own or control the means of production – such as factories, equipment, machines – constitute the capitalist class. Those who must sell their labor in order to survive constitute the working class. Marx reasoned that capitalism is inherently exploitative, as the select few accumulate the surplus value generated by the work of the many. Thus, classes remain in a structural condition of inherent conflict.[4] The implications of the Marxist

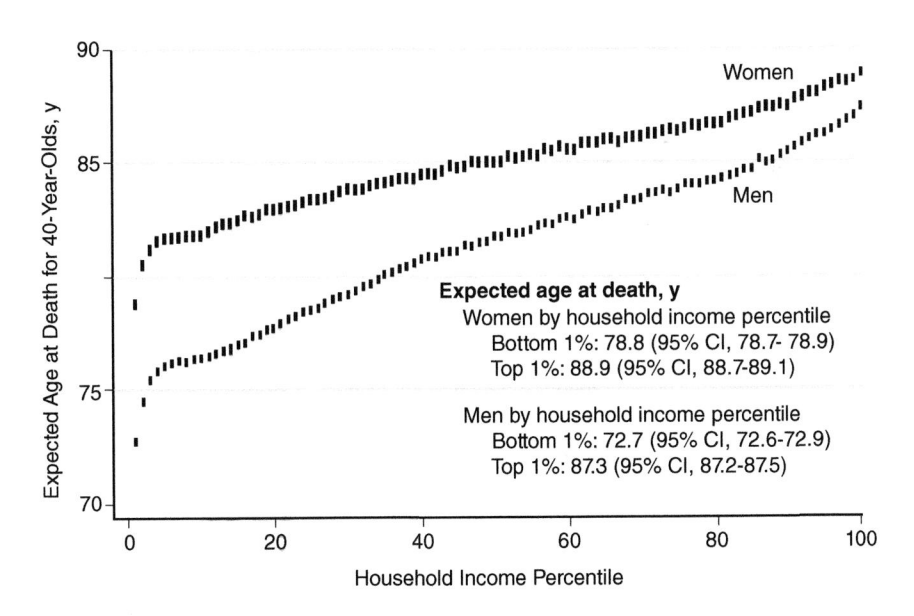

Figure 4.1 Income inequality and life expectancy in the United States.
Source: Chetty, Stepner, Abraham, et al. 2016 (note 3). When adjusted for self-reported race/ethnicity, life expectancy in the United States rises with household income.

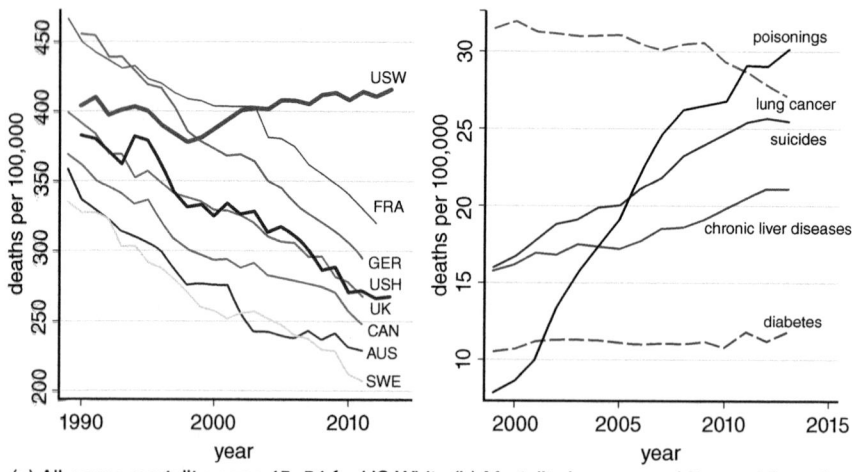

(a) All-cause mortality, ages 45–54 for US White non-Hispanics (USW), US Hispanics (USH), and six comparison countries: France (FRA), Germany (GER), the United Kingdom (UK), Canada (CAN), Australia (AUS), and Sweden (SWE).

(b) Mortality by cause, white non-Hispanics ages 45–54.

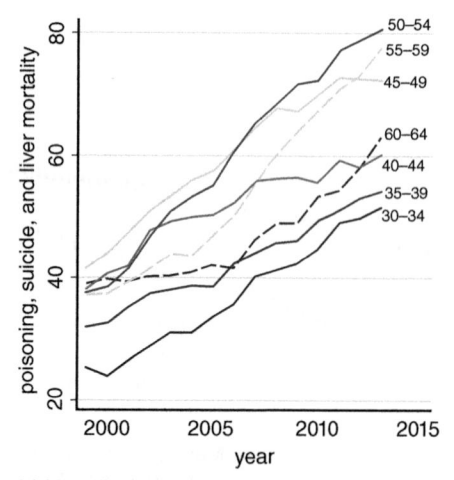

(c) Mortality by poisoning, suicide, chronic liver disease, and cirrhosis, white non-Hispanics by 5-y age group.

Figure 4.2 Changing mortality patterns in the United States.
Source: Case and Deaton 2015, note 3. Mortality has been deteriorating for the mid-life population in the United States, especially because of self-destructive behaviors like poisonings, suicides, and alcoholism and drug abuse contributing to chronic liver disease.

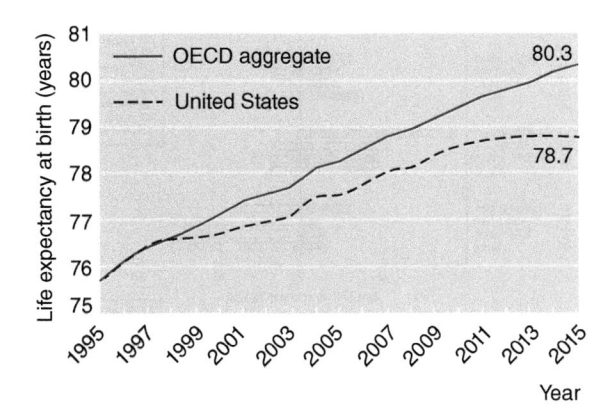

Figure 4.3 Changing life expectancy in the United States and the Organisation for Economic Cooperation and Development, 1995–2015.
Source: Woolf and Aron 2018 (note 3). Overall life expectancy in the United States has been deteriorating when compared to other economically developed countries.

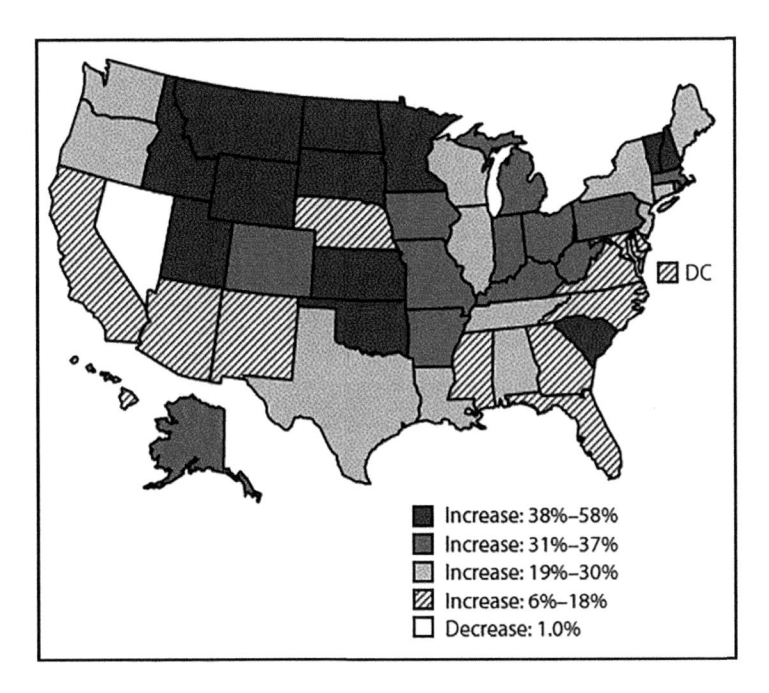

Figure 4.4 Suicide rates in the United States.
Source: Stone, Simon, Fowler, et al. 2018 (note 3). Suicide rates have been increasing throughout the United States.

84 Inequality, Class, Race, Ethnicity, Gender

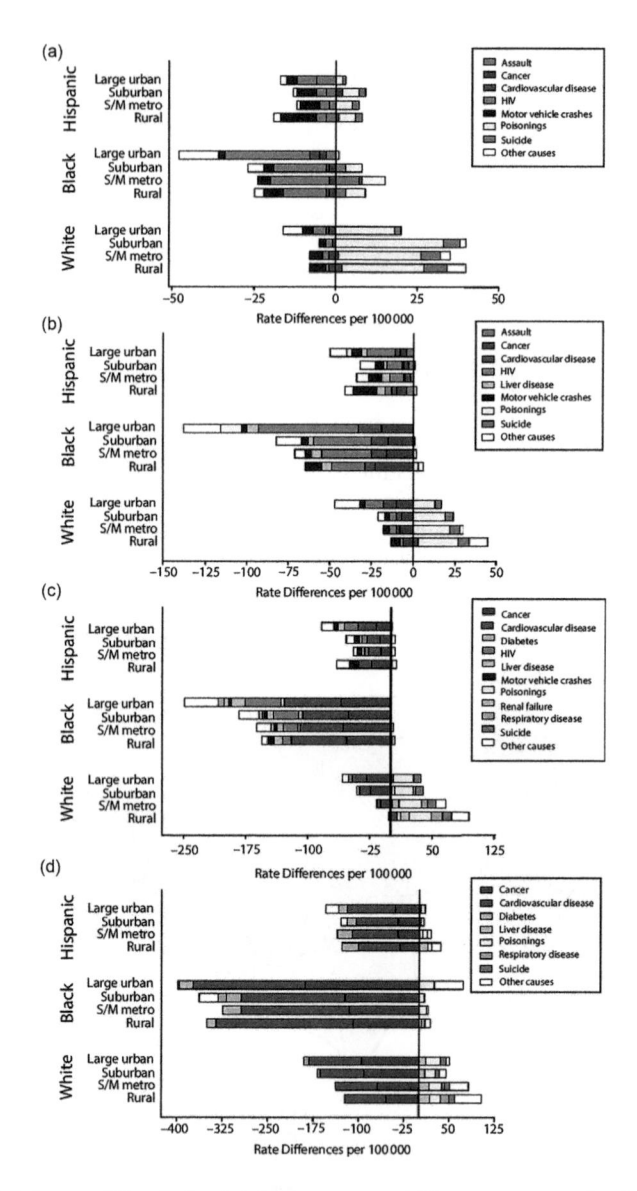

Figure 4.5 Inequalities in health indicators and life expectancy in the United States. Leading causes of mortality rate differences (per 100 000) between 1999–2001 and 2013–2015 among those aged (a) 25–34 years, (b) 35–44 years, (c) 45–54 years, and (d) 55–64 years: trends in the leading causes of premature death, United States, 1999–2015.

Source: Stein, Gennuso, Ugboaja, and Remington 2017 (note 3). Despite inequalities in health indicators and life expectancy that generally favor whites in the United States compared with minorities, mortality among whites has been deteriorating, especially in rural areas.

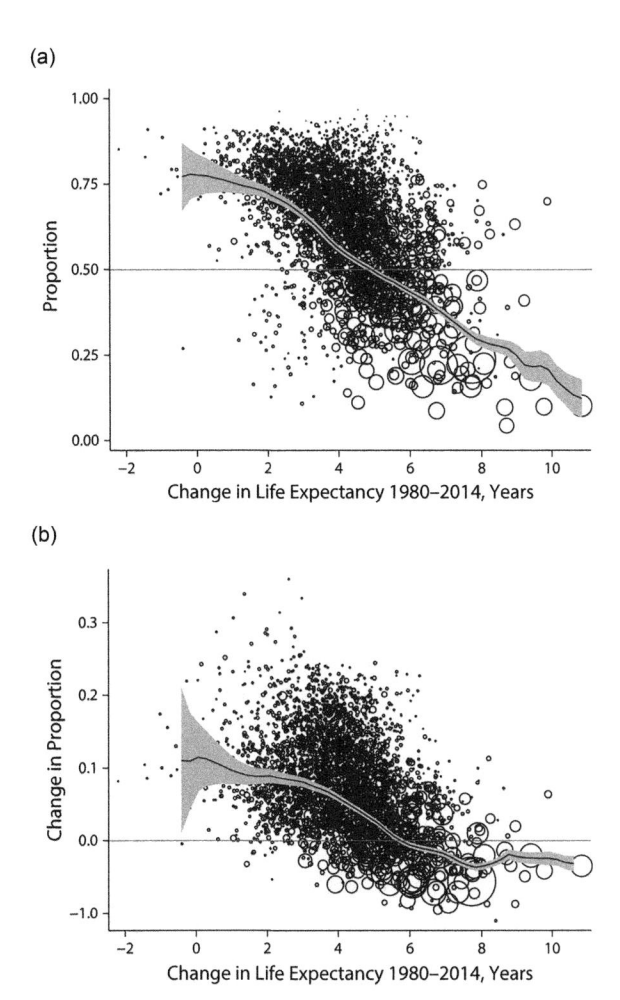

Figure 4.6 Life expectancy by county and voting pattern in the 2016 presidential election (proportion of votes for Donald Trump in (a); change in Republican vote share from 2008 to 2016 in (b)).
Source: Bor 2017 (note 3). Voters in U.S. counties experiencing deterioration or lack of improvement in life expectancy voted disproportionately for Donald Trump.

theory of social class, for health, have been widely discussed. Perhaps most poignantly, Vicente Navarro maintained that there must be a minimum level of health for the working class to ensure that they *can* work. Navarro contended that an alliance therefore may arise between the capitalist class and the medical profession, as physicians perpetuate the belief that the principal causes of ill health are personal and physical rather than social.[5]

Max Weber and Weberian theory tell a different side of the story. Instead of focusing on the sources of social class in economic production,

Weber theorized that individuals clustered into similar classes because they shared similar circumstances, or "life chances." For example, Weber believed that some people remained in a lower economic class because they experienced a "competitive disadvantage" due to lack of abilities and skills, reflecting the circumstances of the families into which they were born. Those people who learned talents related to family background were able to maintain their class position or rise to a higher one. In other words, Weber acknowledged that the distribution of wealth followed certain predictable patterns based on the individual's talents linked to early advantages in the family.[6]

Some of these concepts readily apply to health and health care, including the medical profession itself. In the United Kingdom, a study found that most medical students came from wealthy households – approximately 80 percent of students had a parent in a high-paying professional career. Meanwhile, in some of the poorer secondary schools, a student never had applied to medical school.[7] In the United States, the proportion of medical students from low-income families has remained at about 12 percent for more than a century.[8] Differences in class origins contribute to access and communication barriers that impact physicians and patients in their encounters, and the cycle continues.

The Marxist and Weberian theories are still helpful, but data produced in censuses and surveys rarely provide information about respondents' relationship to the means of production. Instead, information about social stratification, health, and illness deals with demographic variables such as income, education, and occupational prestige. To some extent, these variables parallel the relationships of production but differ in subtle and important ways, especially concerning strategies to change the stratified nature of society. The poor, as defined by these demographic variables, suffer much worse overall mortality than the wealthy. While the impacts of poverty and inequality on health continue to receive wide attention in research, public policies have changed very little.

As mentioned earlier, Marx believed that inequality was due to the unequal ownership of capital. However, in recent years, this concept has received criticism for being overly simplistic and out of date. In social medicine, Carles Muntaner and his colleagues have published several articles that refined the Marxist concept of class by somewhat shifting the focus to several other economic measures related to wealth that show concrete effects on health outcomes (in developing this approach, Muntaner adapted theory and methods from neo-Marxist researchers such as Erik Olin Wright).[9] For example, during the nineteenth century, material conditions referred to housing, adequate nutrition, a safe water supply, and reduction of environmental hazards through waste removal. These social conditions do exert an important impact on public health in poor and developing countries. However, in developed economies, where these basic necessities are more frequently (although not always) met, a set of "neo-material" conditions affect health and longevity in the twenty-first century. Such conditions include living in a safe neighborhood, having easy access to transportation, owning a home, exercising, and eating a reliable and nutritious diet.

The concept of inequality – and what to do about it – remains a key political issue today and one that fluctuates with every election season. The right-wing position is that individual initiative and market forces are the key reasons for income inequality and that government intervention should be kept at a minimum. In contrast, a centrist position calls for raising enough taxes so that government will be able to provide needed health care, education, transportation, and other public services for the needy. A left-wing position argues that the poorest members of a capitalist society are trapped there, and the only ways to change their economic position involve at least partially socializing the means of production and redistributing wealth. In the 2016 presidential election, the Republican and Democratic candidates predictably followed the right wing and centrist political positions, respectively. Republican nominee Donald Trump favored cutting taxes as well as reducing government spending; in contrast, Democratic nominee Hillary Clinton was in favor of raising taxes on the financial elite to fund government spending in public programs such as education.

Inequality of both income and accumulated wealth has increased during recent decades. Current tax rates for the very rich are relatively low compared with rates of the previous century. After World War II, the top income tax bracket was higher than 90 percent, meaning that very rich people paid 90 percent of their income as income taxes. As tax brackets were lowered later in the twentieth century (with maximum taxes about 25–40 percent of income in recent years), and the wealthy got to keep more of their income, the inequality gap widened.[10]

When we consider inequality in accumulated wealth as opposed to inequality in income, by recent estimates, the concentration of wealth has increased in the United States to the point that the three richest men in the United States (Jeff Bezos, Bill Gates, and Warren Buffett) controlled as much wealth as the bottom 50 percent. Considering the world, as Oxfam has reported, eight men recently have controlled the same wealth as the bottom half of the world's population. During the COVID-19 pandemic, wealth became even more concentrated; during a 11-week period, as the U.S. unemployment rate increased to its worst level since the Great Depression of the 1930s, U.S. billionaires' wealth increased by 19.15 percent.[11]

One influential researcher on inequality and social class is Thomas Piketty, a French economist. Piketty analyzes changes in inequality and wealth over time. Through theorizing and data analysis, Piketty argues that a progressive income tax, in which rich people pay proportionately more of their income, is a necessity for reducing inequality. However, the components of the tax rate should be different for different social classes. For example, the top echelon should be taxed at a rate also based on their wealth rather than their income. This change would help reduce tax fraud and loopholes for the very wealthy. For the majority of the population, taxable wealth would be based on the market value of personal assets such as stocks, bonds, and real estate. Piketty argues that without this "global tax," the top 1 percent will continue to accumulate wealth at the expense of everyone else. Other economists have argued for a very small tax on international electronic currency transactions as a simple and relatively painless method to reduce poverty through a slight redistribution of wealth (see box on Tobin tax).[12]

ONE WAY TO REDISTRIBUTE WEALTH THROUGH A SMALL TAX ON INTERNET TRANSACTIONS: THE "TOBIN TAX"

The Nobel Prize winning economist James Tobin has proposed taxing international electronic currency transactions at a rate of 0.5%. In Tobin's view, the main purpose would be to reduce the risk of economic crises that result from over-speculation by investors to earn rapid profits. Advocacy groups and activists have pointed out that the Tobin tax, more recently named the "Robin Hood Tax" by some groups, would generate about $260 billion each year. If this money were redistributed from wealthy investors to the poor worldwide, world poverty could be eradicated. This effect would generate very favorable effects for health. Even this tiny tax or similar proposals like the Robin Hood tax to redistribute wealth have not received support from the political and financial elite. See note 12. We talk more about policies and actions to redistribute wealth in the last chapter.

Piketty is one of several mainstream economists who argue for reducing inequality as one way to save the capitalist economic system in an era of chronic crises and decline. From this perspective, less inequality will help restore some of the lost legitimacy of the capitalist system and also will enhance consumers' ability to purchase the goods and services that capitalism produces. Economists influenced by Marxist thought argue that trying to save capitalism by reducing inequality will not succeed for two reasons: (1) Capitalism depends on the accumulation of surplus value through the exploitation of workers who produce more value than they receive as pay and (2) capitalism requires economic growth through unsustainable use of natural resources that, due to devastating effects on our environment, is threatening the survival of humanity and other life forms.[13]

The data about poverty and inequality are readily available, and the conclusion is always the same: The poor suffer. Especially in terms of health and well-being, the poor remain at the highest risk for morbidity and mortality. To lower that risk, concerted action must change the concentration of wealth that benefits the political and financial elite while perpetuating poverty and inequality. Then will we be able to use data about the health effects of poverty and inequality to improve social conditions for those who live their lives low in the social hierarchy of wealth and power. The health impacts of those improvements in social conditions will be greater than anything we can hope to accomplish if we limit our work to the medical realm alone.

Race and Racism

Often connected to social class, "race" also remains a major predictor of adverse outcomes. In Harlem, survival until 65 years of age for people identified as African American males in the 1980s was worse than for males living in Bangladesh, one of the poorest countries in the world.[14] While the mortality rate for the black population has declined since that shocking article, the net improvement did not match that for whites. As a result, the mortality ratio for young black men as opposed to white men was the same or higher in the 2000s than it was in the 1980s. As of 2000, average life expectancy at birth for African American men in the United States was about seven years shorter than for white men. Similarly, the life expectancy for black females was 3.3 years lower than that of white females, mainly due to higher death rates from heart disease, cancer, diabetes, perinatal conditions, and stroke. These differences in life expectancy and other health outcomes have narrowed since 2000, although the gaps remain large and part of the improvement comes from a recent deterioration of health and life expectancy for whites (in particular among whites in mid-life and in rural areas who experience economic distress).[15]

The concept of race is very controversial. This controversy became especially poignant during and after the 2016 U.S. presidential election, when white privilege became part of the national discourse. However, extensive biological and anthropological research shows that race is a socially constructed concept rather than a biological phenomenon. This work consistently has demonstrated that there is more variability in biological characteristics within socially constructed racial groups than between those groups.[16] Summarizing this research in an interview, Alan Goodman, a biological anthropologist, discussed the problem with classifying race by observable, or "phenotypic," characteristics of an individual:

> But think about race and its universality or lack thereof. Where is your measurement device? There is no way to measure race first. We sometimes do it by skin color. Other people may do by hair texture. Other people may have the dividing lines different in terms of skin color. What is black in the United States is not what's black in Brazil or what's black in South Africa. What was black in the 1940s is different from what is black in 2000. Certainly, with the evolution of whiteness, what was white in 1920 – as a Jew I was not white then, but I'm white now, so white has changed tremendously.[17]

Yet, after decades of research showing that race is a socially constructed concept, claims still arise about the biology of race. In the United States, for instance, African Americans show a very high rate of hypertension. Although some might argue that is due to the genetics of race, people in West Africa have one of the world's lowest rates of hypertension.[18]

Despite the extensive evidence that race holds little or no biological basis, the impact of racism on health care and health outcomes is very real biologically. Socially constructed "race" remains a major predictor of adverse outcomes. The traumas and stresses of racism, rather than the biology of race, account for this profound effect. Several examples show how racism affects health.

People identified by others as black become the targets for police violence and brutality much more often than people identified as members of other socially constructed racial groups, especially whites. Police have killed people identified as black more than five times more frequently, considering their proportion of the U.S. population, as people identified as white; lower reported rates probably are under-estimates due to underreporting by police agencies.[19] Inequalities in mortality due to police brutality led to worldwide protests after the police in Minneapolis killed George Floyd in May 2020, following similar killings by police over many years before that.

Fear, vigilance, arousal, and the stress of living while black, Latinx, or indigenous set in motion an interconnected series of physical and emotional responses. Neurological and endocrine activation generated by stress-inducing lived experiences lead to chronic physical states of over-stimulation. These conditions lead to cardiovascular activation and immunological dysfunctions that "embody" the discriminatory and injurious practices of racism.[20] Higher rates of hypertension (Figure 4.7), other cardiovascular diseases, diabetes, some forms of cancer, and blunted immunological protection against infections such as tuberculosis, HIV, and COVID-19 become manifestations of racism's embodiment.

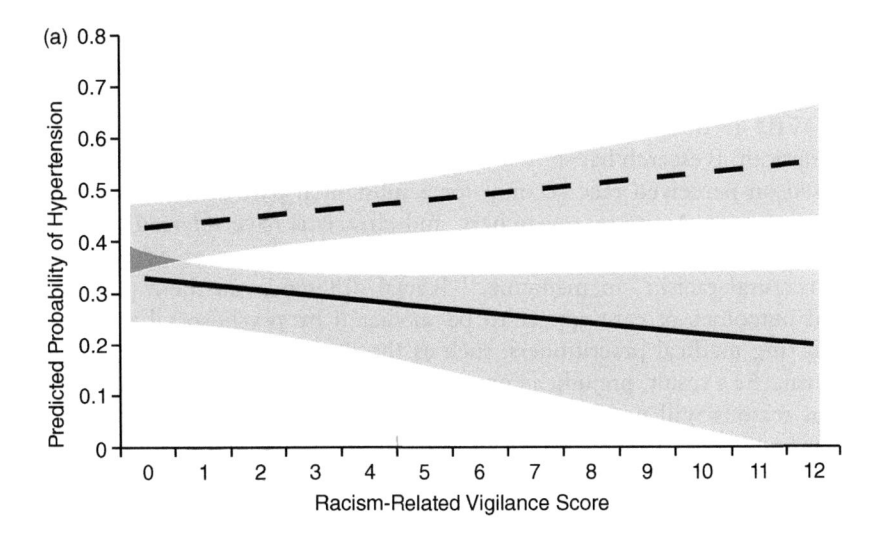

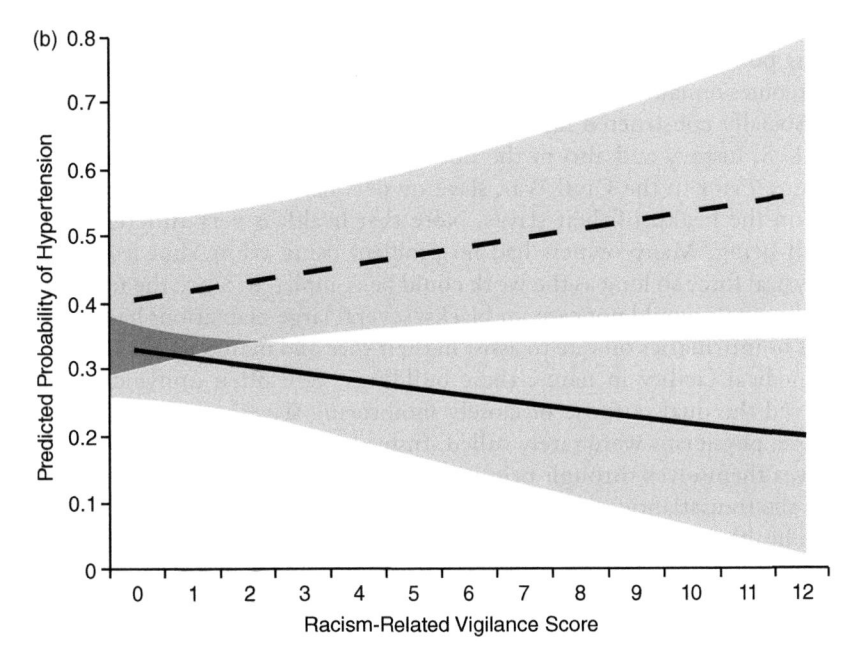

Figure 4.7 Hypertension and racism-related vigilance for (a) non-Hispanic Black versus non-Hispanic White adults, and (b) Hispanic versus non-Hispanic White adults.
Source: Hicken, Lee, Morenoff, et al. 2014 (note 20). Blacks and Hispanics showed an association between hypertension and racism-related vigilance.

Physicians also exert more extensive diagnostic and therapeutic efforts for patients identified as white than for those identified as African American with similar medical conditions. For example, outcomes for cardiovascular disease, cancer, AIDS, and (as discussed in prior chapters) COVID-19 became markedly worse among people identified as African American. Research has shown that such differences in medical treatment based on perceived race account for a substantial part of the differences in outcomes. Activists, researchers, and clinicians have referred to these patterns of unequal treatments based on perceived race as examples of "structural racism" in medicine.[21] Racial differences in these processes and outcomes of care appear to be mediated by psychosocial processes affecting medical practitioners, such as the disrespect that is inherent in racism. As a result, prejudiced expectations that minority patients for various reasons will not be able to tolerate more technologically advanced diagnostic and therapeutic procedures lead to clinical decisions not to initiate these procedures.

Because poverty rates are higher among African Americans, the impact of social class discussed earlier also contributes to adverse health outcomes. Recent research indicates that stressful experiences of racism, lower social class position, and financial inequality are some key reasons that health outcomes remain so much worse for African Americans than for whites.[22]

Socially constructed race has played a central role in the development of U.S. history and also in the development of medicine in the United States. Prior to the Civil War, slave owners had a financial direct interest in the health of their slaves. Note that health is very different from well-being: Many owners had no problem using whips, hot irons, and physical force so long as the work could be completed. Since the few public hospitals would not care for blacks, several large plantations had hospitals or infirmaries on-site to assist in their care and maintenance. Though a medical facility in name, these buildings were often unhygienic and served the dual purpose of closely monitoring slaves' activity. Furthermore, physicians were rarely called. Instead, the slave owners treated the slaves themselves through primitive practices, such as bloodletting. After the transatlantic slave trade declined in the early nineteenth century, the health care of slaves became a lucrative business. A medical provider would often need to notarize a slave's health before he or she could be sold or traded, so the medical system became an important component of the slave market network.[23]

Physicians played a key role in legitimizing the oppression of slaves by claiming to prove scientifically that they were inferior. For example, the physician and natural scientist Samuel Morton, based in Philadelphia, amassed the largest collection of skulls in the world to prove that Caucasians – with their larger skull size – were superior. The Alabama physician Josiah Nott published an article in the *American Journal of Medical*

Sciences on the topic of mulattoes, or individuals with mixed-race parents, who he claimed were "intermediate in intelligence between the whites and blacks." Meanwhile the New Orleans physician Samuel Cartwright studied the livers and lungs of black cadavers to "prove that African American slaves consumed less oxygen than white people, which made their movements slower." This widely held belief echoed writings by early political leaders in the United States.[24]

By the turn of the twentieth century, African Americans were poorer and less healthy than other population groups, sparking a debate that remains with us today. Behavioral explanations spoke of the black family's dysfunction, based on unfounded theories popularized over time by Hollywood, which featured "black mamas… as predictable villains who are often at the center of the families' deep cycle of dysfunction."[25] Meanwhile, scholars and social activists, such as W.E.B. DuBois, linked differences in health to exploitation and racial oppression.[26] DuBois, and other scholars influenced by him, showed that slavery and racism supported the successful growth of capitalism in the United States and Europe. Racialization and slavery benefited not only people who owned slaves but also banks that made loans with slaves as collateral; insurance companies that insured slave ships and slaves themselves; manufacturers of cloth, machinery, and other products made possible by the work of slaves; and other economic elites. These prominent businessmen (they were almost always men) lived and worked not only in the U.S. South but also in the North as well as in northern Europe. Wealth accumulated through slavery funded important institutions of "western civilization," including museums, libraries, Ivy League universities, and medical schools. These linkages between racism and capitalism have become clear through extensive research by Afro-American, Afro-Caribbean, Afro-Latin American, and African scholars, as well as researchers from non-African origins.[27]

Recently, the term "structural racism" has become more widely used, including within medicine and public health. Here is an influential definition:

> "Structural racism" refers to the ways in which historical and contemporary racial inequities in outcomes are perpetuated by social, economic, and political systems, including mutually reinforcing systems of health care, education, housing, employment, the media, and criminal justice. It results in systemic variation in opportunity according to race or ethnic background – for example, in racial differentials in access to health care.[28]

This definition is helpful, because it focuses on the institutions that foster racism and adverse health outcomes rather than only on the racist behaviors of individuals in health care, such as doctors and health administrators.

One problem with the definition, however, is that it does not name capitalism, the political economic system that benefits from and maintains structural racism. The connections between structural racism, as usually defined, and capitalism remain vague and usually unspoken in discussions about structural racism in medicine and public health. As a result, strategies to confront and change structural racism continue to miss some of the most important sources of social determination in the capitalist political economic system, as though structural racism can be transformed without transformation of its capitalist underpinnings. For these reasons, scholars and activists in social medicine increasingly use the term "racial capitalism" to encompass the overall political economy in addition to the institutions to which "structural racism" refers.[29]

Besides adverse health outcomes linked to racial capitalism, African Americans also have faced struggles in becoming doctors, for some of the same structural reasons. Even in the antebellum South, some white physicians began to seek legal means to prevent African American physicians from practicing medicine. The effort continued into the twentieth century. In 1910, the Flexner Report, produced by Abraham Flexner and commissioned by the Carnegie Foundation, called for an overhaul of the medical educational system and closing most medical schools, to be replaced by more scientifically based institutions. With a justification of establishing a higher educational standard, the Flexner Report aimed to limit the "medical education of the Negro." The report stated that better medical schools were needed, and as a result five of the seven African American medical schools in operation at that time were deemed "ineffectual." This effort led to devastating consequences for access to care among the African American population.[30]

African Americans who did become physicians faced additional barriers, particularly in the South. They often could not admit patients to hospitals because local medical societies refused African American physicians as applicants. Occasionally, an African American patient would refuse an African American physician because of the widely held belief that white doctors were superior. This climate persisted even during World War II, when African American doctors "were continuously humiliated by [white] workers in the War Department."[31]

By the 1950s, African American physicians were advocating for change. In 1956, three African American physicians, for whom hospitals had denied admitting privileges, filed a lawsuit. The physicians argued that because the hospitals received federal funds, this discrimination was illegal. While this lawsuit lost in court, other lawsuits soon followed. Finally, in 1964, President Lyndon B. Johnson signed the Civil Rights Act. Title VI stated: "No person in the United States shall, on the ground of race, color, or national origin, be excluded from participation in, be denied benefits of, or be subjected to discrimination under any program or activity receiving federal financial assistance." Despite this legal change, which achieved integration of hospitals receiving Medicare and Medicaid funds, the proportion of African Americans entering medicine has increased very little, and inequalities of health outcomes persist.[32]

To summarize: According to recent research, race is a socially constructed concept rather than a biological phenomenon. There is more variability in biological characteristics within socially constructed racial groups than between those groups. The apparent association between adverse health outcomes and socially constructed race reflects racism more than biological differences. Racial differences in disease outcomes appear to be mediated by psychosocial processes, such as the reaction to the disrespect inherent in racism. And the impact of racism on health outcomes is often difficult to separate from the impact of social class.

Gender and Sexism

Although the women's health movement has been going on for over half a century, the term "women's health" tends to refer only to the traditional model of obstetrics and gynecology while glossing over the whole person, a whole person who has multiple differences in well-being from male counterparts. Inequalities in medical treatment according to gender constitute another injustice in the era of modern medicine, although injustice by gender frequently associates with class and race. Historically, in cancers of the breast and cervix, indicators such as rates of diagnosis, screening procedures (including mammograms and pap smears), and survival rates were all worse for poor than for wealthy women, and for African American women than for white women.[33]

While women continue to show overall mortality advantages compared with men in economically developed countries, age-adjusted outcomes in some situations become more unfavorable. For example, cardiovascular outcomes for postmenopausal women are similar to or worse than those of men. Women have been more likely to die in the year after a heart attack, possibly due to gender bias in diagnostic procedures and treatments. Updates in guidelines for common health problems affecting women also have lagged behind. The American Urological Association published a guideline for the surgical management of stress urinary incontinence in 1997, but it was not updated until 2009 and again in 2017, despite an estimated one in three women suffering from the condition. In contrast, a guideline for management of erectile dysfunction in men was published in 1996 and updated in 2000, 2005, and 2018.[34]

Like race and racism, gender and sexism have played a fundamental role in the development of modern medicine. The traditional convention of lady nurse, gentleman physician has permeated our culture. Studies of preschool-aged children in the 1970s suggested that these kids "knew" that females were nurses and males were doctors and would even change the characters shown to fit that perception. This model can be traced back to the Victorian era, as Vanessa Heggie explains:

> Nursing was both a problem and a pathway for women's entry into professionalized medicine. On the one hand nursing provided a direct route into medicine for many women.... On the other hand the professionalization and gentrification of the nursing role in the second half of the nineteenth century meant that nurses became increasingly idealized as the archetypal, acceptable, and middle-class ideal of femininity. The question "why not be a nurse" was therefore a constant threat to the precarious identity and existence of women doctors.[35]

The same Flexner Report that limited the entry of African American students into medical schools restricted the presence of female students as well. While two schools dedicated to African Americans would meet the revamped criteria, only one school dedicated to women would remain open: the Women's Medical College of Pennsylvania. This remained the only all-female medical school in the United States for 60 years. While other medical schools would accept women, it was at the average of only 6 percent of each entering class until the 1970s. Minimal among students, the female presence was even rarer among faculty and medical school leadership roles.[36]

During the late 1960s and early 1970s, the new feminist movement aimed to end gender stereotypes in medicine. Women argued that they should have control over their own bodies and reproductive health, and they fought against the traditional paradigm of legal and medical institutions that limited their choices. The movement was so sweeping that when the Supreme Court decided *Roe v. Wade* in 1973, granting the right of abortion, the decision did not lead to much resistance.[37] Later, more women began to apply to medical school, until schools were enrolling more women than men. Threats to these legal protections for women, especially regarding reproductive rights like abortions, have increased markedly during recent years, especially since the U.S. presidential election of 2016.

Despite the advances in some arenas of women's health, certain problems unique or more common among women continue to be underaddressed. Diseases that more frequently affect women than men include eating disorders, fibromyalgia, and sexual dysfunction. Misconceptions about "women's issues" also continue to predominate in medicine and the media. For instance, while concussions are typically thought of as a problem more common in young men playing football, an early study of all organized sports in high school and college, confirmed more recently, found that concussions and head injuries are actually more common in women.[38]

The effects of violence on women's health, finally, have received more attention. Women have struggled to overcome the belief that domestic violence is a normal part of women's lives. Approximately one-quarter of women become victims of domestic violence sometime in their lives, with significant implications for health and needed services. In comparison with women who have not been victims of domestic violence,

> abused women have nearly a 6-fold increased risk of substance abuse, a 5-fold greater risk of family or social problems, and a 3-fold greater risk of depression... Women who were physically abused also used more emergency, outpatient, pharmacy, and specialty services.[39]

Then there are the shocking statistics of women subjected to unwanted sexual contact. In a study by the Association of American Universities, over a quarter of female seniors reported that in their four years of college, they had experienced some kind of sexual assault, with approximately 14 percent experiencing penetration or attempted penetration.[40] Violence against women remains a fixture of culture in the United States and some other countries, especially among celebrities and professional athletes. Yet, the consequences have been minimal. Among many examples, one famous celebrity allegedly abused his then equally famous wife for nine straight hours by tying her to a chair, forcing her to perform sexual acts on him, and beating her with a baseball bat. This actor continued an illustrious career with hardly any mention of the violent incident. Similarly, a college athlete received no punishment for rape allegations and went on to become a top professional draft pick.[41]

College students' reports of assault have been repeatedly ignored. In the book to accompany the documentary *The Hunting Ground,* the authors suggested that Stanford University had 259 sexual assault cases reported in 17 years, but only one student had been expelled. Meanwhile, while the problem appeared to be widespread, a report commissioned in 2014 by Senator Claire McCaskill suggested that almost half of all colleges had not conducted a single sexual assault investigation in the previous five years. The issue reached a fever pitch in 2016, when a Stanford athlete was sentenced to only six months in jail for a witnessed assault on an incapacitated female. Vice President Joe Biden wrote a scathing letter in response to the judge's verdict, voicing the overall opinion of the Obama White House administration. Biden went so far as to suggest that federal funding would be discontinued for those universities that failed to address sexual assault allegations appropriately – a policy that the Trump administration did not pursue.[42]

Are women in medicine and other health professionals protected against sexism, harassment, and violence? Definitely not. Research spanning several decades has shown that women health professionals and those in training continue to endure tremendous challenges in this arena. An important study in 1993 showed that 73 percent of female internal medicine residents had experienced at least one episode of sexual harassment. As of 2000, sexual harassment had affected about half of women faculty members. And in 2014, 66 percent of women faculty members stated that they had experienced such harassment (Table 4.1).[43]

Table 4.1 Self-reported Experiences of Gender Bias, Advantage, and Sexual Harassment of National Institutes of Health K08 and K23 Career Development Awardees

	Reporting, No. (%) [95% CI]		Estimate Difference, % (95% CI)	
	Women (n = 493)	Men (n = 573)	Women vs Men	P Value[a]
Respondents who perceived gender-specific bias in the academic environment[b]	343 (69.6) [65.3–73.6]	125 (21.8) [18.5–25.4]	48.0 (42.7–53.3)	<0.001
Respondents who reported they personally experienced gender bias in professional advancement[c]	327 (66.3) [62.0–70.5]	56 (9.8) [7.5–12.5]	57.0 (52.1–61.8)	<0.001
Respondents who reported they personally experienced gender advantage in professional advancement[d]	129 (26.2) [22.3–30.3]	118 (20.6) [17.4–24.1]	5.6 (0.5–10.8)	0.08
Respondents who reported they personally experienced harassment[e]	150 (30.4) [26.4–34.7]	24 (4.2) [2.7–6.2]	26.5 (22.1–30.9)	<0.001

Source: Jagsi, Griffith, Jones, Perumalswami, Ubel, and Stewart 2016 (note 44).

a P value adjusting for specialty, race (majority versus minority), and years in faculty position.
b This item asked, "Do you perceive any gender-specific biases or obstacles to the career success or satisfaction of faculty by gender in your work environment (ranging from 1 [no, never] to 5 [yes, frequently])?" Responses of 3, 4, and 5 were considered affirmative.
c This item asked, "In your professional career, have you ever been left out of opportunities for professional advancement based on gender (1, yes; 2, probably; 3, possibly; 4, probably not; 5, no)?" Responses of 1, 2, and 3 were considered affirmative.
d This item asked, "In your professional career, have you had increased opportunities for professional advancement based on gender (1, yes; 2, probably; 3, possibly; 4, probably not; 5, no)?" Responses of 1, 2, and 3 were considered affirmative.
e This item asked, "In your professional career, have you encountered unwanted sexual comments, attention, or advances by a superior or colleague (yes or no)?" Responses of "yes" were considered affirmative.

While some progress has occurred, it has remained limited and impermanent. Women's health continues to be a political issue, and subject to new policies during every presidential cycle. The Trump administration has put forth plans to defund Planned Parenthood if its professionals continue to perform abortions and also to relax enforcement of laws and regulations to reduce sexual harassment in education.[44] Allegations of sexual assault on college campuses, at medical education institutions, and in Hollywood continue to increase. Like the health effects of classism and racism, the pervasive impacts of sexism, gender discrimination, and violence against women remain problems that cry out for action.

Social Origins, Social Reconstruction

Epidemiological research has documented again and again how the impact of inequality exerts adverse effects on health outcomes. For instance, a series of studies at the University of Wisconsin found that communities with higher income inequality, higher poverty rates, and higher levels of unemployment showed worse health outcomes.[45] Indeed, the research is so consistent that mammoth social policy initiatives designed to redistribute income – such as those proposed by Tobin, Piketty, and others – appear to be completely warranted, if we are serious about addressing the social determination of illness and mortality. The World Health Organization report on the SDOH called for such redistributional tax policies but exerted little effect on subsequent policies about taxation in countries around the world.[46] Measures such as new tax policies, welfare payments, family allowances, and food subsidies would probably exert very favorable effects on the adverse mortality patterns and health outcomes that so many studies have reported. But because income inequality is so firmly rooted in the political structure of the United States and some (but not all) other advanced capitalist countries, such drastic policy changes remain a daunting task.

The improbability of basic change in income inequality has led some researchers, as well as agencies of the U.S. government, to emphasize policies that aim to improve the "social capital" of low-income communities, rather than policies to achieve income redistribution. Social capital in communities involves higher levels of social support, cohesiveness, networking, and friendships. Such characteristics do appear to be associated with improved health outcomes, but much less so than reduced inequality.[47] Although interventions to increase social capital predictably will not improve outcomes to a similar extent as policies to reduce inequality, such interventions have attracted support, since they appear easier to achieve in the political context of the United States. It will be unfortunate if the worthwhile concern about social relationships within communities diverts attention in policy away from the importance of inequality itself.

While access to health care services remains an important goal in the United States, it is very unlikely that improved access alone will lead to substantial improvements in outcomes linked to social class, race, and gender. The evidence for this claim has become clear from countries with national health programs that provide universal access to health care services. This evidence of important differences in outcomes that persist despite universal access again leads to a conclusion that much more fundamental change in the structure of society is required, in addition to national policies that assure access.

For example, in the United Kingdom, social class differentials in mortality and health outcomes have persisted despite the improvements in access achieved by the British National Health Service. As an example of research in this area, the Whitehall study of British civil servants assessed mortality, overall health status, and outcomes from cardiovascular and other specific diseases during the 1960s and again during the 1990s. In this research, the subjects all held jobs in the British civil service but ranged from highly paid administrators to lowly paid clerical and manual workers. For overall mortality and outcomes in nearly all the diseases studied, workers from the lower income levels did much worse than workers at the higher income levels. In fact, for most conditions, a gradient appeared that indicated a direct correlation between outcomes and social class, as measured by income and position in the hierarchy of civil service jobs.[48]

Class and ethnic differentials have appeared in Canada, whose national health program has won wide international admiration. Again, studies of overall mortality and outcomes for specific diseases show worse results for lower income groups. Further, Canada manifests regional variations, with adverse outcomes in rural, economically underdeveloped areas, especially in the northern part of the country with its largely indigenous population. In short, despite Canada's overall prosperity and a national health program that has improved access for people throughout the country, evidence of social class inequalities in health outcomes persists.[49]

The maladies that workers in social medicine have described for more than one and a half centuries remain with us. Even in rich nations that have achieved high levels of economic development, wide inequalities in mortality and key indicators of health outcomes reflect the characteristics of social class, structural racism, and sexism within those societies. In the United States, national health policies cannot afford to overlook the problems that have remained when other countries have enacted successful programs to improve access. The persistence of social determination, despite universally accessible health services, implies that broader changes in society are required for meaningful improvements in health outcomes.

Social pathologies – those that distressed Engels, Virchow, Allende, and more recent researchers on the social determination of health outcomes – continue to create suffering and early death. Inequalities of class, exploitation of workers, and conditions of capitalist production cause disease now as previously. Likewise, the constraints of profit and lack of societal responsibility for individual economic security still inhibit even incremental reforms. The links between social structure and disease become ever more urgent as economic instability, unreliable food supplies, depletion of petroleum, nuclear and toxic chemical wastes, global warming, and related problems threaten humanity's very survival. Understanding these roots of illness also reveals the scope of reconstruction that is necessary for meaningful solutions. We return to the question of "what is to be done" about social determination in the chapters that follow, especially the last chapter.

Notes

1 Several classical publications address the responsiveness of infectious diseases to improved social and economic conditions: John Powles, "On the Limitations of Modern Medicine," *Science Medicine & Man* 1 (1973): 1–30; Archie L. Cochrane, *Effectiveness and Efficiency: Random Reflections on Health Care* (London: Nuffield Hospitals Trust, 1972); John B. McKinlay and Sonja M. McKinlay, "The Questionable Contribution of Medical Measures to the Decline of Mortality in the United States in the Twentieth Century," *Milbank Memorial Fund Quarterly* 55 (1977): 405–28; Thomas McKeown, *The Role of Medicine: Dream, Mirage, or Nemesis?* (Princeton: Princeton University Press, 1979); Thomas McKeown, *The Modem Rise of Population* (New York: Academic Press, 1977); Edward H. Kass, "Infectious Diseases and Social Change," *Journal of Infectious Diseases* 123 (1971): 110–14. For further critical discussions: Howard Waitzkin, *The Second Sickness: Contradictions of Capitalist Health Care*, 2nd ed. (Lanham, MD: Rowman & Littlefield, 2000), chapter 1; Stephen Frankel, "Commentary: Medical Care and the Wider Influences upon Population Health: A False Dichotomy," *International Journal of Epidemiology* 30/6 (2001): 1267–68; Sheldon J. Watts, *Epidemics and History: Disease, Power, and Imperialism* (New Haven: Yale University Press, 1997); James Colgrove, "The McKeown Thesis: A Historical Controversy and its Enduring Influence," *American Journal of Public Health* 92/5 (2002): 725–29; and especially Carles Muntaner and Rob Wallace, "Confronting the Social and Environmental Determinants of Health," in Howard Waitzkin and the Working Group on Health Beyond Capitalism, *Health Care Under the Knife: Moving Beyond Capitalism for Our Health* (New York: Monthly Review Press, 2018), chapter 14.
2 The following writings give helpful introductions to these inequalities in health outcomes and their social causes: Commission on Social Determinants of Health, World Health Organization, *Closing the Gap in a Generation: Health Equity Through Action on the Social Determinants of Health: Final Report of the Commission on Social Determinants of Health* (Geneva: World Health Organization, 2008); Michael Marmot, *The Health Gap: The Challenge of an Unequal World* (London: Bloomsbury Publishing, 2015); Ichiro Kawachi, Maria M. Glymour, and Lisa F. Berkman, *Social Epidemiology* (Oxford: Oxford University Press, 2014); Richard Wilkinson and Kate Pickett, *The Spirit Level: Why Equality Makes Societies Stronger* (New York: Bloomsbury, 2011), and *The Inner Level: How More Equal Societies Reduce Stress, Restore Sanity and Improve Everyone's Well-being* (New York: Penguin, 2019); Donald A. Barr, *Health Disparities in the United States: Social Class, Race, Ethnicity and Health* (Baltimore, MD:

Johns Hopkins University Press, 2014). These sources on social determinants, however, generally report associations between inequalities and health outcomes without clarifying the deeper mechanisms by which social determination exerts its effects.

3 Regarding the worsening mortality and morbidity trends in the United States for self-identified white people in mid-life, see Anne Case and Angus Deaton, "Rising Morbidity and Mortality in Midlife among White Non-Hispanic Americans in the 21st Century," *Proceedings of the National Academy of Sciences* 83 (2015): 15078–83. Other alarming research studies on poverty, inequality, and deteriorating health, mental health, and life expectancy in the United States include: Raj Chetty, Michael Stepner, Sarah Abraham, et al., "The Association between Income and Life Expectancy in the United States, 2001–2014," *JAMA* 315 (2016): 1750–66; Steven H. Woolf and Laudan Aron, "Failing Health of the United States: The Role of Challenging Life Conditions and the Policies Behind Them," *BMJ* 360 (2018), doi:10.1136/bmj.k496; Elizabeth M. Stein, Keith P. Gennuso, Donna C. Ugboaja, BS, Patrick L. Remington, "The Epidemic of Despair among White Americans: Trends in the Leading Causes of Premature Death, 1999–2015," *American Journal of Public Health* 107 (2017): 1541–47; Deborah M. Stone, Thomas R. Simon, Katherine A. Fowler, et al., "Trends in State Suicide Rates—United States, 1999–2016 and Circumstances Contributing to Suicide—27 States, 2015," *Morbidity and Mortality Weekly Report (MMWR)* 67 (2018): 617–24. For studies about the health characteristics of counties that voted predominantly for Donald Trump in the 2016 presidential election, see: Jacob Bor, "Diverging Life Expectancies and Voting Patterns in the 2016 US Presidential Election," *American Journal of Public Health* 107 (2017): 1560–62; James S. Goodwin, Yong-Fang Kuo, David Brown, David Juurlink, and Mukaila Raji, "Association of Chronic Opioid Use With Presidential Voting Patterns in US Counties in 2016," *JAMA Network Open* 1 (2018): e180450. doi:10.1001/jamanetworkopen.2018.0450.

4 Although the concept of class in relation to production pervades Marx's work, he expressed this concept clearly and concisely in: Karl Mark, *Capital*, volume 3, chapter 48 ("The Trinity Formula"), www.marxists.org/archive/marx/works/1894-c3/ch48.htm.

5 Vicente Navarro, *Crisis, Health and Medicine: A Social Critique* (New York: Tavistock, 1986).

6 For more on Weber's concept of class: Max Weber, *The Theory of Social and Economic Organization* (New York: Free Press, 1964); *From Max Weber* (New York: Free Press, 1946); Charles Camic, Philip S. Gorski, and David M. Trubeck, *Max Weber's Economy and Society: A Critical Companion* (Stanford, CA: Stanford University Press, 2005).

7 Kathryn Steven, Jon Dowell, Cathy Jackson, and Bruce Guthrie, "Fair Access to Medicine? Retrospective Analysis of UK Medical Schools Application Data 2009–2012 Using Three Measures of Socioeconomic Status," *BMC Medical Education* 16 (2016): 11, doi:10.1186/s12909-016-0536-1.

8 Data on the social class backgrounds of medical students are much more difficult to obtain in the United States than in the United Kingdom. The rare estimates, based on inference from incomplete data, have found that approximately 12 percent of U.S. medical students come from working-class backgrounds. For instance: Grace Ziem, "Medical Education since Flexner," *Health/PAC Bulletin* 8, no. 76 (1977): 8–14, 23, www.healthpacbulletin.org/CompleteBulletinRun/Health%20PAC%20Bulletin%201977%20%20

%2376%20May-Jun.pdf#search=%22ziem%22; Editors, "Bakke-ing Up the Wrong Tree," *Health/PAC Bulletin* 11, no. 3 (January–February 1980): 1–2, 7–16, 25–28, www.healthpacbulletin.org/CompleteBulletinRun/Health%20 PAC%20Bulletin%201980%20Vol%2011%20%233%20Jan%20-%20Feb.pdf#search=%22ziem%22. Although self-identified race and ethnicity are easier to track in the United States and continue to show much lower recruitment of minorities than their proportions in the U.S. population, these data are not controlled by medical students' social class of origin: American Association of Medical Colleges, *Diversity in Medical Education: Facts & Figures 2019* (Washington, DC: AAMC, 2019), https://www.aamc.org/data-reports/workforce/report/diversity-medicine-facts-and-figures-2019.

9   Carles Muntaner et al., "Two Decades of Neo-Marxist Class Analysis and Health Inequalities: A Critical Reconstruction," *Social Theory & Health* 13, no. 3–4 (2015): 267–87; Carles Muntaner, "On the Future of Social Epidemiology—A Case for Scientific Realism," *American Journal of Epidemiology* 178, no. 6 (2013): 852–57. Wright has synthesized his work on social class: Erik Olin Wright, *Understanding Class* (London, New York: Verso, 2015).

10 For an historical overview of changes in tax rates, see: The Tax Foundation, "Federal Individual Income Tax Rates History, Nominal Dollars, Income Years 1913–2013," https://files.taxfoundation.org/legacy/docs/fed_individual_rate_history_nominal.pdf. In its policy recommendations, the Tax Foundation generally takes a conservative positive against proposals that would raise taxes on the wealthy. For a comprehensive assessment of taxes and inequality with proposals for change, see Emmanuel Saez and Gabriel Zucman, *The Triumph of Injustice: How the Rich Dodge Taxes and How to Make Them Pay* (New York: W.W. Norton, 2019), as well as the discussion that follows about the work of Thomas Piketty.

11 "Just 8 Men Own Same Wealth as Half the World," January 15, 2017, www.oxfamamerica.org/press/just-8-men-own-same-wealth-as-half-the-world/, and "An Economy for the 99%," January 15, 2017, www.oxfamamerica.org/explore/research-publications/an-economy-for-the-99-percent/); six months later, five men controlled this amount of wealth (Paul Buchheit, "Now Five Men Own Almost as Much Wealth as Half the World's Population, Nation of Change, June 12, 2017, www.nationofchange.org/2017/06/12/now-five-men-almost-much-wealth-half-worlds-population/. Wealth concentration has increased further since then. For a helpful overview see: Michael Yates, *The Great Inequality* (New York: Routledge, 2016). Regarding greater concentration of wealth during the COVID-19 pandemic, see: Institute for Policy Studies, "Updates: Billionaire Wealth, U.S. Job Losses and Pandemic Profiteers," June 4, 2020, https://inequality.org/billionaire-bonanza-2020-updates/ (this website continues to update).

12 Thomas Piketty, *Capital in the Twenty-First Century* (Cambridge, MA: Harvard University Press, 2014). Regarding the Tobin tax on international electronic currency transactions and similar small tax schemes to address world poverty, see: Tony Colman, "Funding a Global War on Poverty," Global Policy Forum, February 24, 2002, www.globalpolicy.org/component/content/article/216/45934.html; "Tobin Tax Initiative," 2019, http://www.tobintax.org; "Why We Need Robin," 2018, www.robinhoodtax.org; "The Robin Hood Tax," 2020, https://www.robinhoodtax.org.uk.

13 For further substantiation of these themes, see Waitzkin and the Working Group on Health beyond Capitalism, *Health Care Under the Knife*, and Howard Waitzkin, *Rinky-Dink Revolution: Moving Beyond Capitalism by Withholding*

Consent, Creative Constructions, and Creative Destructions (Ottawa, Canada: Daraja Press, and New York: Monthly Review Essays, 2020), https://darajapress.com/publication/rinky-dink-revolution-moving-beyond-capitalism-by-withholding-consent-creative-constructions-and-creative-destructions, https://mronline.org/2020/05/19/rinky-dink-revolution/#gsc.tab=0.

14 Colin McCord and Harold P. Freeman, "Excess Mortality in Harlem," *New England Journal of Medicine* 322 (1990): 173–77.

15 Arline T. Geronimus, John Bound, and Cynthia G. Colen, "Excess Black Mortality in the United States and in Selected Black and White High-Poverty Areas, 1980s–2000s," *American Journal of Public Health* 101 (2011): 720–29; U.S. Centers for Disease Control and Prevention, *Health, United States, 2016* (Washington, DC: CDC, 2017), Table 15, www.cdc.gov/nchs/data/hus/hus16.pdf#015. See note 3 for recent research on deteriorating health indicators for white people in the United States.

16 Helpful studies about the social construction and biology of "race" include: Patricia H. Collins, *Black Feminist Thought: Knowledge, Consciousness, and the Politics of Empowerment* (New York: Routledge, 2009); Troy Duster, *Backdoor to Eugenics* (New York: Routledge, 2004); Joseph L Graves, Jr., and Joseph L. Graves, *The Emperor's New Clothes: Biological Theories of Race at the Millennium* (New Brunswick, NJ: Rutgers University Press, 2003); Michael Omi and Howard Winant, *Racial Formation in the United States* (New York: Routledge, 2020); Audrey Smedley and Brian D. Smedley, *Race in North America: Origin and Evolution of a Worldview*, 4th ed. (New York: Routledge, 2018). Despite problems of racism in this magazine's history, the following publication gives a helpful overview about the social construction of race: "The Race Issue," *National Geographic*, April 2018.

17 Alan Goodman, "Race – The Power of an Illusion," Public Broadcasting System, 2003, www.pbs.org/race/000_About/002_04-background-01-07.htm.

18 Richard Cooper, Charles Rotimi, Susan Ataman, et al., "The Prevalence of Hypertension in Seven Populations of West African Origin," *American Journal of Public Health* 87, no. 2 (1997): 160–68. Other studies have confirmed similar findings about hypertension and socially constructed race.

19 Nancy Krieger, Jarvis T. Chen, Pamela D. Waterman, Mathew V. Kiang, and Justin Feldman, "Police Killings and Police Deaths Are Public Health Data and Can Be Counted," *PLoS Medicine* 12, no. 12 (2015): e1001915. doi:10.1371/journal.pmed.1001915; Justin M. Feldman, Sofia Gruskin, Brent A. Coull, and Nancy Krieger, "Police-Related Deaths and Neighborhood Economic and Racial/Ethnic Polarization, United States, 2015–2016," *American Journal of Public Health* 109, no. 3 (2019): 458–64, doi:10.2105/AJPH.2018.304851.

20 Margaret T. Hicken, Hedwig Lee, Jeffrey Morenoff, James S. House, and David R. Williams, "Racial/Ethnic Disparities in Hypertension Prevalence: Reconsidering the Role of Chronic Stress," *American Journal of Public Health* 104 (2014): 117–23; Nancy Krieger, "From Structural Injustice to Embodied Harm: Measuring Racism, Sexism, Heterosexism, and Gender Binarism for Health Equity Studies," *Annual Review of Public Health* 2020, in press.

21 Kristen Pallok, Fernando De Maio, and David A. Ansell, "Structural Racism—A 60-Year-Old Black Woman with Breast Cancer," *New England Journal of Medicine* 380, no. 16 (2019): 1489–92; Garth H. Rauscher, Jenna A. Khan, Michael L. Berbaum, and Emily F. Conant, "Potentially Missed Detection With Screening Mammography: Does the Quality of Radiologist's Interpretation Vary by Patient Socioeconomic Advantage/Disadvantage?"

Annals of Epidemiology 23, no. 4 (2013): 210–14, doi:10.1016/j.annepidem.2013.01.006; LaPrincess C. Brewer and Lisa A. Cooper, "Race, Discrimination, and Cardiovascular Disease," *American Medical Association Journal of Ethics* 16, no. 6 (2014): 455–60.

22 For research that clarifies the health impacts of racism and linkages with social class, see especially the work of David Williams and colleagues, for instance: Hicken, Lee, Morenoff, House, and Williams, "Racial/Ethnic Disparities in Hypertension Prevalence: Reconsidering the Role of Chronic Stress"; Tené T. Lewis, Courtney D. Cogburn, and David R. Williams, "Self-Reported Experiences of Discrimination and Health: Scientific Advances, Ongoing Controversies, and Emerging Issues," *Annual Review of Clinical Psychology* 11 (2015): 407–40; David R. Williams, Naomi Priest, and Norman Anderson, "Understanding Associations between Race, Socioeconomic Status and Health: Patterns and Prospects," *Health Psychology* 35 (2016): 407–11; Cynthia G. Colen, David M. Ramey, Elizabeth C. Cooksey, and David R. Williams, "Racial Disparities in Health among Nonpoor African Americans and Hispanics: The Role of Acute and Chronic Discrimination," *Social Science & Medicine* 199 (2018): 167–80; Jennifer Malat, Sarah Mayorga-Gallo, and David R.Williams, "The Effects of Whiteness on the Health of Whites in the USA," *Social Science & Medicine* 199 (2018): 148–56. Nancy Krieger and colleagues also have contributed crucial work on racism and health, as well as mechanisms by which racism becomes "embodied." See chapter 3, note 3; Nancy Krieger, "From Structural Injustice to Embodied Harm"; Nancy Krieger, "Methods for the Scientific Study of Discrimination and Health: From Societal Injustice to Embodied Inequality – An Ecosocial Approach," *American Journal of Public Health* 102 (2012): 936–45.

23 The following are two among many accounts of medicine in the service of slavery: Mitchell F. Rice and Woodrow Jones, *Public Policy and the Black Hospital: From Slavery to Segregation to Integration* (Westport, CT: Greenwood, 1994); Executive Committee of the American Anti-Slavery Society, *Slavery and the Internal Slave Trade in the United States of North America*, volume 3 (London: Thomas Ward & Co., 1841).

24 Thomas, James G., Jr., and Charles Reagan Wilson, *The New Encyclopedia of Southern Culture, Volume 22: Science and Medicine* (Chapel Hill: University of North Carolina, 2012); Eugene Perry Link, *The Social Ideas of American Physicians (1776–1976): Studies of the Humanitarian Tradition in Medicine* (Cranbury, NJ: Susquehanna University Press, 1992); Dea H. Boster, *African American Slavery and Disability: Bodies, Property, and Power in the Antebellum South, 1800–1860* (New York: Routledge, 2014).

25 TreaAndrea M. Russworm, *Blackness Is Burning: Civil Rights, Popular Culture, and the Problem of Recognition* (Detroit, MI: Wayne State University Press, 2016).

26 Daniel Levering Leis, *W.E.B. DuBois: A Biography* (New York: Henry Holt, 2009); W.E.B. DuBois, "Negroes and the Crisis of Capitalism in the U.S.," *Monthly Review* 4, no. 12 (April 1953): https://monthlyreview.org/2003/04/01/negroes-and-the-crisis-of-capitalism-in-the-united-states/; *Black Reconstruction in America: 1860–1880* (New York: Free Press, 1935, 1962), chapters 1, 2, 10–12.

27 From a long and worthy list of scholars and activists with African origins, we would like to cite just a few luminaries, in addition to DuBois, who have influenced our thinking about the connections among racism, capitalism, and imperialism, especially regarding impacts on health and mental health:

Frantz Fanon, on colonialism and its effects on health and mental health: *The Wretched of the Earth* (New York: Grove Press, 1963); C.L.R. James, on slavery and revolution in Haiti and elsewhere: *The Black Jacobins: Toussaint L'Ouverture and the San Domingo Revolution* (New York: Vintage, 1938, 1989); Kwame Nkrumah, on neocolonialism: *Neo-Colonialism: The Last Stage of Imperialism* (Moscow: International Publishers, 1965); Harry Haywood, "On Afro-Americans' Confrontation with Capitalism in the United States: For A Revolutionary Position on the Negro Question," 1959, www.marxists.org/history/erol/1956-1960/haywood02.htm; Malcolm X, on the structural components of racism: "Afro-American History," *International Socialist Review* (March–April 1967): 3–48; and Chokwe Lumumba and Kali Akuno, on Co-operation Jackson, emerging from Pan-Africanism, the work of Malcolm X, and the Mississippi Freedom Party: Kali Akuno and Ajamu Nangwaya, *Jackson Rising: The Struggle for Economic Democracy and Black Self-Determination in Jackson, Mississippi* (Montreal: Daraja Press, 2017). Our intention in presenting this brief and incomplete listing is that these scholars and activists explicitly trace the deep linkages between structural racism and capitalism; the social determination of illness and early death emerges from these linkages.
28 Pallok, De Maio, and Ansell, "Structural Racism."
29 See for instance the work of the Social Medicine Consortium and the Campaign against Racism: https://www.socialmedicineconsortium.org, http://www.socialmedicineconsortium.org/campaign-against-racism. For more on the conceptual and political framework of racial capitalism, see for instance: Cedric Robinson, *Black Marxism: The Making of the Black Radical Tradition* (Chapel Hill, NC: University of North Carolina Press, 2000).
30 Rice and Jones, *Public Policy and the Black Hospital*; Abraham Flexner, *Medical Education in the United States and Canada: A Report to the Carnegie Foundation for the Advancement of Teaching* (Boston: Merrymount Press, 1910); G.A. Johnston, Jr., "The Flexner Report and Black Medical Schools," *Journal of the National Medical Association* 76 (1984): 223–25; Louis W. Sullivan and Ilana Suez Mittman, "The State of Diversity in the Health Professions a Century after Flexner," *Academic Medicine* 85 (2010): 246–53.
31 Thomas J. Ward, *Black Physicians in the Jim Crow South* (Fayetteville, AR: University of Arkansas Press, 2003).
32 David Barton Smith, *The Power to Heal: Civil Rights, Medicare, and the Struggle to Transform America's Health Care System* (Nashville, TN: Vanderbilt University Press, 2016). For a moving account of the continuing challenges that face black medical students in the era of COVID-19, police brutality, and racial capitalism, see: LaShyra "Lash" Nolen, "This Is What I Want To Tell My White Professors When They Ask, 'How Are You Today?'" *Huffington Post*, June 8, 2020, https://www.huffpost.com/entry/black-medical-student-wants-white-professors-to-know_n_5ed91238c5b6e0feefc26315.
33 For a historical review of these inequalities for women mediated by social class and racism: Howard Waitzkin, *At the Front Lines of Medicine* (Lanham, MD: Rowman & Littlefield, 2001), chapter 3. More recently, Nancy Krieger and colleagues have contributed important conceptual and empirical perspectives to the embodiment of sexism and how sexism relates to social class and racism; for instance: Krieger, "From Structural Injustice to Embodied Harm"; Nancy Krieger, "Genders, Sexes, and Health: What Are the Connections—and Why Does It Matter?," *International Journal of Epidemiology* 32 (2003): 652–57; Nancy Krieger, *Epidemiology and the People's Health: Theory and Context* (New York: Oxford University Press, 2013).

34 A.H.E.M. Maas and Y.E.A. Appelman, "Gender Differences in Coronary Heart Disease." *Netherlands Heart Journal* 18 (2010): 598–603; "Guideline for the Surgical Management of Female Stress Urinary Incontinence," American Urological Association, 2017, https://www.auanet.org/guidelines/stress-urinary-incontinence-(sui)-guideline ; "Erectile Dysfunction: AUA Guideline," American Urological Association, 2018, https://www.auanet.org/guidelines/erectile-dysfunction-(ed)-guideline; Marlene B. Goldman, Rebecca Troisi, and Kathryn M. Rexrode, *Women and Health* (Amsterdam: Elsevier/Academic, 2013).

35 Vanessa Heggie, "Women Doctors and Lady Nurses: Class, Education, and the Professional Victorian Woman," *Bulletin of the History of Medicine* 89 (2015): 267–92. Further helpful studies of sexism in the history of medical education include: Rebecca J. Tannebaum, *The Healer's Calling: Women and Medicine in Early New England* (Ithaca, NY: Cornell University Press, 2009); Barbara Ehrenreich and Deidre English, *Witches, Midwives and Nurses: A History of Women Healers* (New York: State University of New York Press, 1996).

36 Delese Wear, *Women in Medical Education: An Anthology of Experience* (New York: State University of New York Press, 1996).

37 Marian Faux, *Roe v. Wade: The Untold Story of the Landmark Supreme Court Decision That Made Abortion Legal* (New York: Cooper Square, 2001).

38 Tracey Covassin, C. Buz Swanik, and Michael L. Sachs. "Sex Differences and the Incidence of Concussions among Collegiate Athletes." *Journal of Athletic Training* 38 (2003): 238–44; Avinash Chandran, Mary J. Barron, Beverly J. Westerman, and Loretta DiPietro, "Multifactorial Examination of Sex-Differences in Head Injuries and Concussions among Collegiate Soccer Players: NCAA ISS, 2004–2009," *Injury Epidemiology*, December 2017, doi:10.1186/s40621-017-0127-6.

39 Goldman, Troisi, and Rexrode, *Women and Health*; Anita Reicher-Rössler and Claudia García-Moreno, *Violence against Women and Mental Health* (Basel, Switzerland: Karger, 2013).

40 Association of American Universities, "AAU Climate Survey on Sexual Assault and Sexual Misconduct (2015)," www.aau.edu/key-issues/aau-climate-survey-sexual-assault-and-sexual-misconduct-2015.

41 Zeba Blay, "Why Do Famous Men Keep Getting Away with Violence Against Women?" *Huffington Post,* September 8, 2015, www.huffingtonpost.com/entry/why-do-famous-men-get-away-violence_us_55e70283e4b0aec9f35534bf.

42 Kirby Dick, Amy Ziering, and Constance Matthiessen, *The Hunting Ground: The Inside Story of Sexual Assault on American College Campuses* (New York: Hot Books, 2016); Juliet Eilperin, "Biden and Obama Rewrite the Rulebook on College Sexual Assaults," *Washington Post,* July 3, 2016, www.washingtonpost.com/politics/biden-and-obama-rewrite-the-rulebook-on-college-sexual-assaults/2016/07/03/0773302e-3654-11e6-a254-2b336e293a3c_story.html?utm_term=.d9064fed4533.

43 Miriam Komaromy, Andrew B. Bindman, Richard J. Haber, and Merle A. Sande, "Sexual Harassment in Medical Training," *New England Journal of Medicine* 328 (1993): 322–26; Phyllis L. Carr, Arlene S. Ash, Robert H. Friedman, et al., "Faculty Perceptions of Gender Discrimination and Sexual Harassment in Academic Medicine," *Annals of Internal Medicine* 132 (2000): 889–96; Reshma Jagsi, Kent A. Griffith, Rochelle Jones, Chithra R. Perumalswami, Peter Ubel, and Abigail Stewart, "Sexual Harassment and Discrimination Experiences of Academic Medical Faculty," *JAMA* 315 (2016): 2120–21.

44 Pam Belluck, "Trump Administration Blocks Funds for Planned Parenthood and Others Over Abortion Referrals," *New York Times*, February 22, 2019, https://www.nytimes.com/2019/02/22/health/trump-defunds-planned-parenthood.html; Erica L. Green, "DeVos's Rules Bolster Rights of Students Accused of Sexual Misconduct," May 6, 2020, https://www.nytimes.com/2020/05/06/us/politics/campus-sexual-misconduct-betsy-devos.html.

45 County Health Rankings and Roadmaps, University of Wisconsin, "2018 County Health Rankings: Key Findings Report," March 2018, www.countyhealthrankings.org/explore-health-rankings/rankings-reports/2018-county-health-rankings-key-findings-report.

46 Commission on Social Determinants of Health, World Health Organization, *Closing the Gap in a Generation*.

47 Simon Szreter and Michael Woolcock, "Health by Association? Social Capital, Social Theory, and the Political Economy of Public Health." *International Journal of Epidemiology* 3 (2004): 650–67.

48 Michael G. Marmot, George Davey Smith, Stephen Standsfeld, et al., "Health Inequalities among British Civil Servants: The Whitehall II Study," *Lancet* 337 (1991): 1387–93; Caroline T. M. van Rossum, Martin J. Shipley, Hendrike van de Mheen, Diederick E. Grobbee, and Michael G. Marmot, "Employment Grade Differences in Cause Specific Mortality: A 25 year Follow Up of Civil Servants from the First Whitehall Study," *Journal of Epidemiology & Community Health* 54 (2000): 178–84.

49 For instance: Kip Brown, Alex Nevitte, Betsy Szeto, and Arijit Nandi, "Growing Social Inequality in the Prevalence of Type 2 Diabetes in Canada, 2004–2012," *Canadian Journal of Public Health* 106 (2015): e132–39; Noemie Savard, Nathalie Auger, Alison L. Park, Ernest Lo, and Jerome Martinez, "Educational Inequality in Stillbirth: Temporal Trends in Quebec from 1981 to 2009," *Canadian Journal of Public Health* 104 (2013): e148–53.

Chapter 5

Social Medicine in the United States

Can One Speak of a U.S. Social Medicine?

We can find evidence of social medicine ideas and initiatives throughout U.S. history. This story begins with the creation of the first modern factories in Massachusetts during the early 1800s and continues to the present moment. Most of the story did not happen explicitly under the banner of "social medicine." But the themes are similar to those addressed elsewhere in the book: the health and safety of workers, the promotion of sanitation, efforts to bring health care to working-class communities, working against the destructive effects of racism and political repression, the struggle for a national health care system (or at least national health insurance), and political activism. The history of U.S. social medicine leaves us with a large unfinished agenda.

The First U.S. Factories, Struggles for Workers' Health, and the Labor Movement

Industrialization started later in the United States than it did in Europe, but as in Europe, it began in the textile factories. Francis Cabot Lowell, a Bostonian who was familiar with English textile mills, created one of the first U.S. factories in 1814, on the banks of the Charles River in Waltham, Massachusetts. Lowell's factory combined both spinning (turning cotton into thread) and weaving (turning thread into cloth), thus allowing the factory to turn raw cotton into finished cloth.

Most of the workers in the mills were women, typically farm girls. To make it socially acceptable for women to work in the foreign environment of a mill (far from farm and family), factory owners developed what was known as the Waltham System. Female workers lived in boarding houses supervised by female chaperones. Lowell's Boston Manufacturing Company also created the country's first industrial hospital in 1840.

Over time, disputes arose regarding the benefits and damages caused by factory life, echoing earlier disputes that had arisen in Europe during its earlier Industrial Revolution. After Lowell's death, his business partners started a new factory town in Massachusetts, named it after Lowell, and expanded the model of factory labor on a much larger scale. The conditions affecting workers in Lowell, Massachusetts, worried many observers in addition to the workers themselves. For instance, Orestes Brownson, a New England intellectual, argued in 1840 that factory women worked for miserly wages and they

> wear out their health, spirits, and morals, without becoming one whit better off than when they commenced labor. (...) The average life, working life we mean, of the girls that come to Lowell, for instance, from Maine, New Hampshire, and Vermont, we have been assured, is only about three years. What becomes of them then? Few of them ever marry; fewer still ever return to their native places with reputations unimpaired. "She has worked in a Factory," is almost enough to damn to infamy the most worthy and virtuous girl. We know no sadder sight on earth than one of our factory villages presents, when the bell at break of day, or at the hour of breakfast, or dinner, calls out its hundreds or thousands of operatives. We stand and look at these hard-working men and women hurrying in all directions, and ask ourselves, where go the proceeds of their labors?[1]

Elisha Bartlett, MD, a former Mayor of Lowell, countered Browson's critique in another article.[2] Bartlett employed a numerical analysis to show that the workers suffered no ill-health from their work in the factory:

> More than one half of our population are between the ages of 15 and 30 years, and a great proportion of these are employed in the mills. In the year 1830, the population stood, by an actual census, at 6477; the number of deaths was 114, and of this whole number only seven occurred among the persons employed in the mills! In the year 1828, the population was 3500; girls in the mills, 1500. During that whole year, there was not a single death, in the city, among these 1500 girls. I ask those who are versed in the lore of medical statistics to match these two facts. Even if they were picked facts, they would be none the less extraordinary.

Bartlett brought statistics into the discussion. While statistics often can clarify a situation, they can also confuse things if not used properly. Bartlett tells us that there were many young workers in the mills, but they count for only a small number of deaths in Lowell, that is, 7 deaths among 114 total deaths in 1830. He considers this to be convincing evidence that the factory girls were healthy. Are there other possible explanations for these numbers? In his article essay, Brownson had offered a potential reason why mortality statistics might be misleading: Women who get sick in the factories would usually go home to convalesce (or die), thus artificially raising the mortality in their hometowns and decreasing mortality rates in Lowell.

The discussion over these numbers was taken up in 1846 by the Bostonian Lemuel Shattuck, one of the leading figures in U.S. public health and the development of statistics. Shattuck pointed out that comparing raw statistics for two very different communities could lead to misleading conclusions. As he noted: "The principle of taking the average age of death alone as a measure of the health of places, is incorrect, and even absurd, when applied to places affected by immigration and other circumstances as are Boston and Lowell."[3]

The workers in Lowell were not passive in this dispute. One of the workers, Sarah George Bagley (1806–1883), emerged as a leading figure in the early U.S. labor movement. In 1845, she was part of an organized attempt to petition the Massachusetts legislature to investigate the factory system and to limit the workday to ten hours. This would be the major demand of the labor movement throughout the rest of the century. The petition campaign was initially successful in so far as the legislature agreed to establish a committee that would look into the matter. Ultimately, it was decided that the length of the workday was a matter to be worked out between workers and employers, and not by the state. The workers continued to petition the legislature; a second commission was appointed but came to the same conclusions. By this time, however, the mill owners had agreed voluntarily to reduce the workday by 30 minutes.

Lowell, Massachusetts, the first major U.S. factory town, shows us the key elements of social medicine as it emerged in Europe. These elements included a concern for the working class, a focus on the effects of industrialization, social approaches to improving health, the role of the labor movement, and the use (and abuse) of medical statistics.

DISCUSSION QUESTION: WHAT IS THE ROLE OF "SCIENTIFICALLY NEUTRAL" PROPOSALS FOR CHANGE

Orestes Brownson was clearly an open advocate for the workers of Massachusetts, whose demands centered on a ten-hour workday. This proposal was rejected initially for political reasons: The legislature felt it should not intervene. Lemuel Shattuck took a more conservative approach, offering "scientifically neutral" suggestions. What are the advantages and disadvantages of each approach?

Shattuck (1793–1857) became a central figure in the "sanitary movement," which influenced that later development of U.S. public health, but his focus included some key themes of social medicine. Early in his career he worked as a schoolteacher, a Boston bookseller and publisher, and later a Massachusetts legislator. Concerned with the collection and proper analysis of health data, he helped started the American Statistical Society (1839) and advocated in favor of a Massachusetts law for compulsory collection of vital statistics such as births, deaths, and marriages.

The *Report of a General Plan for the Promotion of Public and Personal Health*, published in 1850, became Shattuck's best-known accomplishment.[4] In 1849, he had been appointed by the Massachusetts legislature (along with N.P. Banks and Jehiel Abbott) to lead a study about the health conditions in the state. Their report has been compared to Edwin Chadwick's 1842 report on the health of the British working class, which played a central role in English public health and influenced Friedrich Engels's studies on the occupational and environmental conditions that affected the English working class (as we discussed in Chapter 2).[5] Shattuck and colleagues began by reviewing the public health systems in Europe, particularly in France, Germany, and England. They argued for the creation of a strong public health infrastructure, including both local and state health authorities, for disease prevention and health education. The report also suggested a model health law and proposed a "sanitary survey" of Massachusetts, which in 1869 became the first state to establish a statewide health department.

Social Medicine Centered in the "Little Germany" of New York City

Known as the Gilded Age in the United States, the period from the 1870s to roughly 1900 became a time of rapid industrialization and economic growth. This growth happened in large part due to the massive influx of mainly poor European immigrants looking for work. Drawn by the higher wages offered in the United States, the immigrants typically formed enclaves in big cities within which they attempted to recreate their home environments.

The leading example of such an enclave was Kleindeutschand (literally "little Germany"), or Dutchtown, as non-Germans called it. Kleindeutschland was located on New York's lower east side. Beginning in the 1840s hundreds of thousands of German immigrants began arriving in New York City. By 1855, only Berlin and Vienna had more German citizens than New York. Most of these immigrants were well educated and/or highly skilled artisans. Once in New York, they worked in German businesses, worshiped in German churches, banked in German banks, read German newspapers, and participated in local political parties that were extensions of German political parties. Their active social life was centered on beer halls, saloons, shooting galleries, plays, concerts, and mutual aid societies. These mutual aid societies played an important role in the development of health insurance by German and other immigrant communities.

> The stories of Abraham Jacobi and his wife, Mary Putnam Jacobi, illustrate the challenges of this period and the development of a social medicine model based on the principles Jacobi had learned in Germany as a student of Virchow. Despite its sometimes technical appearance, the model also was highly political and informed by socialist values. A woman middle aged has the following story: Seven children, one husband, one basement grocery store; she opens the store at five; she closes it at eleven; she does her washing and housekeeping in a few what are called rooms behind the store, attends to six children, has no time to sit down to a meal, and – wants a prescription to make her feel strong, and well and cheery. I know of only one prescription; that is a different configuration of human society, with less individualism, more solidarity, and more sense of responsibility on the part of society and state. I know also that there are many hundreds of just such grocery women in New York city.[6]

Abraham Jacobi's life (1830–1919) bridged the radical German politics of 1848 with the U.S. Progressive Era of the early twentieth century. Trained as a physician, he actively participated in the revolution of 1848, joining Karl Marx's underground Communist League in 1851. That same year he was arrested for subversion, and during the infamous Cologne Communist Trial, he was one of 12 people accused of plotting to overthrow the Prussian King. He was released after 18 months in jail but was imprisoned later for another 6 months because of his "seditious activities" at the University of Bonn. All of this led him to seek refuge first in Britain and then in New York, where he arrived in November 1853.[7]

Jacobi set up a medical office in his one-room apartment within a tenement in one of the poorer sections of Kleindeutschland. He had achieved a certain notoriety for having been involved in the Cologne trials and received a small amount of financial support, which other immigrants provided in solidarity. In addition to his private practice, he worked as a charity doctor (*Armenartz*) in the tenements.

Jacobi (Figure 5.1) eventually became one of the leading academic physicians in New York and was key in the establishment of several of New York's most important medical institutions. These included the German Dispensary, the New York Academy of Medicine, and the Medical Society of the County of New York. He was the first president of the American Pediatrics Society and also became president of the American Medical Association (AMA).

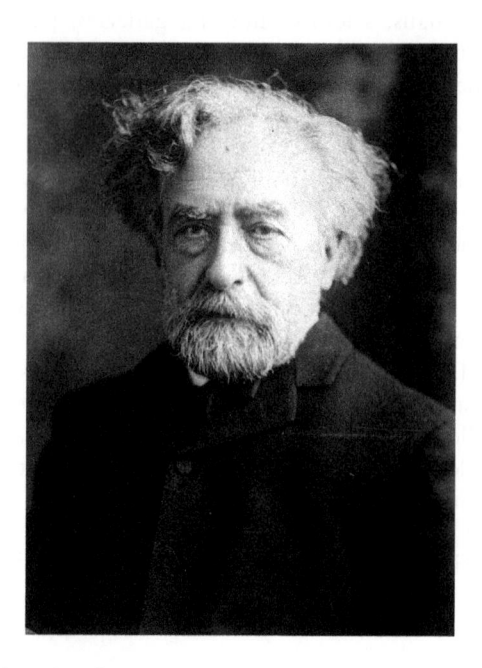

Figure 5.1 Abraham Jacobi.

After studying under Virchow in Germany, Jacobi brought with him many of the key concepts of Virchow's social medicine. He was fortunate to find in New York a community of like-minded, radical, German expatriate physicians. Let us look at some examples of how their ideas, developed initially in Germany, influenced their work in New York.

A sense of injustice as the root of ill-health. In discussing the problems of the middle-aged grocery woman who visited him for something to make her "feel strong," Jacobi relates her problems not to a physical illness but rather to an oppressive social structure that must be changed. This sense of social injustice is quite distinct from Shattuck's somewhat paternalistic concern for the poor and the technical means of improving their lot.

The mission of medicine to promote democratic social reform. Jacobi and his colleagues saw medical reform as a means of promoting a broader social reform based on democratic principles. This led them to put great emphasis on education of both patients and other doctors and professionals. This vision was embodied in the German Dispensary.[8] Jacobi was unhappy with the existing medical establishment and, together with six other radical physicians, he established the German Dispensary of New York. This free clinic provided care to the needy poor of Kleindeutschland and officially functioned according to democratic principles. Regular educational seminars were held for the New York medical community, and a reference library was created.

An academic model of medical care. In accordance with German models of teaching polyclinics, the dispensary did not just provide medical care but was also a center for research and teaching. Jacobi's interest in both children and research were manifested in investigations of pediatric therapeutics, a topic he created. For this work, Jacobi is often considered as the founder of modern pediatrics. This model strongly influenced U.S. medicine, which was still struggling after the Civil War to develop a scientific and clinical basis.

A particular concern for the working class. Because of his special role in founding the specialty of pediatrics, it is understandable that Jacobi advocated to limit and ultimately abolish child labor. In a comprehensive review of child labor laws, Jacobi brought a distinctly political vision (what he refers to as a "calculating business point of view") to the problem:

> ... to look upon the laboring children with merely a sympathetic eye and a warm heart does not cover the case at all. The question can be approached both with a sympathetic warm heart and from a calculating business point of view. In America the legislative interference with the old way of brutally abusing children was first launched against the manufacturers, to protect the young against the physical dangers resulting from premature and protracted work, confinement, bad air, and its consequences; also deformities, losses of limbs and lives. But the study of the discussions of legislative bodies and of the numerous annual reports of factory inspectors ... has taught me that the laws enacted, one by one, with progressive improvements in their tendencies and results, were less the results of warm hearted impressions than of clear-sighted statesmanship. Early child labor interferes with schooling and education. Child labor means ignorance; ignorance means helplessness and poverty; poverty means, or may mean, and does mean in a hundred thousand cases, shiftlessness and poorhouse, crime and prison.[9]

Jacobi also contributed to the adult labor movement in the United States and its fight to reduce working hours. He wrote movingly of the difficulties faced by women who worked with tobacco:

> I wish you to follow me into my office where amongst others I see a goodly number of young girls who work at tobacco mostly in shops, many at home. The latter are worse off than the former, for to them there are no regular hours at all. To them their cramped living and sleeping quarters are also their shops, filled day and night with tobacco odor and dust. All of these patients are anaemic, sallow, thin, underweight. They are poorly paid, poorly nourished, early risers – for they

begin their work at seven.... Tuberculosis of the lungs is very frequent among these young tobacco workers, who are carried off in great numbers between the fifteenth and twenty-fifth year.[10]

Some have argued that the spirit of community activism within pediatrics reflects Jacobi's legacy to the field.[11] In 1963, the American Academy of Pediatrics and the American Medical Association (AMA) jointly sponsored a yearly Abraham Jacobi award that reflects part of the living legacy of 1848 in modern day medicine.

Mary Corrinna Putnam Jacobi (1842–1906) grew up in a privileged New York family. Her father was George Putnam, who founded G.P. Putnam's Sons publishing house in 1838. Mary Jacobi became interested in religion but gradually abandoned the church and turned to science as a way of understanding the world. Eventually, she decided to enter medicine and graduated from the Female Medical College of Pennsylvania in 1863 (Figure 5.2).

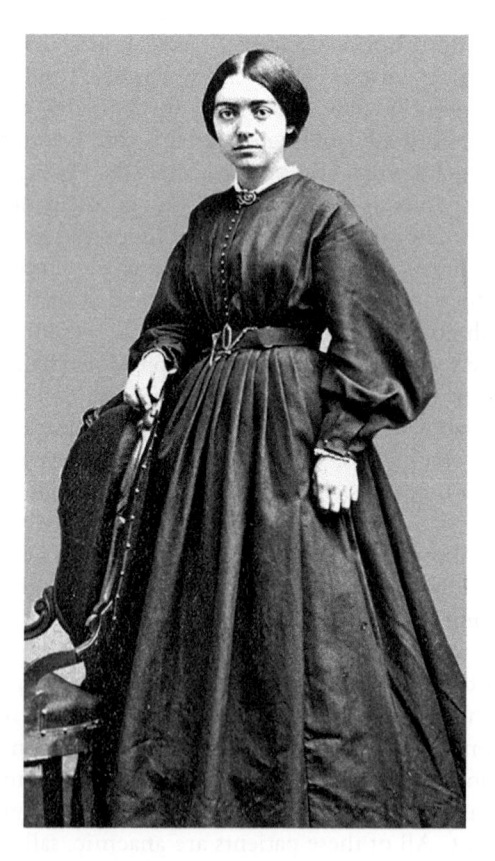

Figure 5.2 Mary Putnam Jacobi.

Unsatisfied with the quality of medical education for women in the United States, she moved to Paris in 1866 with thoughts of further pursuing her medical education there. At the time French attitudes toward women physicians were in a state of flux. Some supported the entry of women into the profession, while others saw it as a man's field. Accepted as the École de Médicine's first female student in 1868, Putman graduated in 1871.[12] Putnam's acceptance and the subsequent acceptance of Elizabeth Blackwell, another woman from the United States, opened the doors of the École to women, a major accomplishment. As students, the two women were required to enter the school through a side door.[13]

As the sixth woman in the country with a medical degree, Putnam returned to the United States with more than just an excellent European medical education – she had also become a researcher and a committed socialist. She was still living in France when the French government declared war on Germany in July 1870. The Germans quickly invaded northeastern France and laid siege to Paris, which fell in January 1871. In response, there was a popular uprising and the creation of a revolutionary socialist government called the Paris Commune. The commune survived a little more than two months before the French military suppressed it in what became known as "the bloody week." Mary Putnam lived through all these events, and they would leave a mark on her future work.

Upon her return to New York in 1871, Putnam set up a medical practice and took a position as professor at the New York Women's Medical School. A year later she helped establish the Women's Medical Association of New York City; she was president of the organization from 1874 to 1903. After she married Abraham Jacobi in 1875, the couple had three children, only one of whom survived to adulthood. (In Germany, Abraham Jacobi already had lost a prior wife during childbirth.) Despite their many differences (gender, country of origin, family background, social status), the couple were both social medicine radicals who were highly successful in advocacy work. Let us see how Mary Jacobi's independent work echoed the ideals of her husband:

Medicine as a tool for social change. The center of Mary Jacobi's work was the demonstration that women were men's equals both intellectually and in the workplace. She brought to this project the rigor of European medical education, a focus on research that was unusual in the education of women physicians, and her political experiences during the Paris Commune. Her approach was not necessarily appreciated at the time.

One example of her advocacy was the essay "The Question of Rest for Women during Menstruation," which won the Harvard Boylston Prize in 1876.[14] She wrote this essay to rebut Harvard Professor Edward Clarke, who had observed: "There have been instances, and I have seen such, of females... graduated from school or college excellent scholars, but with undeveloped ovaries. Later they married, and were sterile."[15]

In her essay, Jacobi responded with a mountain of data showing that these concerns were false. For example, she assembled data from 268 women who completed a 16-question survey on symptoms associated with menstruation. Of this group 94 women (35 percent) reported no menstrual symptoms. She went on to make a careful analysis of how school, physical activity, occupation, family history, general health, and childbirth were related to menstruation. She concluded that "immunity from menstrual suffering" was related to the "vigor of health during childhood and the soundness of family history" as well as the "degree of exercise taken during school life" and "the thoroughness and extension of the mental education." Of course, this was exactly the opposite of what Clarke had asserted. It also supported Jacobi's concern that young women get adequate physical activity and adequate education. This survey was just one of five lines of research reported in Jacobi's essay.

Advocacy for democracy. Mary Jacobi became involved in the women's suffrage movement. As one of many examples, she gave a well-publicized speech at a New York state convention in 1894 that attracted wide attention to the importance of extending the vote to women. Her speech there later came out in book form as *Common Sense Applied to Woman Suffrage.*[16]

Activities with the labor movement. Mary Jacobi also connected herself closely to the labor movement. She took part in the New York Consumer's League, a group formed in 1890 to improve conditions for working women in the city. The league took particular interest in women working in department stores. They were poorly paid and had to work long hours, often without overtime pay. The league published a white list of establishments that treated employees well and a black list of stores that should be avoided for their poor labor practices. Jacobi served as a medical consultant and testified in Albany for the right of store workers to unionize.[17]

Health Initiatives during the Progressive Era

During the so-called Progressive Era (roughly 1890 through the 1920s), there was an explosion of social activism that tried to address some of the major problems created in the Gilded Age: the growing inequities in wealth and political power, governmental corruption, and the power of large trusts. In many ways, the concerns of the Progressive Era mirror concerns today that government has become the tool of the wealthy and that our present democratic structures no longer serve the people. Much of Progressive Era activism centered on health issues and emphasized non-medical interventions, thus, reflecting social conceptions of illness.

While some have traced the community health center (CHC) movement to the 1960s, the roots of CHCs are much older than that. The German Dispensary (1857) already included some essential elements of modern CHCs: location and service within a given locality, concern for population health, attention to social determinants, care for the poor, emphasis on preventive care, a concern for education, and an interest in democratic structures. All these components mark CHCs as a different model from the typical doctor sitting in his or her office and seeing individual patients on a fee-for-service basis.[18]

Kleindeutschland was somewhat exceptional among immigrant communities because most of the arriving Germans had marketable skills and a language that was not completely unrelated to English. Subsequent waves of immigrants were poorer and often lacked the skills needed to learn English quickly and integrate into the so-called melting pot. The result was a growing number of slums and conditions of extreme poverty, amply documented in books like Jacob Riis's *How the Other Half Lives*.[19]

The settlement movement, closely tied to the CHCs of the Progressive Era, tried to overcome the barriers of class, religion, national origin, and language by creating a space within poor urban communities where volunteers, typically middle class, would live and work with the poor. Settlement houses typically involved providing services such as education and health care. The settlement houses also played an important role in promoting women's rights – establishing a settlement house offered women a structure in which they could educate themselves and take part in economic activities largely independent of men.

During the mid-1890s Lillian Wald and Mary Brewster created the Nurses Settlement on Henry Street, one of the first settlement houses in the United States. Their plan was simple: "We were to live in the neighborhood as nurses, identify ourselves with it socially, and, in brief, contribute to it our citizenship. That plan contained in embryo all the extended and diversified social interests of our settlement group to-day."[20]

The two nurses moved into the top floor of a tenement on Jefferson Street, chosen because it was one of the few places that had an indoor bathtub. As Wald noted: "The mere fact of living in the tenement brought undreamed-of opportunities for widening our knowledge and extending our human relationships. That we were Americans was wonderful to our fellow-tenants. They were all immigrants Jews from Russia or Roumania."[21] In 1895, the program would move to its long-term location on Henry Street. At various times, Emma Goldman, a nurse and influential anarchist, collaborated in the Henry Street effort (Figure 5.3).

The year 1893, however, witnessed an important economic downturn in the United States, and conditions became very bad on New York's lower east side, especially during the winter. Wald and Brewster soon developed a practice that Wald called "public health nursing." The nurses literally would walk over the rooftops and up and down the fire escapes to visit their patients. They met initially with some opposition from the medical profession, but over time, they managed to establish themselves independently.

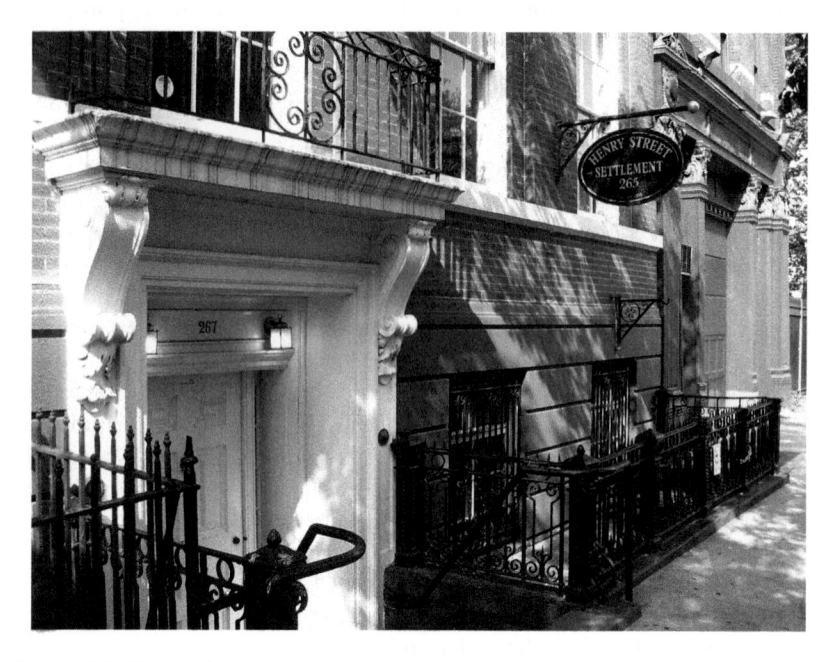

Figure 5.3 Henry Street settlements.

Wald kept statistics about the impact of the program, noting that they were particularly effective in keeping children out of the hospital (where they were often exposed to diseases). In 1914, nurses from the settlement house treated 3,535 cases of pneumonia from all age groups; this total contrasted with that of "four large New York hospitals," which had treated only 1,612. Mortality for the patients treated at home was 8.05 percent; in the hospital it was 31.2 percent. The statistics for children under two were even more striking: Mortality for those treated at home was 9.3 percent versus 38 percent for the hospitals. The original settlement house grew over the years to provide coverage in several parts of the city, and in 1944, the original nursing service became the current Visiting Nurse Service of New York.

The settlement house involved itself in activities other than simply clinical care. It established a small theater, worked to improve educational opportunities for adolescents by offering them scholarships, and developed a nursing program in the schools to recognize children with health problems. The settlement house's participants sought to expose city children to country life during the summers: City children would go to live with farmers' families in a sort of "reverse" settlement program. New York's Fresh Air Fund, founded in 1877, continues this tradition today. Another program from this period, the New York Milk Committee, struggled to find a way to provide fresh milk. While nurses set up feeding stations where they provided education about nutrition and parenting, mothers often avoided them because of stigma and distrust, unless a child was sick.

Wald was a complex thinker inspired by a broad vision of social justice. She clearly understood the social and political context that controlled much of tenement life. As a result, she was an advocate for limiting or abolishing child labor, for women's suffrage, for unionizing the thousands of "informal" workers in the tenements, and for racial integration. She was a socialist and a founding member of the National Association for the Advancement of Colored People (NAACP), as well numerous other organizations dedicated to justice.

The settlement movement remained popular during the first few decades of the twentieth century. In 1911, a handbook listed 413 settlement houses in 34 states (including Hawaii).[22] But the movement became a victim of its own success as more and more social service agencies began to address the problems of poor communities. Eventually, complaints arose about the lack of coordination among the multiple organizations working in these areas.

In response to these concerns, new types of CHCs arose, with a variety of names and functions. Despite this variety, several common themes characterized these centers. First, they usually took responsibility for the health needs of a geographically defined population. Clinics were located near the people they served. Second, the center recognized the primacy of social issues by incorporating social work and welfare services. Ideally, co-location of these services in the clinic would simplify coordination. Third, the CHCs provided services in poor, often immigrant neighborhoods and saw their role partly as integrating these groups into U.S. society. They considered education and health as key elements in this integration. Fourth, they often led advocacy campaigns to address social problems in their neighborhoods, such as food distribution and garbage collection. Many of the centers conducted research or social experimentation. Finally, the CHCs tried to involve the community in the activities of the clinic and even in some measure of self-government.

Several programs put the concepts into action. For instance, the Milbank Memorial Fund was established in 1905 by Elizabeth Milbank Anderson and Albert G. Milbank and financed by funds from the Borden Milk Company. From 1923 to 1934, the Milbank Memorial Fund sponsored three "health demonstrations" in three different communities of New York state: Cattaraugus County (1923–1931), Syracuse (1923–1931), and the Bellevue–Yorkville area of New York City (1926–1934). In Cattaraugus County, the fund's participation allowed existing work of the county health department to be expanded and better coordinated.

These projects were designed to "demonstrate the benefits of offering integrated health and social services to entire communities in New York State." The demonstrations "emphasized the prevention and treatment of TB but also included care for pregnant women, preventive services for infants and children, and the early discovery of cancer and what they called 'cardiac difficulties.'"[23] Such projects helped foster the further development of public health departments and the division of large cities into smaller health districts.

In New York City, the Bellevue–Yorkville demonstration project served the eastern side of Manhattan and ran from 1926 to 1931. A large CHC became the hub for the program. This building's design conveyed the concepts behind the demonstration project: The first floor contained an auditorium and the top (fifth) floor an assembly room. These spaces were designed for educational purposes, such as popular lectures and the screening of films about health. Additional space was provided for the training of nurses and "special courses for small lay groups, such as mothers' clubs, and teachers' and children's clubs."[24] In 1928, the center was used for a course in public health organized by Columbia University.[25]

In addition to education, the first two floors were dedicated primarily to the provision of clinical care: "model tuberculosis, baby health, dental, and venereal disease clinics maintained by the New York City Department of Health, with reception, consultation rooms, and administrative offices for the clinics."[26] The building's third and fourth floors housed the social services, administrative offices for the health demonstration, and the district offices of the Henry Street Visiting Nurse Association, the Kips Bay Neighborhood Association, the New York Association for Improving the Condition of the Poor, and the Charity Organization Society, which were collaborating agencies in the demonstration.[27]

But the vision of these clinics went beyond the strictly medical to include actions that facilitated participation in political life. In 1937, C.E.A. Winslow, founder of Yale's School of Public Health (1915), outlined the aspirations of the Bellevue–Yorkville clinic as a vehicle for promoting democracy in a fast-paced urban community where "knowledge of each other is chiefly derived from jostling in the subway, [the] primary participation in the tasks of government, the pulling of a lever in a voting booth."[28] Winslow hoped to use the clinic to promote "liberal democracy." Writing in 1937, he noted:

> It may be that such an ideal is essentially unattainable and that the vision of liberal democracy is only a dream as the leaders of Italy and Germany declare. [...] Can we take such a district as Bellevue-Yorkville, in the heart of a great commercial metropolis and develop within it the consciousness of mutual interests, the sense of mutual responsibility...?[29]

Was it possible within the context of a health center to achieve the lofty democratic goals that Winslow voiced? George Rosen, historian of social medicine, did not think so and argued:

> ... despite the often expressed aim of involving the local population in the neighborhood health program, this goal was hardly realized and remained more of a pious intention. Although Bellevue-Yorkville in New York City may have been envisaged as an experiment to crystallize community consciousness around health as a center, the demonstration was actually run by a group of voluntary health and welfare agencies, financed by a foundation in collaboration with the municipal health department.[30]

When the Bellevue–Yorkville project ended in 1931, it had accomplished its goal of encouraging the city to create similar centers. In 1929, New York City had decided to build 16 additional clinics, located throughout the city's health districts.

Let us examine an important experience outside New York that promoted democracy through a health program and centers.

Experiments in Social Medicine outside New York

Wilbur C. Phillips, a socialist, had participated in milk distribution programs in New York City and grew interested in creating self-governing bodies within communities. When in 1910 Emil Seidel was elected as the first socialist mayor of Milwaukee, Phillips saw a chance to put his ideas into action. He and his wife, Elsie, also a socialist, were able to convince the city government to support a child welfare commission and to name Phillips as secretary. His goal was to find a neighborhood "small enough to enable our child welfare nurses to reach *every* home easily and quickly and keep in constant contact with every mother."[31]

Acting as a community organizer, Phillips convinced a Catholic priest, Father Szukalski, to use his parish, composed largely of Polish immigrants, as a testing ground. Phillips's program set up tents where mothers could bring their newborns for care by nurses and local doctors. When no one came, Phillips organized a women's committee composed of the community's most influential women. As he worked with this committee, women with newborn children began to arrive at the tents. Phillips eventually convinced one woman from each block to run a block committee. Their goal was to educate the women on the block and to report back to the committee. Phillips reported that infant mortality dropped during the first year by one-half. Later, a new city government decided to incorporate these activities into the local health department.

The Phillipses remained committed to their vision of community democracy and spent much of the next four years developing a more sophisticated version of their original plan. Their work in Milwaukee became nationally recognized, which led to funding from several wealthy donors. In 1916, they established the National Social Unit Organization (NSUO), designed to support their model of participatory democracy.

In 1917, they arrived in Cincinnati, where they had received an invitation to implement their program in the Mohawk–Brighton district. The program involved three councils: a citizen's council composed of 31 women chosen to represent their blocks and led by an elected chairman; an occupational council formed by representatives of different occupational groups (physicians, social workers, clergy, etc.), who also would elect a chairman and function as a de facto technical committee; and a general council that would incorporate both the other two councils and make decisions on financial and budgetary matters. These groups tried to work in collaboration with city agencies.

As in Milwaukee, the entry project for this "social unit" was infant care. The staff set up stations to see newborns, to provide screening exams to infants, and to refer for medical care when needed. Nurses visited all newborn children in their homes. Since organizers created the block structure first, they later could obtain 100 percent coverage.

The project emphasized education and capture of information. Doctors learned about infant care and trained nurses, who taught block workers, and the block workers taught patients. Information flowed back up the chain as block workers reported to nurses, who then reported to doctors. Statistical data helped monitor the program's progress, and a regular bulletin kept everyone in the neighborhood informed. When the influenza pandemic of 1918 arrived in Cincinnati, the social unit immediately printed and distributed 3,500 leaflets with advice on how to avoid infection. Phillips reported that influenza fatalities in Mohawk–Brighton were 2.4 per 1,000 in comparison with 4.1 per 1,000 for the rest of the city.

Despite a hopeful beginning, the Cincinnati social unit closed in 1920, and the NSUO later went bankrupt. The proximal causes for this disappointing end involved the 1919 Red Scare, when anti-communists slandered the program as a radical, Bolshevik movement. Phillips also noted the suspicion of the business community:

> These prominent businessmen ... had been growing more and more suspicious of our demonstration, more and more restive under its success and the keen and growing interest it was arousing not only in Cincinnati but in the country at large. Their suspicions had not been allayed as they watched our non-partisan block elections, with

political alignments utterly ignored and with voters selecting councils and executives solely on the basis of their ability and integrity as servants of the public good. Nor had this uneasiness been quieted by the spectacle of a solid district of citizens showing the results of functional education in a growing habit of considering all plans on the basis of common needs and accurate facts, of taking counsel from skilled groups not from ward bosses and heelers![32]

Its organizers did not intend the NSUO primarily as a health intervention, but it shared characteristics common to the experiences we have seen before: use of public health as a means of promoting community development, interest in population health, emphasis on teaching and gathering data, and promotion of participatory political values. Some historians have seen the NSUO's failure as resulting from U.S. attitudes favoring individualism over community, as well as an emphasis on privatization of public services that discourages citizen participation.[33]

The Contested Status of Social Insurance in the United States

Discussions of U.S. health care reform often, if not always, invoke the fact that the United States is very much an international outlier. This orientation is also sometimes referred to as "American exceptionalism." The United States has the costliest health care system in the world, it does not cover the entire population, and its population's health outcomes are not stellar. (See Chapter 4 for more information about nonstellar U.S. health outcomes.) While most countries have adopted some recognition of a right to health in their constitutions, the United States treats health care as a commodity, not as a right. But health care simply represents just one example of a broader ambivalence toward social insurance in the United States.

What is social insurance? Most societies recognize that people face unavoidable risks that are best managed, or can only be managed, through a government-sponsored insurance program. The term "social insurance" is unfamiliar to most people; yet, everybody is impacted and protected by a variety of social insurance programs. Social security is the most well-recognized type of social insurance. Marmor has described social insurance as "a set of interventions designed to reduce the impacts of common threats across each person's life cycle, threats that simply cannot be countered effectively by individual prudence or private markets." With his colleagues Marmor has created a typology of such risks.[34] Several social insurance programs in the United States protect people against these risks.

> **TYPES OF RISKS THAT REQUIRE SOCIAL INSURANCE (MARMOR AND COLLEAGUES)**
>
> - The threat of being born into a poor family
> - The threat of early death of a breadwinner
> - The threat of ill-health
> - The threat of involuntary unemployment
> - The threat of disability
> - The threat of outliving one's savings

Social Security: protecting against the threats of disability, outliving one's savings, and early death of a breadwinner. Historically, the elderly were the poorest segment of the adult population since they no longer worked. As early as 1797, Thomas Paine recognized this problem and published a plan to provide annual payments to persons over 50 years of age, with money originating from an inheritance tax.[35] In addition, all citizens would get a one-time payment when they turned 21, so they could start their adult life.

Paine justified this plan based on human rights. He argued that while the earth was given to all, the human creation of land ownership displaced large parts of the population and divided society into rich and poor. Societies should compensate this dispossession of people from land, according to Paine:

> In advocating the case of the persons thus dispossessed, it is a right, and not a charity, that I am pleading for. But it is that kind of right which, being neglected at first, could not be brought forward afterwards till heaven had opened the way by a revolution in the system of government. Let us then do honour to revolutions by justice, and give currency to their principles by blessings.[36]

Needless to say, the United States did not act on Paine's proposal. However, during the Civil War the federal government set up an extensive disability and survivors' program. These pensions either compensated soldiers for disabling wounds or provided equivalent funds to family if soldiers died. Qualification for these pensions expanded over time so that by 1910 nearly all Civil War veterans, including former Confederate soldiers, were receiving pensions and death benefits.

In his speech to Congress on June 8, 1934, President Franklin D. Roosevelt discussed his plans for creating a Social Security System. He described the purpose of this system as "the security of the men, women, and children of the Nation against certain hazards and vicissitudes of life."[37]

Earlier, Roosevelt had set up a Committee on Economic Security, and he wanted to turn its recommendations into law. This process resulted in the system we now know as Social Security, a key component of our social insurance system. Social Security protects against three of the key threats in Marmor's typology: becoming disabled, outliving one's savings, and losing the family breadwinners.

Workers and their employers pay into this system with the expectation that when they become elderly or disabled, the system will offer them some financial security. The program also provides benefits for the widows and survivors of workers when the family breadwinner passes away. Participation in the program is compulsory, thus assuring that the wealthy have an interest in supporting the system. The system is also redistributive, since higher paid workers pay more into the system than lower paid workers. This redistribution is somewhat restrained by placing a cap on the contributions of wealthy workers. In addition, the system is not exclusive since there is a commercial market where individuals can obtain similar benefits through pensions; savings plans, such as individual retirement accounts (IRAs); and life insurance and disability plans that provide benefits to family members.

Medicare and Medicaid: protecting against the threat of becoming ill. Initially, the Social Security System covered only a limited number of federal employees, but over the years, it expanded to cover nearly everyone over age 65. What it did not provide was easy access to health care. This lack was obviously a major concern for older people.

After World War II the government imposed wage freezes but still allowed unions to negotiate with employers for health care benefits. This period strengthened the association of health care benefits with employment and with unions. Many have suggested that this pattern dampened the union movement's interest in government-sponsored health plans because workers' health insurance paid partly by employers had become a focus for union organizing and expansion: A universal system would make employment-based health insurance, which had become a major union goal, unnecessary.

The AMA was also adamantly against any compulsory health insurance or national health plan, calling any such plans "socialist." So opposed was the AMA to Medicare that it hired a conservative actor to make an 11-minute speech entitled "Ronald Reagan Speaks Out against Socialized Medicine."[38] This speech became available as a vinyl record. The wives of AMA physicians were supposed to organize coffee klatches with their friends to listen to the speech. In it, Reagan made dire warnings about the future if "socialized medicine" (i.e., Medicare) were enacted:

> One of the traditional methods of imposing statism or socialism on a people has been by way of medicine.... The doctor begins to

lose freedoms; it's like telling a lie, and one leads to another. First you decide that the doctor can have so many patients. But then the doctors aren't equally divided geographically, so a doctor decides he wants to practice in one town and the government has to say to him you can't live in that town, they already have enough doctors.[39]

Later, in 1965, despite organized medicine's opposition, President Lyndon Johnson – in the context of a militant civil rights movement and a growing antiwar movement – pushed Medicare and Medicaid through Congress and signed them into law. Medicare was a federal program that paid for medical services for those over 65, while Medicaid was a joint federal and state program to cover medical services for the poor. These programs continue to provide two of the most important pillars for the U.S. social insurance system.

The structures of Medicare and Medicaid differ markedly. Medicare is virtually a universal system for the elderly. It is financed by payroll deductions shared between employees and employers. Since Medicaid is a joint federal–state program, there is no "one" Medicaid program, because Medicaid differs across the 50 states. This arrangement has created great variation in the benefits provided to Medicaid patients, depending upon the state plan. Activists who support universal health insurance for children have achieved notable success in using the Medicaid program to provide insurance to everyone under 18 through the Child Health Insurance Program (CHIP).[40]

Temporary Assistance for Needy Families (TANF): protecting against the threat of being born into a poor family. The English poor laws of 1601 strongly influenced early approaches in the United States to deal with poverty. Poor relief was considered a local problem to be managed by town officials using local tax money. A distinction was made between the "worthy" and the "unworthy" poor. Eventually almshouses (also known as poor houses) were created, where conditions were deliberately harsh to discourage people from entering.

As part of the New Deal of the Roosevelt presidency, the government had set up the Aid for Families with Dependent Children (AFDC) program, which provided cash benefits to poor families. In 1996, President Clinton announced his plan to "end welfare as we know it," which ended AFDC. Critics of the program, such as the Cato Institute, had argued: "The primary way that those with low incomes can advance in the market economy is to get married, stay married, and work – but welfare programs have created incentives to do the opposite."[41]

To replace AFDC, President Clinton and a Republican Congress created the TANF program. By design, TANF ended entitlements to cash payments and conceptualized government assistance as a "work-focused, time-limited program." TANF functioned as a block grant: States received a set amount of money and enjoyed wide latitude on how they spent those funds. Welfare rolls dropped dramatically in the years immediately following its implementation. Many considered this change as an effect of a growing economy.[42] Most of the jobs obtained by mothers on TANF were very low-paid, low-skilled jobs. Critics of the program, such as Professor Frances Fox Piven, argued that despite its "moral preoccupation," the program put more poorly paid workers on the market, thus, depressing wages generally:

> The gist of my argument today is that throughout this campaign, this national revival movement to restore moral compulsion to the lives of poor women, we were encouraged to look at the wrong issues. The American public become preoccupied with the morality of the personal choices of poor women. We were preoccupied with whether women who confronted very limited and bad alternatives were choosing the more moral of those alternatives. Was it right for poor mothers to take welfare? What we should have looked at instead was the impact of welfare cutbacks on the institutional arrangements that generate the choices which confront poor women. We should have focused on the bearing of welfare and welfare reform on labor markets ... the moral issues have to do with the distribution of economic well being in our society, as well as the distribution of opportunity and hope.[43]

Concerns over the deficiencies of the TANF program arose particularly during and after the 2009 recession, a time when poor people and poor families were particularly vulnerable. As noted by the Center on Budget and Policy Priorities:

> In 2014, for every 100 families in poverty, only 23 received cash benefits from TANF. This is down from the 68 families for every 100 in poverty that received cash assistance when TANF was first enacted in 1996. This ratio, which we call the TANF-to-poverty ratio (TPR), has declined nearly every year since 1996 and reached its lowest point in 2014.
> ... this ratio varies widely among states, ranging from a low of 4 to a high of 78. In 12 states, the ratio is less than 10, meaning that for every 100 families living in poverty, fewer than 10 receive TANF cash assistance. Many states have made policy and administrative changes that have significantly cut their TANF caseloads, even as families struggled financially during and after the Great Recession.[44]

EVALUATING THE IMPORTANCE OF SOCIAL INSURANCE: A TALE OF TWO SINGLE MOTHERS IN THE UNITED STATES VERSUS 16 OTHER HIGH-INCOME COUNTRIES.[45]

Consider the hypothetical single mother, Theresa. For simplicity's sake, assume that she has only one child, Daniel. Suppose first that Theresa and Daniel live in one of the comparison countries outside the United States. If employed at Daniel's birth, Theresa would have been entitled to a period of paid parental leave ranging from 9 to 46 weeks and averaging over 20 weeks. While employed, Theresa would typically be entitled to paid sick leave and to at least four weeks of paid annual leave. Whether or not Theresa was employed, she and Daniel would be guaranteed health care coverage. Theresa would likely have access to public education for Daniel from the age of three on, or even sooner in some of the countries. She would typically be entitled to a monthly child allowance benefit to help her provide for some of Daniel's basic needs. In the majority of the countries, she could also be entitled to "advance maintenance" benefits if Daniel's father neglected to pay child support or was unable to do so. If Theresa lost her job and had been employed long enough to satisfy the Unemployment Insurance (UI) employment history requirement, she would on average be entitled to up to 57 weeks of UI benefits. If she and Daniel were in financial need, she would be entitled to social assistance ("welfare"), which in the majority of the comparison countries would raise family income close to or above the poverty line.

Now, suppose instead that Theresa and Daniel live in the United States.
Theresa would have no entitlement under national law to paid parental leave, paid annual leave, or paid sick leave. She might be without health care coverage for herself or Daniel, whether employed or not. She would be unlikely to have access to public education for Daniel until Daniel was five. She would not receive child allowance or advance maintenance. If Theresa lost her job, she might not qualify for UI, as single mothers in the United States are very often in low-wage jobs and, thus, less likely to qualify for UI benefits if they lose a job. If she did qualify for UI, she would typically receive benefits for a maximum of 26 weeks unless Congress renewed the temporary extensions of UI benefit weeks enacted in response to the "Great Recession." If Theresa and Daniel were in financial need, the family might be ineligible for social assistance because of "time limits," or might be unable to access benefits because U.S. social assistance enrolls only a minority of eligible families. If eligible for and able to enroll in social assistance, the meager social assistance benefit would leave the family income far below the poverty line.

Why the Weakness of U.S. Social Insurance Compared with Those of Other Countries?

The United States has a "patchwork" social insurance system and one that is particularly punitive to the poor. The contrast between being a single mother in the United States and a single mother in other countries with similar levels of economic development highlights the ways in which social context exerts dramatic effects on health and well-being, one of the key concerns of social medicine. This comparison suggests that strengthening the U.S. social insurance system is a key goal for progressive reform with consequences far beyond health.

Failure of the Progressive Era to promote a social insurance program. The Progressive Era (1890–1920s) seemed a good moment for the United States to move toward a national health program. In 1912, the widely popular Theodore Roosevelt decided to challenge his former protégé, President Taft, for the Republican nomination. Upset over Taft's tactics at the June 1912 Republican convention, Roosevelt and his supporters walked out and two weeks later formed the Progressive (Bull Moose) Party. A "single national health service" was part of the new party's platform.[46] And Roosevelt, an admirer of the German social insurance system, included the following in his "Declaration of Faith" speech:

> It is abnormal for any industry to throw back upon the community the human wreckage due to its wear and tear, and the hazards of sickness, accident, invalidism, involuntary unemployment, and old age should be provided for through insurance. This should be made a charge in whole or in part upon the industries, the employer, the employee, and perhaps the people at large to contribute severally in some degree. Wherever such standards are not met by given establishments, by given industries, are unprovided for by a legislature, or are balked by unenlightened courts, the workers are in jeopardy, the progressive employer is penalized, and the community pays a heavy cost in lessened efficiency and in misery. What Germany has done in the way of old-age pensions or insurance should be studied by us, and the system adapted to our uses, with whatever modifications are rendered necessary by our different ways of life and habits of thought.[47]

Indeed, by the early twentieth century, many European countries had adopted programs of social insurance that included sickness insurance, workmen's compensation, disability insurance, and old-age pensions.[48] Following the German model, most of these programs were compulsory and most expanded over time to encompass the entire population.[49]

Another source of support for social insurance was the Socialist Party of America, which had formed in 1901 from the union of two small parties:

the Social Democratic Party of America and the Socialist Labor Party. German immigrants had founded the Socialist Labor Party and, at least for the first few years, they held meetings in German. The new Socialist Party of America grew rapidly over the next two decades. Its candidate for president, Eugene V. Debs, ran five times between 1900 and 1920; he was in prison during the 1920 campaign after his conviction for "seditious" activities, specifically because of his opposition to U.S. involvement in World War I. In both his 1912 and 1920 campaigns, he managed to garner over 900,000 votes (about 6 percent of the vote in 1912 and 3.5 percent in 1920). But Debs was not the only socialist candidate who did well in 1912. The party could boast some 1,200 socialists elected at the municipal level.

In this setting, a bill introduced into the New York State legislature in 1916 (the Mills Bill) would have established compulsory health insurance for workers. Sponsors reintroduced the bill in 1917, 1918, and 1919, when the legislature finally voted on it. After passing the Senate in April 1919, the bill died in the Assembly, where the Speaker, John B. Andrews, refused to release the bill (along with several other pieces of social legislation), and a vote to overrule this decision was defeated. A similar California bill sponsored during November 1918 by the California Social Insurance Commission lost in a public referendum.

Defeat of the New York bill reflected fierce opposition by a number of interest groups (organized medicine, the commercial insurance industry, and some sectors of organized labor). The political environment of the Red Scare, at its height in 1919 after the Russian Revolution, also weakened the bill's support. The fact that compulsory health insurance for workers had originated in Germany, once seen as a positive factor, further alienated a nation that had recently been at war with that country.[50]

The first Red Scare describes a period in the late 1910s when fears of foreign subversion helped justify U.S. entry into World War I and to suppress forcefully leftist and, particularly, socialist activities and organizations. Several conditions fed paranoia among the public. Large numbers of immigrants had been entering the United States, leading to anti-immigrant sentiments. Strikes, such as the Seattle general strike in February 1919, which involved some 60,000 peaceful workers, fed anti-union sentiment. General strikes were portrayed as foreign imports, involving either Russian Bolsheviks or German subversives, whose goal was violent revolution. The victory of the Bolsheviks in the Russian Revolution of 1917 concerned the very capitalistic U.S. ruling class. Several bombings attributed to anarchists also reduced support for the progressive agenda.

Continuing advocacy for national health insurance. Advocacy for compulsory insurance law did not end with the defeat of the New York State law in 1919 and the Red Scare.[51] In 1926, a group of foundations got together to form the Committee on the Costs of Medical Care (CCMC).[52] The committee included some 50 experts who studied the economics of health care provision. The committee continued its work until 1932, publishing 26 volumes of research and 15 reports.

At the end of its work, the committee issued both "majority" and "minority" recommendations. The majority recommendations were well intentioned but not specific. The first read: "Comprehensive medical service should be provided largely by organized groups of practitioners, organized preferably around hospitals, encouraging high standards, and preserving personal relations."[53] The minority report was much clearer. Its first two recommendations were:

> Government competition should be discontinued, restricting activities to the indigent, diseases requiring care in governmental institutions, public health, the Armed Forces, etc., and only service-connected veterans' cases (except tuberculosis and nervous and mental disease). 2. Government care of the indigent should be expanded, ultimately relieving the medical profession of this burden.[54]

The suggestion that care for the indigent represented a burden for doctors indicated how far the social mission of U.S. medicine had deteriorated from the vision of the Jacobis. The AMA attacked the majority report as "socialized medicine," and the national AMA and some of its state affiliates called for a boycott of Borden Condensed Milk, the Milbank Foundation's source of income.

For international comparison, at roughly the same time, British socialists were planning what would become the National Health Service. This step essentially would nationalize all health services, converting them into a public service. By 1939, Saskatchewan had passed the Municipal Medical and Hospital Services Act, which established municipal health plans funded by individual contributions. This was one of many provincial experiments in health care provision taking place in Canada at the time.

The second Red Scare and its impact on social medicine. From the late 1940s through the 1950s, the United States experienced a second Red Scare, commonly associated with Senator Joseph McCarthy and the House Un-American Activities Committee (HUAC, 1938–1975). McCarthy made a number of false accusations concerning Soviet "infiltration" of the U.S. government and of various professions, including medicine. The Communist Party USA, which had replaced the Socialists as the main party of the left, faced severe persecution, leading to its virtual destruction.[55]

Progressive physicians were also targeted by the so-called witch hunts, a component of the second Red Scare that has not received much historical attention.[56] The tool typically used to discipline wayward doctors was blacklisting – keeping them from obtaining employment in hospitals or in the U.S. government. This policy derived from the Federal Employees

Loyalty Program, created by President Truman, which allowed "political loyalty" boards to determine if a prospective employee was "Un-American." One such panel rejected the renowned Swiss medical historian Henry Sigerist as unfit for government employment.

Here we will mention just three of these blacklisted doctors.[57] Thomas Perry (1916–1991) was a prominent Los Angeles pediatrician. After a public hearing during 1952 in front of HUAC, he lost his medical school appointments at the University of California Medical School and at several local hospitals. He emigrated eventually to Canada. Lorin E. Kerr (1910–1991) was the director of the United Mine Workers of America Department of Occupational Health for 17 years and produced important research on coal workers' pneumoconiosis (black lung). He lost his position in the U.S. Public Health Service in the late 1940s. He remained active in social causes and, in 1974, became the president of the American Public Health Association (APHA). The APHA named its Occupational Health and Safety Award in his honor. Jeremiah Stamler (1919–) was a noted cardiologist who coined the term "risk factor." He was a prominent Chicago activist in civil rights, and his refusal to participate in an HUAC hearing led to a criminal indictment. In response, a campaign against the work of HUAC led by Dr. Paul Dudley White, President Eisenhower's personal physician, ultimately was successful in getting the committee to drop the indictment and to stop discrediting Stamler's work.[58]

George Rosen, a leading historian of social medicine, worked for the U.S. military during World War II in Germany, where he read multiple European social medicine texts. On his return to the United States, he set about writing a history of social medicine, a project that he largely abandoned because of the anti-communist politics of the late 1940s and 1950s.[59] Instead of a book, he published an essay, "What is Social Medicine: A Genetic Analysis of the Concept," with which we began this book.[60] In addition to this briefer than intended essay on social medicine, Rosen later wrote an "authoritative history" of public health, which became the standard U.S. text on this topic for many years.[61] The second Red Scare affected Rosen's and also Sigerist's abilities to write and to teach about social medicine in the United States, which became one reason for the lack of a meaningful critical text on social medicine in English until this one that we are trying to create now.

Notes

1 O.A. Brownson, "The Laboring Classes," *Boston Quarterly Review*, 1840, https://goo.gl/DvyEFM. See also: George Rosen, "The Medical Aspects of the Controversy over Factory Conditions in New England, 1840–1850," *Bulletin of the History of Medicine* 15 (1944): 483.

2 Elisha Bartlett, *A Vindication of the Character and Condition of the Females Employed in the Lowell Mills: Against the Charges Contained in the Boston Times, and the Boston Quarterly Review* (Boston, MA: Leonard Huntress, printer, 1841), https://archive.org/details/101161910.nlm.nih.gov.
3 Lemuel Shattuck, *Report to the Committee of the City Council Appointed to Obtain the Census of Boston for the Year 1845: Embracing Collateral Facts and Statistical Researches, Illustrating the History and Condition of the Population, and Their Means of Progress and Prosperity* (Boston, MA: J.H. Eastburn, city printer, 1846), p. 169, https://goo.gl/0yfzaz.
4 Lemuel Shattuck, Nathaniel Prentiss Banks, and Jehiel Abbott, *Report of a General Plan for the Promotion of Public and Personal Health* (Boston, MA: Dutton & Wentworth, state printers, 1850), https://archive.org/details/reportofgeneralp00mass.
5 Edwin Chadwick, *Report on the Sanitary Condition of the Labouring Population of Great Britain. A Supplementary Report on the Results of a Special Inquiry into the Practice of Interment in Towns*, vol. 1 (London: HM Stationery Office, 1842).
6 Abraham Jacobi, *The Physical Cost of Women's Work: Reprinted for the Consumers' League* (New York: Charity Organization Society, 1907).
7 Robert J. Haggerty, "Abraham Jacobi, MD, Respectable Rebel," *Pediatrics* 99 (1997): 462–71. See also Russell Viner, "Abraham Jacobi and German Medical Radicalism in Antebellum New York," *Bulletin of the History of Medicine* 72 (1998): 434–63.
8 The original site of the German Dispensary remains a clinic in New York, as of this writing.
9 Abraham Jacobi, "American Child Labor Laws," Transactions of the Seventh International Congress for Hygiene and Demography, 1891. Reprinted in Abraham Jacobi, *Miscellaneous Addresses and Writings by, Collectanea Jacobi, Volume 8* (New York: The Critic and Guide Company, 1909), p. 158.
10 Abraham Jacobi, "The Physical Cost of Women's Work."
11 Jerome A. Paulson, "Pediatric Advocacy," *Pediatric Clinics of North America* 48 (2001): 1307–18; Committee on Community Health Services, "The Pediatrician's Role in Community Pediatrics," *Pediatrics* 103 (1999), 1304–06.
12 Elizabeth Garret, who was accepted to the École after Mary Putnam, managed to graduate in 1870 and is, thus, the first female graduate of the École de Médicine.
13 Carla Bittel, *Mary Putnam Jacobi and the Politics of Medicine in Nineteenth-Century America* (Chapel Hill: University of North Carolina Press, 2012).
14 Mary Putnam Jacobi, *The Question of Rest for Women during Menstruation* (New York: G.P. Putnam's Sons, 1877), https://archive.org/details/questionofrestfo00jacoiala.
15 Edward H. Clarke, *Sex in Education; or, A Fair Chance for Girls* (Boston, MA: Houghton Mifflin, 1884).
16 Mary Putnam Jacobi, *Common Sense Applied to Woman Suffrage; a Statement of the Reasons Which Justify the Demand to Extend the Suffrage to Women, with Consideration of the Arguments Against Such Enfranchisement, and with Special Reference to the Issues Presented to the New York State Convention of 1894* (New York: G. P. Putnam's Sons, 1894), https://iiif.lib.harvard.edu/manifests/view/drs:2581504$5i.
17 Bittel, *Mary Putnam Jacobi and the Politics of Medicine in Nineteenth-Century America*.
18 George Rosen, "The First Neighborhood Health Center Movement – Its Rise and Fall," *American Journal of Public Health* 61 (1971): 1620–37.

19 Jacob Riis, *How the Other Half Lives* (Mineola, NY: Dover Publications, 1890).
20 Lillian Wald, *The House on Henry Street* (New York: Routledge, 1991), p. 8.
21 Ibid., p. 13.
22 Albert Joseph Kennedy and Robert Archey Woods, eds., *Handbook of Settlements* (New York: Charities Publication Committee, 1911).
23 Daniel M. Fox, "The Significance of the Milbank Memorial Fund for Policy: An Assessment at Its Centennial." *Milbank Quarterly* 84, no. 1 (2006): 5–36.
24 "Bellevue-Yorkville Health Building Dedicated in New York City," *Milbank Memorial Fund Quarterly Bulletin* 5 (1920): 13–20.
25 "News Digest of the New York Health Demonstrations," *Milbank Memorial Fund Quarterly Bulletin* 6 (1928): 101–05.
26 Ibid.
27 Ibid.
28 C.-E. A. Winslow, and Savel Zimand, *Health under the "El": The Story of the Bellevue-Yorkville Health Demonstration in Mid-Town New York* (New York: Harper, 1937), p. 12.
29 Ibid.
30 Rosen, "The First Neighborhood Health Center Movement – Its Rise and Fall."
31 Wilbur Carey Phillips, *Adventuring for Democracy* (New York: Social Unit Press, 1940).
32 Ibid., p. 323.
33 Robert Blundo, "Social Unit Plan (1916–1920): An Experiment in Democracy and Human Services Fails," *Journal of Sociology and Welfare* 24 (1997): 169–91.
34 Theodore R. Marmor, Jerry L. Mashaw, and John Pakutka, *Social Insurance: America's Neglected Heritage and Contested Future* (London: CQ Press, 2013).
35 Thomas Paine, *Agrarian Justice, Opposed to Agrarian Law, and Agrarian Monopoly: Being a Plan for Ameliorating the Condition of Man, by Creating in Every Nation a National Fund* (London: Evans and Bone, 1797).
36 Ibid.
37 Franklin Delano Roosevelt, "Message to Congress on Social Security," January 17, 1935, www.ssa.gov/history/fdrstmts.html#message2.
38 "Ronald Reagan Speaks out Against Socialized Medicine," 1961, www.youtube.com/watch?v=BnLa1BvtaxM.
39 Ibid.
40 "Children's Health Insurance Program Overview," January 10, 2017, www.ncsl.org/research/health/childrens-health-insurance-program-overview.aspx.
41 Michael Tanner and Tad DeHaven, "TANF and Federal Welfare," September 2010, www.downsizinggovernment.org/hhs/welfare-spending.
42 Peter Germanis, "TANF Is Broken! It's Time to Reform "Welfare Reform,'" unpublished manuscript, July 25, 2015, https://mlwiseman.com/wp-content/uploads/2013/09/TANF-is-Broken.072515.pdf.
43 Frances Fox Piven, "The Link between Welfare Reform and the Labor Market," 1999 Sparer Conference Keynote Address, http://scholarship.law.upenn.edu/cgi/viewcontent.cgi?article=1041&context=jlasc.
44 Ife Floyd, Ladonna Pavetti, and Liz Schott, "TANF Reaching Few Poor Families," *Center for Budget Policies and Priorities*, www.cbpp.org/research/family-income-support/tanf-reaching-few-poor-families.

45 Timothy Casey and Laurie Maldonado, "Worst Off: Single-Parent Families in the United States: A Cross-National Comparison of Single Parenthood in the US and Sixteen Other High-Income Countries," *Legal Momentum* (New York), December 2012, www.legalmomentum.org/sites/default/files/reports/worst-off-single-parent.pdf. Comparison countries were: Australia, Austria, Belgium, Canada, Denmark, Finland, France, Germany, Ireland, Italy, the Netherlands, Norway, Spain, Sweden, Switzerland, and the United Kingdom.
46 "Progressive Party Platform of 1912," August 7, 1912, http://teachingamericanhistory.org/library/document/progressive-platform-of-1912/.
47 "Address by Theodore Roosevelt before the Convention of the National Progressive Party in Chicago, August, 1912," Social Security History, www.ssa.gov/history/trspeech.html.
48 Britain, for example, had passed the National Insurance Act in 1911.
49 Abe Bortz, "Social Security: A Brief History of Social Insurance," *VCU Libraries, Social Welfare History Project*, www.socialwelfarehistory.com/social-security/social-security-a-brief-history-of-social-insurance/.
50 Congress had declared war in April 1917, and the Armistice was signed in November 1918. Between those dates, however, some 2.8 million men were drafted.
51 Karen S. Palmer, "A Brief History: Universal Health Care Efforts in the US," Physicians for a National Health Program, www.pnhp.org/facts/a-brief-history-universal-health-care-efforts-in-the-us.
52 The Carnegie Endowment for the Advancement of Teaching; the Commonwealth, Milbank, and Rosenwald Funds; and the Josiah Macy New York, Russell Sage, and Rockefeller Foundations.
53 Joseph S. Ross, "The Committee on the Costs of Medical Care and the History of Health Insurance in the United States," *Einstein Quarterly* 19 (2002): 129–34.
54 Ibid.
55 The many helpful sources on McCarthyism and the second Red scare include the following: Ellen Schrecker, *Many Are the Crimes: McCarthyism in America* (Boston: Little, Brown, 1998), and *Age of McCarthyism: A Brief History with Documents* (Boston: Bedford, 1994); Landon R. Y. Storrs, *The Second Red Scare and the Unmaking of the New Deal Left* (Princeton, NJ: Princeton University Press, 2012); Gerald Horne, *The Final Victim of the Blacklist: John Howard Lawson, Dean of the Hollywood Ten* (Berkeley: University of California Press, 2006); Jeff Woods, *Black Struggle, Red Scare: Segregation and Anti-communism in the South, 1948–1968* (Baton Rouge: Louisiana State University Press, 2004); and George Lewis, *The White South and the Red Menace: Segregationists, Anti-communism, and Massive Resistance, 1945–1965* (Gainesville: University Press of Florida, 2004). A helpful brief overview appears in: Landon R. Y. Storrs, "McCarthyism and the Second Red Scare," Oxford Research Encyclopedias, July 2015, doi:10.1093/acrefore/9780199329175.013.6, https://oxfordre.com/americanhistory/view/10.1093/acrefore/9780199329175.001.0001/acrefore-9780199329175-e-6.
56 Jane Pacht Brickman, "'Medical McCarthyism': The Physicians Forum and the Cold War," *Journal of the History of Medicine and Allied Sciences* 49 (1994): 380–418.
57 The Editors, "An Interview with Dr. Walter Lear," *Social Medicine* 4 (2009): 70–79, https://www.socialmedicine.info/index.php/socialmedicine/article/view/296.

58 Paul Buhle, "Halting McCarthyism: The Stamler Case in History," *Monthly Review* 51, no. 5 (October 1999): 44–49, https://archive.monthlyreview.org/index.php/mr/article/view/MR-051-05-1999-09_5.
59 Elizabeth Fee and Edward T. Morman, "Doing History, Making Revolution: The Aspirations of Henry E. Sigerist and George Rosen," *Clio Medica* 23 (1993): 275–311.
60 George Rosen, "What Is Social Medicine? A Genetic Analysis of the Concept," *Bulletin of the History of Medicine* 21 (1947): 674–733.
61 George Rosen, *A History of Public Health* (New York: MD Publications, 1958).

Chapter 6

Health and Empire, Part I
Empire's Historical Health Component

Imperialism, Medicine, and Public Health

Both historically and in modern times, medicine and public health have played important roles in imperialism. Understanding and changing these roles have become key concerns for social medicine. The connections among imperialism, health, and health services have operated through several key mediating institutions: philanthropic foundations, international financial institutions and trade agreements, and international health organizations. Philanthropic foundations tried to address several public-health challenges faced by capitalist enterprises that were expanding into countries with a high prevalence of infectious diseases; these challenges included the reduced productivity of labor when workers became ill with infections, safety for investors and managers working in those countries, and the costs of care for sick employees. From modest origins, international financial institutions and trade agreements would eventually morph into a massive structure of trade rules that have exerted profound effects on public health and health services worldwide. Last but not least, international health organizations have collaborated with corporate interests to protect commerce and trade. In this chapter, we try to clarify the connections among these mediating institutions and imperialism, and we explain some of the counterintuitive negative effects these connections have exerted on health.

While imperial connections are deeply woven into global economic markets, conditions during the twenty-first century have changed. The outcry for improvements in public health, largely voiced by activists in social medicine, has put a spotlight on organizations that implement a "vertical" approach to health care, which we will explain. Such scenarios convey a picture very different from that of the historical relation between empire and health: one that shows diminishing tolerance among the world's peoples for the public health policies of empire and a growing demand for health systems grounded in solidarity rather than profitability.

Although it is a complex phenomenon, we define "imperialism" in simple terms as expansion of economic activities – especially investment, sales, extraction of raw materials, and use of labor to produce commodities and services – beyond national boundaries, as well as the social, political, and economic effects of this expansion. Empire has achieved many advantages for economically dominant nations. It is important to note, however, that the venture to build and maintain empire is not limited to only capitalist countries. Some socialist superpowers also have sought economic dominance, like the former Soviet Union's so-called social imperialism.

For centuries, to achieve this economic empire required military conquest and the maintenance of colonies under direct political control. The decline of colonialism in the twentieth century led to the emergence of political and economic "neocolonialism," which followed the same pattern: an alliance between colonizing nations and their newly "independent" former colonies that facilitated the colonizing countries' ability to maintain a dominant position.[1]

Colonialism and neocolonialism still exist, as shown by the relationships between the United States and its continuing colonies, such as Puerto Rico, and its former colonies, such as the Philippines. In the Philippines, which the United States ruled as a colony between 1898 and 1946, U.S. leaders granted the island nation a path toward independence, with an official stance that the United States would protect the Philippines until the newly independent country was able to develop political maturity and strengthen its own government. Meanwhile, the United States trained the Philippine armies, sold them U.S. military equipment, supervised their commerce, and educated them about the U.S. government.[2] The idea of freedom was maintained as long as the Filipino people favored these pro-U.S. policies.

Imperialism often has involved military conquest, in addition to economic domination, even after the decline of formal colonialism. Despite its benign profile, medicine has contributed to the military efforts of European countries and the United States. For instance, health workers have assumed armed or paramilitary roles in Indochina, North Africa, Iraq, and Afghanistan. Health institutions also have taken part as bases for counter-insurgency and intelligence operations in Latin America and Asia.[3]

One fundamental characteristic of the empire, including neocolonialism, involves the extraction of raw materials and human capital, which move from less developed nations to economically dominant countries. In less developed countries, the "underdevelopment of health" follows inevitably from this depletion of natural and human resources.[4] Under empire, such extraction of wealth further limits poorer countries' ability to construct their own effective health systems.

These countries also face a loss of health care workers, who migrate to the economically dominant nations after expensive training at home. For example, India is one of the largest exporters of trained physicians. Medical doctors trained in India account for approximately 5 percent of physicians in the United States and 11 percent in the United Kingdom. Through the loss of locally trained medical leaders, especially those who attend more prestigious medical schools (one study showed that more than half the graduates of India's highest ranked school lived and worked outside India), the emigration of medical professionals projects a symbolic image of lower quality practitioners who remain in the former colony and adversely affects the health system of the home country.[5]

Empire also has reinforced international class relations, and medicine has contributed to this phenomenon. As in the United States, medical professionals in less developed countries most often come from higher income families. Even when they do not, they frequently view medicine as a route of upward mobility. As a result, medical professionals tend to ally themselves with the capitalist class – the "national bourgeoisie" – of less developed countries. Health care providers also frequently support cooperative links between the local capitalist class and business interests in economically dominant countries. These economic motivations for health professionals have led them to resist social change that would threaten the current class structure, either nationally or internationally.

Another thrust of empire has involved the creation of new markets for products, including medical products that are manufactured in dominant nations and sold throughout the rest of the world. This process further enhances the accumulation of capital by multinational corporations and has appeared nowhere more clearly than in pharmaceutical and medical equipment industries.[6] The monopolistic character of these industries, as well as the negative impact that imported technology has exerted on local research and development, has hindered access to needed medications for cancer, AIDS, and other important health conditions. Worldwide advocacy and resistance, again involving many social medicine activists, have targeted trade rules that protect patents and, therefore, enhance the financial interests of multinational pharmaceutical and equipment corporations that operate in less developed countries. Yet, these corporations remain very profitable and show little intention to lower prices or ease patent rules to improve access for those countries that need access to medications and medical equipment.[7]

As mentioned earlier, the connections among empire, health, and health services have operated primarily through philanthropic foundations, international financial institutions and organizations that enforce trade agreements, and international health organizations.

Philanthropic Foundations

The concept of charitable contributions by wealthy people to the needy dates back at least to the Greek practice of "philanthropy," but modern practices involving foundations with their own legal status began in the early twentieth century. Andrew Carnegie, who accumulated his fortune mainly through the steel industry, took a leadership role in the creation of philanthropic foundations. His charitable ventures began with the establishment of Carnegie libraries in small U.S. towns and cities. In writings such as "The Gospel of Wealth" published in 1901, Carnegie presented his opinions about the social responsibilities of the wealthy (Figure 6.1).[8]

In his book, speeches, and other efforts to influence his fellow barons of capitalism, Carnegie argued that contributing to the needs of society was consistent with good business practices. By contributing intelligently to address social needs rather than squandering one's wealth, Carnegie argued a businessman could also assure personal entry into the heavenly afterlife – the central theme of "The Gospel of Wealth." Through the Carnegie Endowment for International Peace and other interconnected foundations, Carnegie acted to share his earthly gains in pursuit of his own heavenly future.

Philanthropy related to health soon involved John D. Rockefeller and the Rockefeller Foundation. His fortune based in oil, Rockefeller emulated Carnegie's beneficence, despite their conflicts in the world of monopolistic

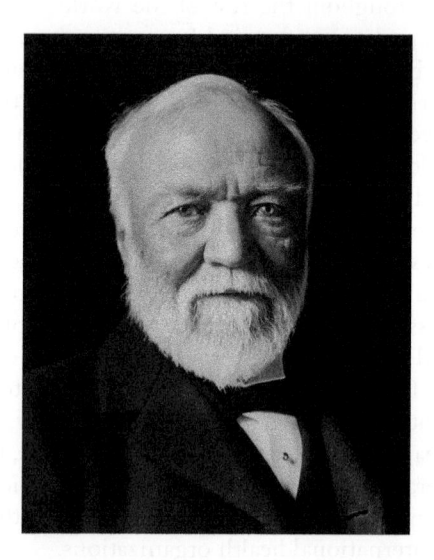

Figure 6.1 Andrew Carnegie.

business practices. Rockefeller and associates moved to support public health activities and services that would benefit the economic interests of Rockefeller-controlled corporations throughout the world. After all, productivity depended on having workers who are "educated, safe, healthy, decently housed, and motivated by a sense of opportunity."[9] This concept of corporate philanthropy persists even now (Figure 6.2).

To foster these goals, the Rockefeller Foundation initiated international campaigns against infectious diseases such as hookworm, malaria, and yellow fever. Between 1913 – the year of its founding – and 1920, the foundation supported the development of research institutes and disease eradication programs on every continent except Antarctica. For capitalist enterprises expanding internationally, infectious diseases proved troublesome for several reasons, which became clear from the writings of Rockefeller and the managers of the Rockefeller Foundation. First, these infections reduced workers' energy and, therefore, their productivity. This relationship was such common knowledge that hookworm became known as the "lazy man's disease." Second, endemic infections in areas of the world designated for such efforts as mining, oil extraction, agriculture, and the opening of new markets for the sale of commodities made those areas unattractive for investors and managerial personnel. Third, when corporations assumed responsibility for the care of workers, the costs of care escalated when infectious diseases could not be prevented or easily treated.

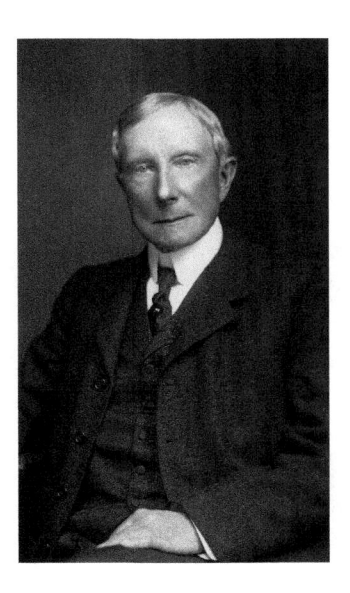

Figure 6.2 John D. Rockefeller.

Addressing these three problems, the Rockefeller Foundation's massive campaigns took on certain characteristics that persist to this day, not only for Rockefeller but also for other foundations, international public health organizations, and nongovernmental organizations. The Rockefeller Foundation emphasized "vertical" programs, initiated by the donor and focusing on specific diseases such as hookworm or malaria. An alternative approach could encourage "horizontal" programs, to provide a broader spectrum of preventive and curative services through a well-organized public health infrastructure of clinics and hospitals. Rather than such broad public health initiatives targeting disadvantaged populations, the Rockefeller Foundation's vertical orientation favored a so-called magic bullet approach, targeting new vaccines and medications that could prevent and treat infectious diseases.

Such a vertical orientation has continued in recent, large-scale efforts by the Rockefeller Foundation, the Gates Foundation, and other philanthropies to address public health problems like AIDS, tuberculosis, malaria, the Ebola crisis, and the COVID-19 pandemic. The foundations often frame their participation as attempts to improve economic development by "investing in health," a term first promoted by the World Bank.[10] These initiatives usually encourage the participation of multinational pharmaceutical companies, which hold the patents for key medications and vaccines used in infectious disease campaigns, and private insurance companies or managed care organizations, which assume responsibility and receive payment for delivering services in "public–private partnerships" (Figure 6.3).

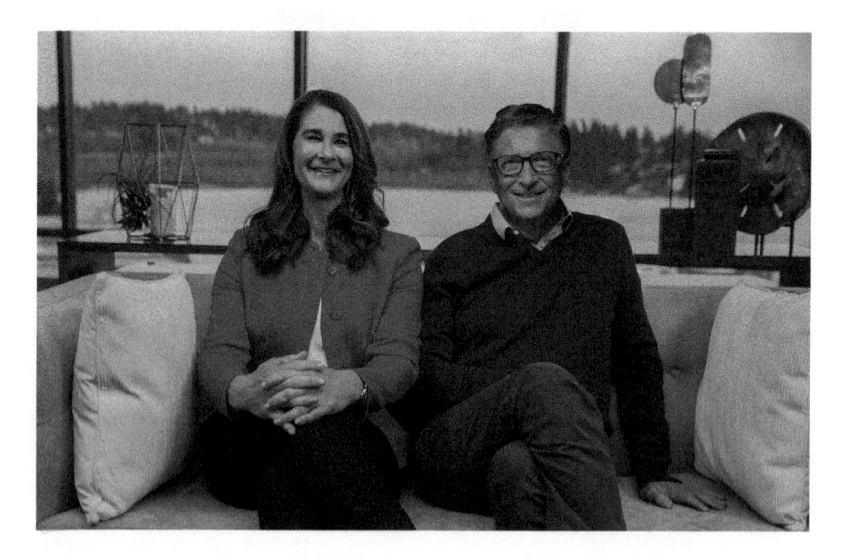

Figure 6.3 Bill and Melinda Gates.

Such dynamics, which involve profit motivation, appear in situations like COVID-19, when the virus in question quickly mutates so prior vaccines lose effectiveness and new vaccines need to be manufactured and sold.

Currently, the Gates Foundation has emerged as the largest philanthropy worldwide focusing on public health. Its efforts continue to target specific infectious diseases, especially AIDS in Africa. Together with the World Health Organization (WHO), whose limited budget the Gates Foundation helps fund, and various nongovernmental organizations also supported by Gates and Rockefeller, philanthropies have invested heavily in the control of infectious diseases through vaccines and other pharmaceutical products. In general, these strategies have left the insufficient public health infrastructures in many countries relatively untouched, while lavish spending has occurred to support programs on AIDS, malaria, tuberculosis, and more recently coronaviruses.

Despite this charity, access to medical and public health facilities remains inadequate for people who often face desperate circumstances. The contradictions of vertical programs, which persist as the legacy of the Rockefeller orientation in philanthropic support, lead to bizarre and tragic situations that have become well known to public health workers in less developed countries. For example, in countries devastated by AIDS, sick patients feign or even intentionally get infected with HIV so they can receive medical care in well-funded AIDS programs for other serious health disorders such as cancer. When severe epidemics like Ebola strike, the vertically oriented investment policies of these foundations leave countries in Africa without an urgently needed infrastructure of primary care clinics and hospitals to care for critically ill patients.

The importance of horizontally focused public health systems became clear once again with the epidemic of Zika virus, which involved a crippling outbreak of microcephaly, a congenital deformation of the skull. In early 2016, WHO declared the surge of brain-damaged infants linked to the virus a worldwide public health emergency, mainly because most affected countries lacked services and facilities that could care adequately for the thousands of affected infants and their families. As we write, there remains no "magic bullet" vaccine or treatment available for Zika. However, the virus has continued to threaten countries throughout the Americas, Africa, and Asia, many of which lack even a basic public health infrastructure to deal with such epidemics.[11]

International Financial Institutions and Trade Agreements

A framework for modern international financial institutions and trade agreements began after World War II, with the "Bretton Woods" accords, a set of agreements that initially focused on the economic reconstruction of Europe. These accords grew from meetings held in Bretton Woods, New Hampshire, involving representatives of the victorious countries. Between 1944 and 1947, the Bretton Woods negotiations led to the creation of the International Monetary Fund (IMF) and the World Bank, as well as the establishment of the General Agreement on Tariffs and Trade (GATT).

By the 1960s, after Europe's recovery, these institutions and agreements gradually expanded their focus to other countries. For instance, the World Bank adopted as its vision statement: "Our dream is a world free of poverty," which later became "to end extreme poverty and promote shared prosperity."[12] However, because the IMF and World Bank provided most of their assistance through loans rather than grants, the debt burden of the poorer countries increased rapidly. As a result, by 1980, many of the poorest countries in the world were spending on average about half their economic productivity, as measured by gross domestic product, on payment of their debts to international financial institutions, even though these institutions' goals usually emphasized the reduction of poverty. During the early 1980s, the international financial institutions embraced a set of economic policies known as "the Washington consensus." These policies, mainly advocated by the United States and the United Kingdom, involved deregulation and privatization of public services, which added to the debt crisis by reducing even further the public health efforts and health services that poorer countries could afford.

GATT initially aimed to reduce trade barriers among its 23 member countries by eliminating or reducing taxes and other fees on exports and imports. This trade agreement's fairly simple principles included "most favored nation treatment," whereby the same trade rules applied to all participating nations, and "national treatment," which required no discrimination in taxes and regulations between domestic and foreign goods.[13] GATT also established ongoing rounds of negotiations concerning trade agreements, which rarely involved health concerns.

Eventually, in 1994, the World Trade Organization (WTO) replaced the loose collection of agreements that constituted GATT. International trade agreements eventually changed into a massive structure of rules that would exert profound effects on public health and health services worldwide. WTO and regional trade agreements aimed to remove both tariff and nontariff barriers to trade. *Tariff barriers* to trade involve financial methods of protecting national industries from competition by foreign corporations, mostly through import taxes. *Nontariff barriers* to trade refer to nonfinancial laws and regulations affecting trade, such as those that pertain to public health, which governments use to assure accountability and quality. The removal of nontariff barriers to trade has affected the ability of national, state, and local governments to implement or protect public health and medical services. The huge array of international trade agreements encompassed under WTO – seen also in recent negotiations concerning regional agreements such as the Trans-Pacific Partnership (TPP, on hold as of the early Trump presidency in the United States, while still actively pursued by other participating countries) and the Trans-Atlantic Free Trade Agreement (TAFTA) – expanded the purview of trade rules far beyond tariff barriers. For example, these new trade agreements interpreted a variety of public health measures, such as environmental protection, occupational safety and health regulations, quality assurance for food and drugs, intellectual property pertaining to patented medicines and equipment, and even health services themselves, as potential barriers to trade.

In over 900 pages of rules, WTO aimed to achieve "free" trade across borders by limiting governments' regulatory authority while enhancing the authority of international financial institutions and trade organizations. WTO rules, under general exceptions of GATT, Article XX, permit national and subnational "measures to protect human, animal or plant life or health." While this orientation seems promising, the additional provisions and requirements make this exception difficult to sustain in practice. For example, a country may be required to prove that its laws and regulations are the best options least restrictive to commerce and are not disguised barriers to trade. Such mandates are difficult to prove as they may be partly subjective, but are also costly and time consuming to fulfill for the country in question. Furthermore, these rules restrict public subsidies – especially those designated for domestic health programs and institutions – as potentially "trade distortive." Therefore, such subsidies have to apply to both domestic *and* foreign companies that provide services under public contracts, preventing public policies from directing subsidies to *domestic* companies and public programs.

Pertinent to public health, a key WTO provision requires "harmonization," which seeks to reduce variation in nations' regulatory standards for goods and services. Proponents argue that harmonization can motivate countries to initiate labor and environmental standards where none previously existed. However, harmonization also can lead to erosion of existing standards, since it requires uniform global standards at the level least restrictive to trade. Regardless, this is a massive undertaking as WTO has encouraged harmonized standards on issues as diverse as truck safety, pesticides, worker safety, community right-to-know laws about toxic hazards, consumer rights regarding essential services, banking and accounting standards, international labeling of products, and pharmaceutical testing standards.

WTO and regional agreements, such as the North American Free Trade Agreement (NAFTA), supersede member countries' internal laws and regulations, including those governing health. Under these agreements, governments at all levels face a loss of sovereignty in policy making pertinent to public health and health services. Traditionally, government agencies at the federal, state, county, and municipal levels maintain responsibility for protecting public health by assuring safe water supplies, controlling environmental threats, and monitoring industries for occupational health conditions. Trade agreements can reduce or eliminate such governmental activities, because the agreements treat these activities as potential barriers to trade.

In disputes, an appointed tribunal instead of a local or national government determines whether a challenged policy conforms to the rules of WTO or a regional trade agreement. The tribunal includes experts in trade but not necessarily in the subject matter of the cases – such as health or safety – or in the laws of the contesting countries. Documents and hearings remain closed to the public, press, and state and local elected officials. Additionally, because trade agreements consider federal governments as the only pertinent level of participation, only representatives of contesting countries can participate in the hearings, in addition to "experts" whose participation the tribunal requests.

If a tribunal finds that a domestic law or regulation does not conform to the rules of WTO or a regional trade agreement, the tribunal can order that the disputed transaction proceed despite the wishes of government officials or public health experts. When a country fails to comply, WTO or the commission with authority, like NAFTA, can impose financial penalties and can authorize the "winning" country to apply trade sanctions against the "losing" country in whatever sector the winner chooses until the other country complies. Therefore, corporations and even individual investors have caused governments to suffer financial consequences and trade sanctions because of efforts to pursue traditional public health functions. As they grapple with such sanctions, losing countries usually give in and eliminate or change the laws or regulations in question, and they rarely enact similar laws in the future.

Table 6.1 gives examples of decisions under trade agreements that have affected public health and health services. The table shows the immense scope of trade agreements' health-related impacts. Trade agreements like the TPP and the TAFTA – the Obama administration's two major trade initiatives that continue to reappear in various formats – contain provisions that similarly remove or constrain governments' ability to protect public health.[14]

Table 6.1 Examples of Actions under International Trade Agreements That Affect Public Health

Occupational and environmental health	Under Chapter 11 of the NAFTA, the Metalclad Corporation of the United States successfully sued the government of Mexico for damages after the state of San Luis Potosi prohibited Metalclad from reopening a toxic waste dump. The Methanex Corporation of Canada sued the government of the United States in a challenge of environmental protections against a carcinogenic gasoline additive methyl-tertiary-butyl-ether (MTBE), banned by the state of California.
Access to medications	Acting on behalf of pharmaceutical companies, the U.S. government invoked the Agreement on Trade-Related Aspects of Intellectual Property Rights (TRIPS) of WTO in working against attempts by South Africa, Thailand, Brazil, and India to produce low-cost, antiretroviral medications effective against AIDS.
Safety and quality of products	Canada challenged France's ban on asbestos imports under WTO's agreement on Technical Barriers to Trade (TBT). Although a WTO tribunal initially approved Canada's challenge, an appeal tribunal reversed the decision after international pressure.
Safety and quality of food	On behalf of the beef and biotechnology industries, the United States and Canada successfully challenged the European Union (EU) ban of beef treated with artificial hormones under the WTO agreement on the Application of Sanitary and Phytosanitary Standards (SPS). The EU had to pay the United States and Canada more than $120 million annually in extra tariffs imposed due to its decision to limit importation of hormone-treated beef.
Medical and public health services	The WTO General Agreement on Trade in Services (GATS) removes restrictions on corporate involvement in public hospitals, water, and sanitation systems. The GATS affects state and national licensing requirements for professionals and can facilitate challenges to national health programs that limit participation by for-profit corporations.

International Health Organizations

An early approach to international public health organizations arose in Europe during the Middle Ages. To prevent people from leaving or entering geographical areas affected by epidemics of infectious diseases, some governments established local, national, and international "cordons sanitaires," or guarded boundaries.[15] Certain governments also imposed maritime quarantines that prevented ships from entering ports after visiting regions where epidemics were taking place. "Sanitary" authorities arose intermittently and remained active when epidemics were present or anticipated.

As international trade expanded during the late nineteenth and early twentieth centuries, conventional maritime public health went into decline. Instead, concerns about infectious diseases as detrimental to trade in the expanding reach of capitalist enterprise became a motivation for international cooperation in public health. An incentive for redesigning international public health emerged from a need to protect ports, investments, and land holdings, such as plantations, from infectious diseases.

After all, even a disease that is relatively commonplace and associated with a usually low mortality rate can cause substantial economic havoc. For example, influenza was the predominant infectious disease to be influenced by the growing global trade network and to display pandemic behavior: Three major pandemics occurred, in 1918, 1957, and 1968, respectively. More recently, in late 2002 to early 2003, a coronavirus causing severe acute respiratory syndrome (SARS) adversely affected global tourism and travel. The economic impact from that outbreak was estimated at over $30 billion.[16] Beginning in late 2019, COVID-19 followed an even more devastating trajectory through its effects on health and mortality, economic insecurity, hunger and malnutrition, and accentuation of inequality and racism.

The first formal international health organization arose in the Americas. Founded in Washington, D.C., explicitly as a mechanism to protect trade and investments from the burden of disease, the International Safety Bureau focused on the prevention and control of epidemics. During the early twentieth century, plans proceeded for the construction of the Panama Canal, the development of agricultural enterprises in the "banana republics" of Central and northern South America, and the extraction of mineral resources as raw materials for industrial production from areas such as southern Mexico, Venezuela, Colombia, and Brazil. Work in the tropics demanded public health initiatives against mosquito-borne diseases like yellow fever and malaria, parasitic illnesses like hookworm, and the more common viral and bacterial illnesses like endemic diarrhea. As a result, mosquito eradication campaigns and the implementation of a vaccine for yellow fever preoccupied health professionals in this organization during that time.

In its role as the first modern international health organization, the International Sanitary Bureau devoted much of its early activities to infectious disease surveillance, prevention, and treatment, largely to protect trade and economic activities throughout the Americas. Later, during the 1950s, the International Sanitary Bureau became the Regional Office for the Americas of WHO and in 1958 changed its name to the Pan American Health Organization (PAHO). Subsequently, PAHO's public health mission broadened. Despite the name change and widened scope, PAHO has retained a focus on the protection of trade until the present day, and in general it supports the provisions of international trade agreements.[17]

In 1948, WHO emerged as one of the key component suborganizations of the United Nations. Prevention and control of infectious disease epidemics remained a vital objective throughout its history, but WHO did not frame its purpose in controlling infectious diseases as a way to protect trade and economic transactions. Instead, during the 1970s, WHO prioritized the improved distribution of health services, such as primary health care. As noted in Chapter 1, this focus culminated in the famous WHO declaration on primary health care issued at an international conference in Alma Ata, USSR, during 1978.[18] As the principle of universal entitlement to primary care services became one of WHO's priorities, the organization advocated programs for improving access to care, especially in the poorest countries. This "horizontal" vision of public health policy gained substantial support worldwide, at least for a brief time.

During the 1980s, however, WHO entered a chronic financial crisis largely due to the fragile financing providing for by its parent organization, the United Nations. Because of ideological opposition to several programs operated by other component organizations of the United Nations – such as the United Nations Educational, Scientific, and Cultural Organization (UNESCO) – the Reagan administration withheld large portions of annual dues from the United States to the United Nations. As a result of these budgetary shortfalls, the United Nations passed on financial cuts to its other component organizations, including WHO.

In the midst of this financial crisis entered the World Bank, which began to provide a large part of the WHO budget. WHO does not release its full budget publicly, so the precise degree of its dependency on the World Bank is difficult to determine. However, the dependency was significant enough that WHO began to transform its policies away from those of the United Nations to more closely resemble those of international financial institutions and trade agreements. The financial crisis that originated in nonpayment of dues by the United States eventually led WHO to a policy perspective regarding international trade that proved similar to PAHO's earlier focus.

Thus, during the 1990s, the pendulum swung back from the horizontal orientation toward the preference for vertical interventions. This renewed stance emphasized "macroeconomic" policies that involved national and international economic relationships instead of "microeconomic" policies pertinent to markets for specific goods and services; there was also a revived priority for the "magic bullet" in public health and health services. This orientation emerged largely from the efforts of the World Bank and affiliated international financial institutions, as well as key private foundations. Attention turned again to vaccines and medications as technological solutions to health problems, which would further facilitate the financial operations of multinational corporations in these countries.

The *Report of the Commission on Macroeconomics and Health: Investing in Health for Economic Development* (hereafter referred to as *Report*), published by WHO in 2001, defined the relationships between health and economy in the context of imperialism.[19] This *Report* led to a series of WHO projects on economic issues in health policy, health services, and public health. Many of the *Report's* conceptual and methodological approaches mirrored the World Bank's orientation to health and economic development.

Partly for that reason, the *Report* gave a revealing picture of the dominant ideology that shaped imperial health policies. For example, most of the commissioners responsible for the *Report* held extensive experience with the World Bank, IMF, or other international financial institutions. The commissioners showed little background in collaborating with other types of social organizations. Notably absent among the commissioners were representatives of political parties, unions, professional organizations in medicine and public health, organizations of indigenous or ethnic-racial minorities, organizations working to improve occupational and environmental health, or members of the worldwide movement targeting economic globalization.

The *Report* emphasized its central theme at the beginning: "Improving the health and longevity of the poor is, in one sense, an end in itself, a fundamental goal of economic development. But it is also a *means* to achieving the other development goals relating to poverty reduction."[20] Indeed, the goal of improving the health conditions of the poor became a key element of economic development strategies. From this viewpoint, reducing the burden of the endemic infections – such as AIDS, tuberculosis, and malaria – that plagued the poorest countries would increase workforce productivity and facilitate investment.

This policy emphasis on "investing in health" (the *Report's* subtitle) echoed the influential and controversial *World Development Report: Investing in Health*, published in 1993 by the World Bank.[21] The terminology of the *Report's* title conveyed a double meaning: investing in health to improve health and productivity while investing capital as a route to private profit in the health sector. These dual meanings of investment are complementary but distinct, and they pervaded the *Report*. As Jeffrey Sachs (an economist previously known for "shock therapy" in the implementation of neoliberal policies leading to public sector cutbacks in Bolivia, Poland, and the Soviet Union), the commission's chair, stated in an address about the *Report's* public health implications at the American Public Health Association's annual meeting in 2001: "What investor would invest his capital in a malarial country?"[22]

In asserting that disease was a major determinant of poverty, the *Report* argued that investments to improve health constituted a key strategy toward economic development, distancing itself from prior interpretations of poverty as a cause of disease. Specifically, the *Report* emphasized various data on the "channels of influence from disease to economic development."[23] Meanwhile, the *Report* de-emphasized social determinants of disease such as class hierarchy, inequalities of income and wealth, and racial discrimination. Although the *Report* referred to health as "an end to itself," the focus on economic productivity diminished the importance of health itself as a fundamental human right.

More recently, WHO has vacillated between two markedly different visions of global health. On the one hand, it has continued to pursue the vertically oriented emphasis on vaccines and medications rather than the horizontally oriented advocacy of comprehensive public health systems and access to services. With this orientation, WHO has collaborated with WTO (with headquarters close to WHO's in Geneva) in trade agreements that limit governments' ability to protect public health and medical services.[24] On the other hand, WHO has responded intermittently to a worldwide constituency calling for greater attention to the social determination of health. As discussed in Chapters 3 and 4, this orientation led to an influential WHO report on social determinants and some suggestions about policy changes that would improve social conditions leading to ill-health and early death.[25] In research and policy analysis, economic inequality consistently has emerged as the most important social determinant crying out for dramatic changes in policy. Meanwhile, existing policies continue to worsen inequality in the United States and other countries.

The Ebola epidemic further epitomizes the shortcomings of WHO's leadership and the vertically oriented policies of the past. Partly due to its underfunded circumstances and dependency on the World Bank and the Gates Foundation, WHO mounted a delayed and inadequate response to the viral epidemic. As usual, a race for the "magic bullet" emerged, with predictable financial bonanzas for the pharmaceutical industry. However, because no effective vaccine or treatment of Ebola yet exists, an infrastructure of clinics and hospitals must provide supportive services like hydration and blood products, educational efforts, and simple supplies such as adequate gloves to block transmission of the virus. This type of infrastructure does not exist in West Africa, largely due to the failure of past public health policies, and very similar problems arose during the COVID-19 pandemic. A change in key goals might prove feasible if the powers that be would recognize the practical benefits of a horizontal approach for the development of public health infrastructure. But that approach contradicts a long tradition of top-down vertical policies that have nurtured the political and economic foundations of empire.

Recycling Public Health Interventions at the End of Empire

Philanthropic foundations, international financial institutions, and international health organizations have operated in distinct but complementary ways as they have supported a vertically oriented focus of public health. Throughout most of the twentieth century, the Rockefeller Foundation sponsored such vertical campaigns against endemic infections such as hookworm, yellow fever, tuberculosis, and malaria. The Rockefeller campaigns interpreted these infectious as impediments to labor productivity, investment, and economic development. Rockefeller-funded programs also recognized that endemic infections blocked efforts to extract raw materials and to transport products and workers throughout the world. However, such campaigns did not foster a broader, horizontal infrastructure that could provide integrated public health and primary care services. Instead, these interventions aimed to improve the economic circumstances of enterprises in the imperial countries by improving the health of the imperialized.

WHO's *Report on Macroeconomics and Health* updated this earlier Rockefellerism. Like the Rockefeller Foundation, its unacknowledged predecessor in macroeconomic thought, the *Report* called for investment to reduce poverty in poor countries while enhancing the economic prospects of the rich in both rich and poor countries alike. This approach also revived a vertical attack on specific diseases, rather than encouraging the development of integrated health care systems. Health as a fundamental human value, worthy of investment for its own sake, slipped from consciousness, as did the vision of redistributing wealth as a worthy goal in macroeconomic policy.

More recent efforts by WHO, the Gates Foundation, the International Fund for AIDS, the World Bank, and other agencies focusing on global health have replicated the failed policies of earlier eras.[26] Such influential programs that link public health, health services, and economic development emphasize vertical interventions based on technological fixes for specific diseases rather than horizontal enhancement of public health infrastructure. This old ideological wine continues to produce a familiar euphoria as it appears in new bottles.

But that age is ending. Conditions during the twenty-first century have changed to such an extent that a vision of a world without imperialism has become part of an imaginable future. In struggles throughout the world, especially in Latin America, a new consciousness rejects the inevitability of imperial power, even in situations when such power resurfaces after it apparently had been defeated. This new consciousness also fosters a vision of social medicine constructed around principles of justice, not capital accumulation. Such a vision differs from the historical relation between imperialism and health. Instead, the new vision reveals a diminishing tolerance among the world's peoples, including practitioners of social medicine, for the public health policies of imperialism, and a growing demand for health systems grounded in solidarity rather than profitability and commodification.[27]

Notes

1 Kwame Nkrumah of Ghana wrote an early, in-depth study of neocolonialism: *Neo-Colonialism, the Last Stage of Imperialism* (London: Thomas Nelson & Sons, 1965). Other useful studies include Jean-Paul Sartre, *Colonialism and Neocolonialism* (London: Routledge, 2001 [published in French, 1964]); and William H. Blanchard, *Neocolonialism American Style, 1960–2000* (Westport, CT: Greenwood, 1996).
2 Blanchard, *Neocolonialism American Style*, chapter 9. See also Benedict Anderson, *Under Three Flags: Anarchism and the Anti-Colonial Imagination* (London and New York: Verso, 2005).
3 See Barry S. Levy and Victor W. Sidel, eds., *War and Public Health* (New York: Oxford University Press, 2008).
4 Vicente Navarro argued this perspective in an important early work, "The Underdevelopment of Health or the Health of Underdevelopment: An Analysis of the Distribution of Human Health Resources in Latin America," *Politics & Society* 4 (1974): 267–93.
5 Manas Kaushik, Abhishek Jaiswal, Naseem Shah, and Ajay Mahal, "High-end Physician Migration from India," *Bulletin of the World Health Organization* 86 (2008): 40–45.
6 Howard Waitzkin, *The Second Sickness: Contradictions of Capitalist Health Care*, 2nd ed. (Lanham, MD: Rowman & LIttlefield, 2000), chapter 4; Milton Silverman, Mia Lydecker, Philip R. Lee, *Bad Medicine: The Prescription Drug Industry in the Third World* (Stanford, CA: Stanford University Press, 1992); Peter Davis, ed., *Contested Ground: Public Purpose and Private Interest in the Regulation of Prescription Drugs* (Oxford: Oxford University Press, 1996).
7 Joel Lexchin, "The Pharmaceutical Industry in the Context of Contemporary Capitalism," in Howard Waitzkin and the Working Group on Health Beyond Capitalism, eds., *Health Care Under the Knife: Moving Beyond Capitalism for Our Health* (New York: Monthly Review Press, 2018).
8 Andrew Carnegie, *The Gospel of Wealth & Other Timely Essays* (New York: The Century Company, 1901).
9 Michael E. Porter and Mark R. Kramer, "The Competitive Advantage of Corporate Philanthropy," *Harvard Business Review*, December 2002, https://hbr.org/2002/12/the-competitive-advantage-of-corporate-philanthropy; see also Howard Waitzkin and Rebeca Jasso-Aguilar, "Imperialism's Health Component," and Anne-Emanuelle Birn and Judith Richter, "U.S. Philanthrocapitalism and the Global Health Agenda: The Rockefeller and Gates Foundations, Past and Present," in Howard Waitzkin and the Working Group on Health Beyond Capitalism, *Health Care Under the Knife: Moving Beyond*

Capitalism for Our Health (New York: Monthly Review Press, 2018). For important early studies of the Rockefeller Foundation, see E. Richard Brown, *Rockefeller Medicine Men: Medicine and Capitalism in the Progressive Era* (Berkeley: University of California Press, 1979); Anne-Emanuelle Birn, *Marriage of Convenience: Rockefeller International Health and Revolutionary Mexico* (Rochester, NY: Rochester University Press, 2006); Anne-Emanuelle Birn, Yogan Pillay, Timothy H. Holtz, eds., *Textbook of Global Health* (New York: Oxford University Press, 2017), chapters 1–4; Marcus Cueto, ed., *Missionaries of Science: The Rockefeller Foundation and Latin America* (Bloomington: Indiana University Press, 1994).

10. Howard Waitzkin, "Report of the World Health Organization's Commission on Macroeconomics and Health: A Summary and Critique," *Lancet* 361 (2003): 523–26, and *Medicine and Public Health at the End of Empire* (Boulder, CO: Paradigm Publishers, 2011); Anne-Emanuelle Birn, "Gates's Grandest Challenge: Transcending Technology as Public Health Ideology," *Lancet* 366 (2005): 514–19.

11. For more on Ebola, Zika, COVID-19, the lack of an effective public health response, and the impact of global capitalist agricultural production on their spread, see Waitzkin and Jasso-Aguilar, "Imperialism's Health Component"; Birn and Richter, "U.S. Philanthrocapitalism and the Global Health Agenda"; Carles Muntaner and Rob Wallace, "Confronting the Social and Environmental Determinants of Health," all in Waitzkin and the Working Group on Health Beyond Capitalism, *Health Care Under the Knife: Moving Beyond Capitalism for Our Health* (New York: Monthly Review Press, 2018), as well as Chapters 1 and 3 of this book.

12. World Bank, "Poverty Overview," www.worldbank.org/en/topic/poverty/overview.

13. Ellen R. Shaffer, Howard Waitzkin, Rebeca Jasso-Aguilar, and Joseph Brenner, "Global Trade and Public Health," *American Journal of Public Health* 95 (2005): 23–34; Waitzkin, *Medicine and Public Health at the End of Empire*.

14. Ronald Labonté, Ashley Schram, and Arne Ruckert, "The Trans–Pacific Partnership Agreement and Health: Few Gains, Some Losses, Many Risks," *Globalization and Health* 12, no. 25 (2016): 1–7, doi:10.1186/s12992-016-0166-8.

15. Rachel Kaplan Hoffman and Keith Hoffman, "Ethical Considerations in the Use of Cordons Sanitaires," *Clinical Correlations*, New York University, February 19, 2015, www.clinicalcorrelations.org/?p=8357.

16. N. J. Cox and K. Subbarao, "Global Epidemiology of Influenza: Past and Present," *Annual Review of Medicine* 51, no. 1 (2000): 407–421; Danuta M. Skowronski, Caroline Astell, Robert C. Brunham, et al., "Severe Acute Respiratory Syndrome (SARS): A Year in Review," *Annual Review of Medicine* 56 (2005): 357–381.

17. Marcos Cueto, *The Value of Health: A History of the Pan American Health Organization*. Washington, DC: Pan American Health Organization, 2007; Elizabeth Fee and Theodore M. Brown. "100 Years of the Pan American Health Organization," *American Journal of Public Health* 92, no. 12 (2002): 1888–1889.

18. World Health Organization, "Declaration of Alma-Ata: International Conference on Primary Health Care," Alma Ata, USSR, September 6–12, 1978, www.who.int/publications/almaata_declaration_en.pdf; Marcos Cueto, "The Origins of Primary Health Care and Selective Primary Health Care," *American Journal of Public Health* 94 (2004): 1884–93. For a comprehensive social history of WHO, see: Marcos Cueto, Theodore M. Brown, and Elizabeth Fee, *The World Health Organization: A History*): New York: Cambridge University Press, 2019.

19 Commission on Macroeconomics and Health, *Macroeconomics and Health: Investing in Health for Economic Development* (Geneva: World Health Organization, 2001); Waitzkin, "Report of the World Health Organization's Commission on Macroeconomics and Health." For WHO's perspective during the shift to the macroeconomic perspective, see Kodjo Evlo and Guy Carrin, "Finance for Health Care: Part of a Broad Canvas," *World Health Forum* 13 (1992): 165–70.
20 Commission on Macroeconomics and Health, ibid., 1.
21 World Bank, *World Development Report: Investing in Health* (New York: Oxford University Press, 1993).
22 Jeffrey Sachs, "The Report of the Commission on Macroeconomics and Health," Paper Presented at the Annual Meeting of the American Public Health Association, Atlanta, Georgia, 2001. See also Japhy Wilson, *Jeffrey Sachs: The Strange Case of Dr Shock and Mr Aid* (London and New York: Verso, 2014), chapter 6.
23 Commission on Macroeconomics and Health, *Macroeconomics and Health*, 30–40.
24 World Trade Organization Secretariat and World Health Organization, *WTO Agreements and Public Health: A Joint Study by the WHO and the WTO Secretariat* (Geneva: World Trade Organization, 2002); "The WTO and the World Health Organization," World Trade Organization, www.wto.org/english/thewto_e/coher_e/wto_who_e.htm.
25 World Health Organization, *Closing the Gap in a Generation. Commission on Social Determinants of Health* (Sterling, VA: Stylus Publishing, 2008); also available at www.who.int/social_determinants/final_report/en/.
26 Anne-Emanuelle Birn, "Gates's Grandest Challenge: Transcending Technology as Public Health Ideology," *Lancet* 366 (2005): 514–19; Birn, Pillay, and Holtz, *Textbook of Global Health*.
27 Rebeca Jasso-Aguilar and Howard Waitzkin, "Resisting Empire and Building an Alternative Future in Medicine and Public Health," *Monthly Review* 67, no. 3 (July–August 2015): 114–29. See update in Chapter 10.

Chapter 7

Health and Empire, Part 2
Resisting Empire, Building an Alternative Future in Medicine and Public Health

A World without Empire

While the vision of an empire-free world is no longer mere utopian fantasy, struggles against the logic of capitalism, imperialism, and privatization continue. One question is how to create a model of social medicine that confronts the adverse effects of imperialism and that tries to create an alternative future. In some Latin American countries, efforts have aimed to move beyond the historical pattern fostered by imperialism. The struggles that we will describe remain in the process of dialectic change, which includes both advances and setbacks. However, these accounts show a common resistance to the logic of capital and a common goal of public health systems grounded in solidarity, not profitability.[1]

People in Latin America have experienced the direct impacts of political and economic imperialism imposed by the United States for nearly two centuries. This conflict can be traced back to 1823, when U.S. President James Monroe and Congress drafted the Monroe Doctrine due to concerns about European interference in the western hemisphere. The document asserted that "the American continents, by the free and independent condition which they have assumed and maintain, are henceforth not to be considered as subjects for colonization by any European powers."[2] Through this doctrine, the young United States was claiming Latin America for itself, embodying the conflicting principles of anti-colonialism and economic growth. Indeed, economic and political elites created a neocolonial environment in which corporations based in the United States could extract raw materials while creating new markets. Throughout the nineteenth and twentieth centuries, the U.S. military protected the expanding empire through a series of invasions and other interventions. Although Latin American countries have achieved varying levels of political independence over the past 200 years, economic independence has proved more elusive.

Between the 1940s and 1970s, these countries tried to establish their own economic paths. During this period, the region experimented with policies that favored state intervention to promote industrialization. These policies allowed for development and expansion of public services such as education and health care. While such policies did little to reduce poverty or inequality, they emphasized the role of the state in national economic policy and its responsibility to provide a social safety net.

Then, in the late 1980s, an ideological shift occurred that allowed Latin America to experiment with the stringent economic policies that would become known as neoliberalism. Neoliberalism seeks to assert the superiority of the market over the state; it aims to reduce the role of the state in the economy by favoring austerity, fiscal discipline, deregulation, privatization, and the dismantling of the welfare state.[3] Neoliberal policies were first imposed under military rule in Chile and were later introduced by elected governments in other Latin American countries. Adoption of neoliberal polices often resulted from pressure by the United States and other economically dominant countries. For example, Bolivia adopted the neoliberal model after the International Monetary Fund (IMF) agreed to forgive some of its crushing foreign debt.[4] The policies were packaged as the "Washington Consensus" and were monitored carefully by the World Bank. Between 1980 and 2010, neoliberal policies led to a massive transfer of resources from the public to the private sector, systematic elimination of the safety net, and worsening social and economic inequalities.

Perhaps due to its long history of confronting imperialism, Latin America became an especially fertile ground for resistance against neoliberalism. As a result, Latin American countries that experienced economic distress due to neoliberal policies later have led a battle against neoliberalism. Social movements in the region have unseated governments, appropriated factories, expelled corporations, sought autonomy and self-determination, engaged in electoral struggles, and shared broad demands of social justice.[5]

On the other hand, national and international elites have pushed back with innovative tactics to maintain their positions of economic and political dominance. These tactics have included military threats and some military actions, but "soft" or "hybrid" wars have become the new norm. Such tactics have affected some countries whose elected governments have resisted neoliberal and imperialist policies and have initiated social medicine programs.

These efforts to overthrow elected governments usually involve funding and logistic support from the United States and other allied countries including Canada and the European Union.[6] Through their embassies and intelligence services, these dominant countries coordinate standard scenarios that include several components: sponsored demonstrations by so-called "democratic" opposition groups that try to disrupt the programs of elected progressive governments; economic interventions such as confiscation of property and embargos that impede economic stability; and actions in national congresses and courts to depose elected national leaders.

Such soft or hybrid wars have led to abrupt ousters for elected heads of governments in Honduras, Paraguay, Brazil, and Bolivia (where a military coup accompanied other destabilization efforts), and similar tactics have affected Venezuela, Nicaragua, and other countries, not only in Latin America but also in other regions of the world. Although these disruptive tactics in many instances have not succeeded, they have emerged as key methods to preserve neoliberal policies and advantages of powerful elites.

We now analyze some of the popular struggles in which we and our colleagues in social medicine have participated during the past decade as researchers and activists. Such struggles have included resisting privatization of health services in El Salvador, blocking privatization of water in Bolivia, and expanding the public health sector in Mexico. These scenarios paint a picture very different from that of the historical relation between imperialism and health – a picture that demonstrates a diminishing tolerance among the world's peoples for the public health policies of imperialism and a growing demand for health care grounded in solidarity.

A dialectic process continues in these countries, in which failures may follow victories and victories may follow failures. For instance, while this book has been in press, the progressive coalition that led the fight against privatization of health services in El Salvador lost an election for president, Bolivia suffered a military coup d'état supported by the United States that threatened advances in water security and other social medicine priorities, and Mexico elected a president who strongly supports social medicine yet has received criticism from representatives of the Zapatista revolution in southern Mexico.

Despite the ebbs and flows of national politics (the realities of which we consider further in Chapter 10), in all these countries organizing on the ground reflects much deeper and ongoing processes of fundamental social change. These examples also reflect a larger phenomenon: popular struggles to facilitate participation by ordinary citizens in social issues usually decided by economic and political elites. In practice, this change has translated into demands to have a say in public-sector policies related to health services, medications, and natural resources such as water.

The Struggle against Privatization of Health Services in El Salvador

An early outbreak of sustained resistance to imperial policies in public health and medicine, emphasizing principles of social medicine, took place during the 1990s in El Salvador. This struggle focused on privatization policies initiated by the World Bank, in collaboration with the right-wing political party that was in power. The efforts to resist the privatization of public health services became so widespread that many people took to the streets in protest, crying out that "health care is a right, not a commodity."[7] As a result, El Salvador has served as a model for similar social movements elsewhere in Latin America.

From 1998 to 1999, the health care sector in El Salvador fell into political turmoil. The reasons were complicated. First, El Salvador had recently emerged from a decades-long civil war. The war had badly damaged the already limited health care facilities, especially in rural areas. Progressive union activists who managed to survive this repressive era formed a new union based at the Salvadoran Institute of Social Security (Instituto Salvadoreño del Seguro Social, ISSS) and mobilized for a salary increase. Second, while an agreement was reached, it was not honored by the ISSS authorities. An unfavorable revision of the collective bargaining contract further strained the relationship between workers and the ISSS administration. And third, the ISSS administration began to contract private entities for the delivery of services such as food, laundry, and cleaning for ISSS hospitals. This outsourcing became the first sign of privatization within the ISSS. In line with this trend, two major public hospitals under renovation remained closed for several months, waiting to outsource their services to private entities rather than be managed by the ISSS.[8]

Such actions were part of a strategy, favored by the World Bank, to privatize public hospitals and clinics. Simultaneously, the government tried to gain public sympathy for privatization of all health services due to alleged corruption and inefficiency within the ISSS, while avoiding the controversial term "privatization." People supporting the public sector challenged the credibility of these allegations. For example, during the previous 13 years, the party in power, the Republican Nationalist Alliance (Alianza Republicana Nacionalista, ARENA) had appointed those directly responsible for the functioning of the ISSS. These appointments included hospital directors as well as ISSS officials. In addition, some ARENA politicians who supported privatization also held a financial stake in this effort. Therefore, the health budget was underspent, creating an artificial shortage of medications and delays in services, which proponents of privatization used to build the case for "modernization" and "democratization" of the health care system.[9]

These issues led to strikes in El Salvador's capital city, San Salvador. Workers mobilized in the vicinity of public hospitals. Those belonging to the Union of Workers of the Salvadoran Institute of Social Security (Sindicato de Trabajadores del ISSS, STISS) began a national strike. The conflict quickly escalated, and negotiations between the ISSS administrative authorities and STISSS workers collapsed. This collapse, combined with a growing concern among doctors about the privatization of health care, provided the ground for an alliance between the STISSS workers and the doctors of the recently created Medical Union of Workers of the Salvadoran Institute of Social Security (Sindicato Médico de Trabajadores del ISSS, SIMETRISS). Together, STISS and SIMETRISS produced a document: "Historical Agreement for the

Betterment of the National Health System" (Acuerdo Histórico por el Mejoramiento del Sistema Nacional de Salud). This document contained several points, including a demand for ending privatization in the national health system.[10]

A government commitment not to privatize health services ended the conflict temporarily. But instead of honoring the commitment, the Ministry of Health and the ISSS authorities continued to outsource hospital services. So for three years, workers from STISS and doctors from SIMETRISS organized strikes and rallies that gradually drew the support from the larger civil society. Supporting organizations included teachers and blue-collar unions, students, feminist and environmentalist groups, bus drivers, market vendors, peasants, and coffee growers – the majority of them affiliated with the umbrella coalition Citizens Alliance against Health Care Privatization.[11] Strikes varied in length, and participants walked a fine line so as not to alienate the population at large. During strikes, doctors took care of acutely ill patients on the sidewalks, a humanitarian action but also a strategy to gain wider support. Another action involved "handing the hospitals to the administrators" and walking out, a symbolic gesture to demonstrate that the hospitals could not run without physicians. The government responded with repression, including tear gas, rubber bullets, and water cannons. Doctors were fired and replaced with new personnel.[12]

Eventually responding to these protest actions, the national Congress passed Decree 1024, in which the federal government guaranteed public health and social security.[13] Decree 1024 assured that health care would remain public, prevented any future outsourcing of public health services, and effectively voided any prior outsourcing the government had authorized since the beginning of the conflict. The then president, Francisco Flores, threatened to veto the decree, but coordinated pressure from Congressional legislators and mass collective actions on the streets forced him to comply.[14]

The victory was short lived. Behind the scenes, Flores's party – ARENA – formed a Congressional alliance that produced enough votes to repeal Decree 1024. The conflict continued for another six months, as more marches and demonstrations took place in San Salvador. These were massive rallies where demonstrators dressed in white as a symbol of peace and a sign of solidarity with the doctors and nurses wearing white coats. The demonstrations drew thousands of participants.

The conflict ended when the World Bank reversed a privatization clause in a loan earmarked for modernizing the public health system. Union leaders and government representatives reached an agreement to stop privatization. Members of STISS and SIMETRISS were reinstated with their previous salaries and seniority, though some doctors who were replaced during the strike were forced to relocate. The agreement also established a Follow-up Commission on Health Reform, which included medical professionals, government officials, and representatives of unions and civil society.

Efforts to maintain and expand public health care have continued, especially after the election in 2009 of leftist Mauricio Funes as president. Funes belonged to the Farabundo Marti National Liberation Front, or FMLN. The military wing of this party had fought against ARENA during the long civil war of the 1980s and 1990s. Dr. María Isabel Rodríguez, a well-known leader of Latin American social medicine who had lived in exile during much of the civil war, returned to direct public health and medical services as national minister of health.[15] Funes markedly increased the government's consultation with civil society in economic and social policies. In health care particularly, this orientation translated into a five-year strategic plan in which the Citizen's Alliance against Health Care Privatization acted as the main consultant. In this way, the Citizen's Alliance became an independent movement engaged in proactive, long-term actions. An independent National Health Forum also emerged, as members of civil society were invited to design and implement health care policies and to hold the government accountable for its commitments. The Funes administration incorporated voices that previously were marginalized, such as those of nurses, who took part with other groups in a new National Labor Roundtable. In addition, Funes brought more women into his cabinet, and these women used their positions to emphasize reproductive health.

Salvador Sánchez Cerén, a former guerrilla leader with the FMLN who won the election for president in 2014, pledged to consolidate the advances in health care that were accomplished during the Funes presidency. The Ministry of Health embarked on other initiatives to strengthen the public health sector in health services. Supporting these efforts from a constructively critical position, a new coalition of health professionals became active. Inspired by the contributions of Salvador Allende to social medicine in Chile, the coalition honored Allende through its name: the Dr. Salvador Allende Movement of Health Professionals. Although the coalition grew from the earlier struggles against neoliberal policies in El Salvador, younger health workers took leadership in the organization. They spearheaded the selection of San Salvador as the site of the November 2014 congress of the Latin American Social Medicine Association, which drew thousands of progressive health care workers to advance the struggle against neoliberal policies on behalf of alternative models that strengthen public health services. Even after the FMLN candidate lost the presidential election of 2019, the vision of social medicine continued through the efforts of activists in the Allende Movement and in the national Ministry of Health.

Resistance to Privatization of Water in Bolivia

Unlike access to affordable health care, there are certain human necessities traditionally recognized as fundamental rights. For example, an Action Plan from the United Nations Water Conference in 1977 declared that "...all people have the right to drinking water in quantities and of a quality equal to their basic needs."[16] Although clean water remains a fundamental goal of public health, the world's declining supplies of fresh water have resulted in major corporations trying to sell water as a commodity. Long-term resistance against the privatization of water in Bolivia shows how a previously marginalized population can organize to win a struggle against powerful corporate forces that seek to sell a critical public health resource.

The climate and environment in the province of Cochabamba, Bolivia, made it a prime agricultural area. However, water availability historically has posed serious challenges. Agricultural workers in charge of irrigation (*regantes*) managed the dwindling water resources through practices rooted in cultural traditions known as *usos y costumbres* (uses and customs).[17] These people believed water to be a right, but more than that it was something sacred: Water belonged to everyone, no one could own it.[18] Urbanization further increased the demand for drinking water and water for other domestic uses. Newer policies depleted underground water resources and favored urban development at the expense of the rural, indigenous population.[19]

In 1997, the World Bank promoted privatization of Cochabamba's public water utility, based on the rationale of eliminating public subsidies, securing capital for water development, and attracting skilled management. In characteristic fashion, the bank pressured the Bolivian government by promising international debt relief in the amount of $600 million, contingent on the privatization of water. New legislation – Ley 2029 – allowed a private corporation, Aguas del Tunari, to lease Cochabamba's public water and sewer company (Servicio Municipal de Agua Potable y Alcantarillado, SEMAPA). The contract effectively awarded Aguas del Tunari monopoly control over water services for 40 years. The terms of the contract also prevented the *regantes* from using water in their traditional ways; the company could appropriate any and all water sources, including neighborhood wells and rain. The contract even prevented rural workers from collecting rainwater. A few weeks after the contract was signed, water bills increased by an average of 200 percent, an action known as the *tarifazo*.

Together, both urban and rural citizens protested the rising water prices. The Water War, a series of collective actions that took place during the year 2000, quickly ensued. The Coalition for the Defense of Water and Life (often just called the "Coordinadora") emerged to coordinate the mobilization of farmers, factory workers, professionals, neighborhood associations, teachers, retirees, the unemployed, and university students. These efforts resulted in roadblocks, strikes, mass demonstrations, and public assemblies. An intensive parallel investigation discovered that, among other things, Aguas del Tunari was a "ghost consortium" of enterprises grouped together under the control of Bechtel, a large U.S.-based corporation. Prominent Bolivian politicians had strong economic interests in this consortium. Once this information became public, the Coordinadora was able to gather additional support.

During these tense months, several developments strengthened the popular mobilization to block the privatization of water. The citizens of Cochabamba refused to pay their water bills, which they burned in public as symbolic acts. Demonstrations, barricades, and strikes paralyzed the city several times, disrupting economic activity. The government responded with police and military actions, forcing protestors to escalate their demands. A referendum showed an overwhelming rejection of the contract with Aguas del Tunari. However, the government dismissed this democratic exercise. Protestors' demands continued to escalate, and mass mobilization intensified. As a result, the government took further repressive actions: a disinformation campaign, martial law, and use of live ammunition in clashes with demonstrators. The protestors responded with citywide blockades, bringing the city to a halt. During a protest at the height of the conflict, military police shot and killed a 17-year-old Bolivian student, and other protestors suffered injuries from the gunfire.[20] The youth's funeral drew tens of thousands of angry protestors. Later that day, Aguas del Tunari announced that it was rescinding the contract and leaving Cochabamba.

Cochabamba's public water and sewer company, SEMAPA, remained a public company, and several policy changes occurred as a result of the struggle. The board of directors implemented community engagement and direct participation through the election of community representatives, who became accountable to social organizations and the population at large. These changes revealed a social reappropriation of SEMAPA – its transformation into a public company under *control social*, meaning control exercised by the community. This effort by civil society to exercise control over public resources produced mixed results over the ten years after the Water War. Nevertheless, the Water War weakened neoliberal ideology, challenged the common sense of privatization policies, and opened the door to new forms of citizens' participation in political life.

The struggle to defeat privatization and to strengthen public water supplies constituted the first of a wave of mobilizations and uprisings that broke the trajectory of neoliberalism in Bolivia. Opposition to the commodification of water and the social reappropriation of SEMAPA signaled people's commitment to a new way of doing politics. Indeed, this new form of political participation characterized the social upheaval that swept

Bolivia. During this period, citizens defeated a tax hike, challenged water policies in El Alto (a suburb of Bolivia's capital, La Paz), unseated the neoliberal president Gonzalo Sánchez de Lozada, and – in what came to be known as the Gas War – participated in the decision-making process regarding the nation's gas resources.[21] This chain of events made the defeat of neoliberalism seem possible. The Water War contributed substantially to this possibility, as it did to the election in 2005 and reelections in 2009, 2014, and 2019 of Evo Morales, a socialist and Bolivia's first indigenous president (Figure 7.1). Morales appointed leaders of social medicine in Bolivia as officials in the national Ministry of Health, responsible for reconstructing the country's health services and public health system.

Novel processes of democracy and participation took place during the Morales administration. At the request of the Coordinadora and other activists representing various social movements, Morales committed to creating a new cabinet position: minister of water. This cabinet post dealt with pressing problems that remained after the water struggles and aimed to encourage popular participation in government. The Ministry of Water included a social–technical commission formed by social movements, social organizations, and academics with expertise in water issues. The commission's charge was to discuss, reach consensus, and approve any projects, plans, and programs of the ministry. Again, the commission was to exercise *control social*. The type of community control involved in the social reappropriation of SEMAPA evolved to a form of co-management between the government and civil society. The commission originally held rights of discussion and voting on any project, plan, or program proposed by the ministry. However, this role was limited from the beginning, and it became gradually more constrained under the argument that

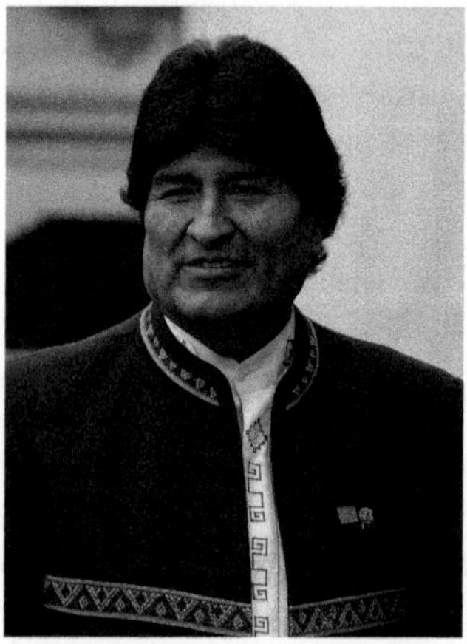

Figure 7.1 Evo Morales.

decisions made by others could not take precedence over the decisions of the minister. Although the commission eventually disbanded, it represented one of the several exercises in community participation to exert control and demand accountability from the Bolivian government, as well as to obtain the right to resources such as water that are critical for public health.

In October 2019, a military coup d'état, supported by the United States, overthrew the coalition government that took power after Morales's re-election as president. Although various claims about electoral irregularities arose, the fact that Morales won the election was not seriously disputed due to his approximately 10 percent lead over the candidate in the second place, and eventually the claimed irregularities were not proven. The coup showed once again that elites tolerate the results of electoral democracy only so far and still do not hesitate to use violent methods to overthrow elected governments when they disagree with those governments' policies. These actions threatened some advances of social medicine accomplished during Morales's presidency. On the other hand, resistance remained widespread. The profound improvements that Bolivia's indigenous populations experienced, especially in practices that honor traditional healing principles, are unlikely to be reversed.[22] In coming years, Bolivia will continue to offer important lessons for social medicine.

Social Medicine's Coming to Power in Mexico City and Mexico

Bold new health policies, linked to the election of a progressive government in Mexico City, further illustrate what an alternative vision can accomplish under conditions of broad sociopolitical change. In the 2000 election, the left-oriented Party of the Democratic Revolution (Partido de la Revolución Democrática, PRD) gained control of the government in Mexico City, while the conservative Party of National Action (Partido de Acción Nacional, PAN) won the presidential election. Thus, political life in Mexico during the first decade of the twenty-first century saw a rivalry between two very distinct political and economic projects: an antineoliberal position in Mexico City, led by Andrés Manuel López Obrador (popularly known as AMLO, Figure 7.2), and a neoliberal one at the federal level, led by President Vicente Fox.

As governor of Mexico City, AMLO initiated wide-ranging reforms of health and human services. To the post of secretary of health, he appointed Asa Cristina Laurell (Figure 7.3), a widely respected leader of Latin American social medicine.[23] Laurell and colleagues began a series of ambitious health programs, modeled according to social medicine principles. They first focused on senior citizens and the uninsured population, with a goal of guaranteeing the right to health protection.[24]

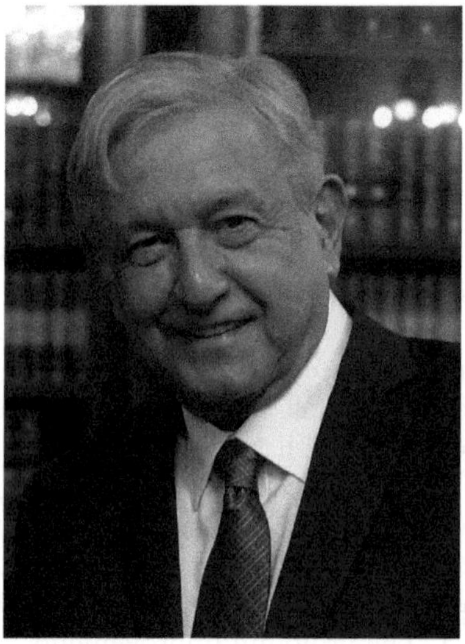

Figure 7.2 Andrés Manuel López Obrador.

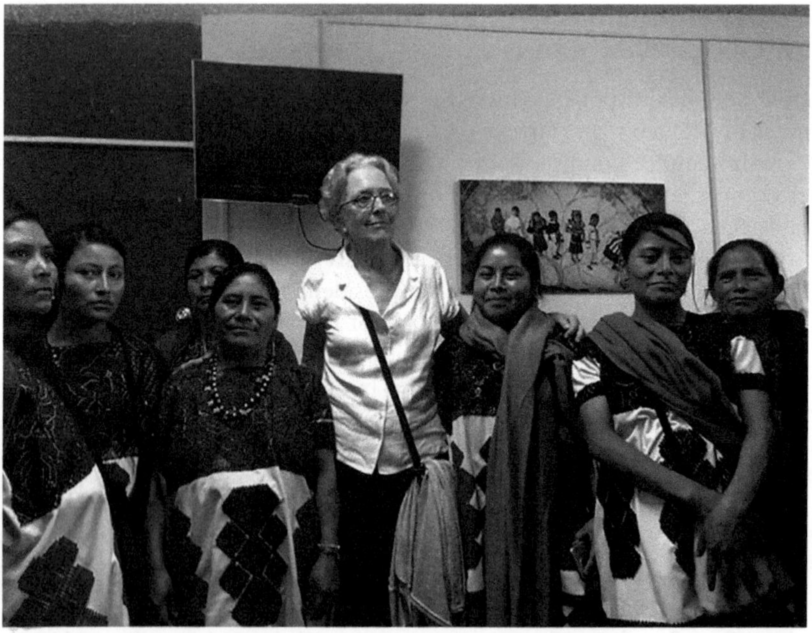

Figure 7.3 Asa Cristina Laurell and colleagues in Chiapas, Mexico.

The Constitution of Mexico and federal health legislation granted this right, as well as universal coverage and free health care throughout public institutions. However, because these documents did not clarify what entity held the obligation to provide health services, the right to health protection often came to be seen as merely "good intentions."[25] An assumption underlying these documents, however, is that public institutions should provide health protection. This assumption offers a legal justification for requiring the state to guarantee the right to health services and other protective measures.[26] The Mexico City Government (MCG) made use of this legal justification to design and implement health and human services policies that targeted vulnerable groups. Laurell described the MCG's goals in health policy:

> To democratize health care, reducing inequality in disease and death and removing economic, social, and cultural obstacles to access; to strengthen public institutions as the only socially just and economically sustainable option granting equal and universal access to health protection; to attain universal coverage; to broaden services for the uninsured population; to achieve equality in access to existing services; and to create solidarity through fiscal funding and the distribution of the costs of disease among the sick and the healthy.[27]

Health policies of the MCG derived from a concept of social rights. Leaders of the MCG saw the creation of social rights – those that the state must guarantee – as one of the Mexican Revolution's most important gains.[28]

Two major programs initiated by the MCG aimed to improve public health and medical services. First, the Program of Food Support and Free Drugs for Senior Citizens created a social institution that granted all seniors a new version of the right to health protection. This program started in February 2001, and by October 2002, it had become virtually universal, covering 98 percent of Mexico City residents aged 70 years or more. Citizens received a monthly stipend amounting to the cost of food for one person (the equivalent of $70) and free health care at the city government's health facilities.[29]

A second initiative, the Program of Free Health Care and Drugs, focused on the uninsured residents of Mexico City. By December 2002, about 350,000 of 875,000 eligible families had enrolled. Later, by the end of 2005, 845,000 family units had registered in the program, effectively amounting to universal coverage of the target population. The health care program provided all personal and public health services, including primary and hospital care for individuals and families.[30]

Financing these programs proved possible because of the MCG's commitment to curb administrative waste and corruption. An austerity program beginning in 2000 implemented a 15 percent pay cut for top government officials and eliminated superfluous expenses. The austerity measures yielded savings of $200 million in 2001, and $300 million in 2002. Simultaneously, the government undertook crackdowns against tax evasion and financial corruption. These savings allowed the government to increase the health budget by 67 percent, meaning that 12.5 percent of the Mexico City budget went for public health and health services.[31]

Such community-oriented initiatives achieved wide admiration and contributed to the PRD's electoral success. In 2000, the PRD victory in Mexico City had been tight. But by April 2003, the approval rate for AMLO reached an unprecedented 80–85 percent. The PRD swept the 2003 midterm election and took control of the Mexico City legislature. AMLO's austere and efficient administration, with zero tolerance for corruption and an emphasis on social programs for the most vulnerable population, earned him the support of Mexico City in his 2006 national presidential bid. It also earned him the wrath of forces that supported the neoliberal status quo, including Mexico's political and financial elites who controlled the country's major media sources. Weeks after the election, the national electoral commission awarded the presidency to the PAN candidate, Felipe Calderón, even after the widespread social mobilization to challenge the election due to extensive evidence of fraud.[32]

The *lopezobradorista* ("López-Obrador-ist") movement that emerged to challenge the election continued despite its failure to reverse the results. This movement led to the formation of the "Legitimate Government of Mexico."[33] In this unofficial government, AMLO served as president and appointed a cabinet of intellectuals, social scientists, and politicians of leftist and anti-neoliberal ideology. Laurell once again became the minister of health. This parallel government kept the social medicine vision alive as a viable policy alternative. According to Laurell, the Legitimate Government was "not a shadow government understood as a reaction to official actions of the other government"; it was "much more proactive," with the capacity "to elaborate and discuss original proposals using as a starting point another idea of what we want our nation to be."[34]

Perhaps prompted by pressure from the Legitimate Government, President Calderón announced that public health would be a priority for his administration. The Popular Insurance Program (Seguro Popular), a federal health coverage program proposed and partly implemented by Vicente Fox's administration between 2003 and 2006, expanded during the Calderón administration from 2006 to 2012. The goal was to increase coverage, especially for the remaining uninsured and people in rural areas. However, this insurance program involved a service package with limited coverage, cost sharing by families, and gradual enrollment of the uninsured population. Limited coverage disrupted the provision of comprehensive care. Cost sharing amounted to 6 percent of family income, a financial burden for poor families. Services not included had to be purchased through private insurance. The latter signaled a further push toward the privatization of health care, which was in line with Fox's and Calderón's neoliberal agendas.

The different ways in which Fox and Calderón on the one hand and AMLO on the other treated public health and health services policies illustrated two discrepant visions of development. In 2006, the Mexico presidential election became so contested because it was a referendum on these different projects with the potential to create two very different countries. As Laurell notes:

> In 2006 what was at play was not just the election of a candidate, the future of the country was at stake... We lost the opportunity to rebuild our country and to make it less unequal, of building a nation for everyone, in which social rights are guaranteed and built, that is what we lost with this electoral fraud... What we are trying to do with the Legitimate Government and with the mobilization of citizens is to keep the hope alive.[35]

The *lopezobradorista* social movement continued to struggle against neoliberalism and for the social, political, and economic transformation of the country. This movement deterred Calderón's efforts to privatize energy during 2008. In 2009, several seats in Congress were gained, representing the only opposition to the neoliberal project. They questioned budgets and reforms, defended the movement's positions, and presented counterproposals.

As the movement continued to organize and promote an alternative national project, AMLO ran for president again in 2012. The 2012 presidential election was a replay of the 2006 struggle between two very different projects. One project attempted to maintain the neoliberal dominance; it was embodied in the candidate of the Revolutionary Institutional Party (Partido Revolucionario Institucional, PRI), Enrique Peña Nieto, and supported by the PAN, the corporate and business class, and the church hierarchy. The other project represented an effort supported by the *lopezobradorista* movement, the PRD, and smaller progressive parties; it posed a substantial challenge to the status quo. Corruption and fraud plagued this election too, through practices such as the use of cash and gift cards in exchange for people's votes in favor of the PRI candidate.[36]

Neoliberal reforms and the repression of social movements became trademarks of Peña Nieto's government. His administration began with a labor reform that further eroded workers' rights and security, and throughout 2012, he pursued regressive reforms in education, energy, and fiscal policy.[37] Yet, the countermovement in Mexico continued, as the leadership (including AMLO, Laurell, and many others) and their constituencies continued the struggle in health and other arenas. AMLO won the

2018 presidential election in a "landslide" victory, as the candidate of the new Movement for National Regeneration (Movimiento Regeneración Nacional, MORENA), and Laurell has continued as one of his main advisors in trying to transform Mexico's national health policies to the model of social medicine.[38]

Despite these important advances in Mexico, tensions have emerged between AMLO's presidential government and the Zapatista revolutionary movement in southern Mexico. Named for Emiliano Zapata, a hero of the Mexican revolution in the early twentieth century, the Zapatista Army of National Liberation (Ejercito Zapatista de Liberación Nacional, EZLN) took control of a large area in the state of Chiapas in southern Mexico on January 1, 1994. This timing coincided with the enactment of the North American Free Trade Agreement (NAFTA), which the Mayan communities of Chiapas opposed due to an expectation that it would increase the exploitation of natural and human resources on indigenous lands.

Since that time, the Zapatistas have self-governed their communities within an "autonomous region." The federal government mostly has relinquished political and economic control to local Mayan communities. In these communities, health centers provide basic services through a collaboration among indigenous healers, doctors, nurses, and other medical personnel.[39] Although AMLO, Laurell, and other leaders of the national government coordinated by MORENA have offered to collaborate, the Zapatista communities usually have decided not to work cooperatively with the federal government.

This lack of collaboration has emerged from several continuing differences in orientation between the Zapatistas and MORENA. Most importantly, AMLO and MORENA have emphasized the consolidation of political power at the federal level. The Zapatistas point out that, despite reforms in government, AMLO and MORENA have not worked out a clear strategy to move beyond the capitalist state and economic system, which is a system that consistently has tried to exploit the human and natural resources of indigenous communities.

For instance, AMLO and MORENA have started to implement strategies that aim toward economic development and growth. These strategies include a high-speed train, *Tren Maya*, which would traverse the tropical forests of the Yucatan Peninsula. Another project involves the conversion of native forests into fruit plantations. The Zapatistas have opposed such projects, arguing that resulting changes will disrupt the traditional homelands and practices of indigenous communities, with economic advantages that will favor outside capitalist investors more than the communities themselves.[40]

So, as in other countries, the situation in Mexico continues to evolve. Aside from electoral victories or losses, however, the social medicine orientation fostered by Laurell and AMLO, as well as the alternative community-based approach pioneered by the Zapatistas, has made an indelible mark on Mexican politics and social policies. This dialectical process will continue to play itself out in Mexico during the coming years.

Sociomedical Activism toward a New Order

The struggles considered here confirm certain core principles of public health: the right to health care, the right to water and other components of a safe environment, and the reduction of illness-generating conditions such as inequality and related social determinants of poor health and early death. Affordable access to health care and clean water supplies provided by the state, for instance, has become the focus of activism throughout the world. Such struggles reinforce grassroots activism and the right to have communities' voices heard and counted in policy decisions. Activism that seeks alternatives to neoliberalism and privatization encourages participation by diverse populations, with an emphasis on solidarity and a rejection of traditional political forms that foster decision making mainly by financial elites.

The challenge is to develop strategies for activism that criticize dominant ("hegemonic") ideologies. Such ideologies favor neoliberalism, the buying and selling of health services within the marketplace, privatization of public services, and the notion that "there is no alternative" to global capitalism. Instead of these hegemonic ideologies, "counterhegemonic spaces" are opening up and creating meaningful possibilities for fundamental social transformation. A goal of the social movements that we have described is not simply to win but also to encourage public debate and to raise the level of political consciousness. A new consciousness rejects the logic of capital and fosters a vision of medicine and public health constructed around principles of justice rather than commodification and profitability. No other path will resolve our most fundamental aspirations for healing.

Notes

1 Rebeca Jasso-Aguilar and Howard Waitzkin, "Resisting the Imperial Order and Building an Alternative Future in Medicine and Public Health," *Monthly Review* 67, no. 3 (July–August 2015). The authors thank Rebeca Jasso-Aguilar for contributing information from her research for our use in this chapter. For further background, see Howard Waitzkin, *Medicine and Public Health at the End of Empire* (Boulder, CO: Paradigm Publishers, 2011), chapter 14 (with Rebeca Jasso-Aguilar).
2 Jay Sexton, *The Monroe Doctrine: Empire and Nation in Nineteenth-Century America* (New York: Hill and Wang, 2011).
3 Susanne Soederberg, "From Neoliberalism to Social Liberalism: Situating the National Solidarity Program within Mexico's Passive Revolution," *Latin American Perspectives* 28 (2001): 104–23; Héctor Guillén Romo, *La Contrarrevolución Neoliberal en México* (México, DF: Ediciones Era, 1997), 13.

4 Jimmy Langman, "Neoliberal Policies – Big Loser in Bolivia," *Global Policy Forum*, July 5, 2002, www.globalpolicy.org/component/content/article/162/27752.html.
5 The work of Samir Amin has influenced our own, for instance, "Popular Movements toward Socialism," *Monthly Review* 66, no. 2 (June 2014): 1–32.
6 The following sources give helpful explanations about "soft" or "hybrid" wars and coups d'état: Tricontinental: Institute for Social Research, "Venezuela and Hybrid Wars in Latin America," June 2019, https://www.thetricontinental.org/wp-content/uploads/2019/06/190604_Dossier-17_EN_Web-Final-2.pdf; Joshua E. Keating, "Coups Ain't What They Used to Be," *Foreign Policy*, June 27, 2012, https://foreignpolicy.com/2012/06/27/coups-aint-what-they-used-to-be/; Andrew Korybko, *Hybrid Wars: The Indirect Adaptive Approach to Regime Change* (Moscow: Peoples' Friendship University of Russia, 2015), https://orientalreview.org/wp-content/uploads/2015/08/AK-Hybrid-Wars-updated.pdf.
7 Paul Almeida, *Waves of Protest: Popular Struggle in El Salvador, 1925–2005* (Minneapolis: University of Minnesota Press, 2008).
8 STISS (Sindicato de Trabajadores del Instituto Salvadoreño del Seguro Social, the Union of Workers of the Salvadoran Institute of Social Security), internal document detailing the chronology of the movement (San Salvador, El Salvador: STISS, 2002); Leslie Schuld, "El Salvador: Who Will Have the Hospitals?" *NACLA Report on the Americas* 36 (2003): 42–45.
9 Schuld, "El Salvador."
10 SIMETRISSS, "Historical Agreement for the Betterment of the National Health System," Working Paper (San Salvador, El Salvador: SIMETRISSS, 2002).
11 Lisa Kowalchuck, "Mobilizing Resistance to Privatization: Communication Strategies of Salvadoran Health-Care Activists," *Social Movement Studies* 10 (2011): 151–73.
12 STISS, internal document.
13 Sandra C. Smith-Nonini, *Healing the Body Politic: El Salvador's Popular Struggle for Health Rights – From Civil War to Neoliberal Peace* (New Brunswick, NJ: Rutgers University Press, 2010).
14 SIMETRISS, "Historical Agreement for the Betterment of the National Health System."
15 Global Health Workforce Alliance, "Alliance Champion Dr. Maria Isabel Rodriguez," www.who.int/workforcealliance/about/spec_advocates/mariaisabelrodriguez/en/.
16 John Scanlon, Angela Cassar, and Noémi Nemes, *Water as a Human Right?* (Gland, Switzerland: IUCN Publications, 2004).
17 Dik Roth, Rutgerd Boelens, and Margreet Zwarteveen, *Liquid Relations: Contested Water Rights and Legal Complexity* (New Brunswick, NJ: Rutgers University Press, 2005).
18 Oscar Olivera and Tom Lewis, *Cochabamba!: Water War in Bolivia* (Cambridge, MA: South End, 2004).
19 Alberto García Orellana, Fernando García Yapur, and Luz Quiton Heras, *La Guerra del Agua, Abril de 2000: La Crisis de la Política en Bolivia* (La Paz, Bolivia: Fundación PIEB, 2003); William Assíes, "David versus Goliath en Cochabamba: Los Derechos del Agua, el Neoliberalismo, y la Renovación de la Protesta Social en Bolivia," *Tinkazos* 4 (2001): 106–31.
20 Camille E. Gaskin-Reyes, *Water Planet: The Culture, Politics, Economics, and Sustainability of Water on Earth* (Santa Barbara, California: ABC-CLIO, LLC, 2016).

21 Graciela Schneier-Madanes, *Globalized Water: A Question of Governance* (Paris, France: Springer, 2014); Charles W. Bergquist, Ricardo Peñaranda, and Gonzalo Sánchez G., *Violence in Colombia, 1990–2000: Waging War and Negotiating Peace* (Wilmington, DE: SR Books, 2001); Benjamin H. Kohl and Linda C. Farthing, *Impasse in Bolivia: Neoliberal Hegemony and Popular Resistance* (Chicago: University of Chicago Press, 2006).

22 Chris Hartmann, "Bolivia's Plurinational Healthcare Revolution Will Not Be Defeated," *North American Congress on Latin America (NACLA)*, December 19, 2019, https://nacla.org/news/2019/12/19/bolivia-plurinational-healthcare-revolution-evo-morales. In the election of October 2020, Morales's party, the Movement for Socialism, recaptured the presidency and both chambers of the Plurinational Legislative Assembly.

23 Howard Waitzkin, Celia Iriart, Alfredo Estrada, and Silvia Lamadrid, "Social Medicine in Latin America: Productivity and Dangers Facing the Major National Groups," *Lancet* 358 (2001): 315–23; Howard Waitzkin, Celia Iriart, Alfredo Estrada, and Silvia Lamadrid, "Social Medicine Then and Now: Lessons from Latin America," *American Journal of Public Health* 91 (2001): 1592–601.

24 Asa Cristina Laurell, "Granting Universal Access to Health Care: The Experience of the Mexico City Government," World Health Organization, Health Systems Knowledge Network, March 2007, http://www.who.int/social_determinants/resources/csdh_media/mexico_universal_access_2007_en.pdf

25 Asa Cristina Laurell, "Interview with Dr. Asa Cristina Laurell," *Social Medicine* 2 (2007): 46–55; Asa Cristina Laurell, "Health Reform in Mexico City, 2000–2006," *Social Medicine* 3 (2008): 145–57.

26 Asa Cristina Laurell, "What Does Latin American Social Medicine Do When It Governs? The Case of the Mexico City Government," *American Journal of Public Health* 93 (2003): 2028–31.

27 Laurell, ibid.

28 Laurell, ibid.

29 Laurell, "Health Reform in Mexico City, 2000–2006."

30 Laurell, ibid.

31 Héctor Díaz-Polanco, *La Cocina del Diablo: El Fraude de 2006 y los Intelectuales* (México, DF: Editorial Planeta Mexicana, 2012).

32 Beldon Butterfield, *Mexico behind the Mask: A Narrative, Past and Present* (Washington, DC: Potomac, 2013).

33 Emily Edmonds-Poli and David A. Shirk, *Contemporary Mexican Politics* (Lanham, MD: Rowman & Littlefield, 2009).

34 Laurell, "Interview with Dr. Asa Cristina Laurell."

35 Laurell, "Interview with Dr. Asa Cristina Laurell."

36 Nick Miroff and William Booth, "Mexico's Presidential Election Tainted by Claims of Vote-buying," *Washington Post*, July 4, 2012, https://www.washingtonpost.com/world/mexicos-presidential-election-tainted-by-claims-of-vote-buying/2012/07/04/gJQAHqTzNW_story.html?noredirect=on&utm_term=.8463338c355c.

37 Robin Alexander and Dan LaBotz "Mexico's Labor Reform: A Workers' Defeat – For Now." *NACLA,* North American Congress on Latin America, April 3, 2014, https://nacla.org/article/mexico's-labor-reform-workers'-defeat%25E2%2580%2594-now.

38 During June 2020, in the context of the COVID-19 pandemic and reduced income from federal taxes due to economic setbacks, AMLO's administration

initiated several organizational changes to reduce administrative costs. Although Laurell resigned as sub-secretary of health, she did not express differences with AMLO concerning social medicine goals or policies. As of this writing, her ongoing relationship with the federal government remains undecided.

39 Andrej Grubacic and Denis O'Hearn, *Living at the Edges of Capitalism: Adventures in Exile and Mutual Aid* (Oakland, CA: University of California Press, 2016), chapter 4; J.H. Cuevas, "Health and Autonomy: the Case of Chiapas – A Case Study Commissioned by the Health Systems Knowledge Network," World Health Organization, 2007, https://www.who.int/social_determinants/resources/csdh_media/autonomy_mexico_2007_en.pdf; Ginna Villarrea, "Health Care Organized from Below: The Zapatista Experience," *Narco News Bulletin*, January 11, 2007, https://www.narconews.com/Issue44/article2502.html.

40 Jerome Baschet, "Zapatistas Take on President AMLO at 25th Anniversary," *Earth First! Newswire*, February 27, 2019, https://earthfirstjournal.org/newswire/2019/02/27/zapatistas-take-on-president-amlo-at-25th-anniversary/; Courtney Parker, "Zapatista Face off with Mexico's New President," *Intercontinental Cry* (Center for World Indigenous Studies), January 21, 2019, https://intercontinentalcry.org/zapatista-face-off-with-mexicos-new-president/; Jared Olson, "Zapatistas Maintain Suspicion of Mexico's President-Elect Andrés Manuel López Obrador, 'AMLO'," Flagler College Gargoyle, December 14, 2018, https://gargoyle.flagler.edu/2018/12/zapatistas-maintain-suspicion-of-mexicos-president-elect-andres-manuel-lopez-obrador-amlo/; Hilary Klein, "A Spark of Hope: The Ongoing Lessons of the Zapatista Revolution 25 Years On," *North American Congress on Latin America (NACLA)*, January 18, 2019, https://nacla.org/news/2019/01/18/spark-hope-ongoing-lessons-zapatista-revolution-25-years.

Chapter 8

Social Medicine in Latin America

Social medicine addresses not only the links among empire, public health, and medical services, but also strategies to move toward a healthier future post-empire. Latin American social medicine (LASM) encompasses research, teaching, clinical practice, and activism toward change[1]. As we noted in Chapter 1, in Brazil "collective health" (*saúde colectiva*) rather than social medicine became the preferred term, to emphasize collective actions that focus on enhancing health rather than actions focusing mainly on medicine and medical services. Partly through its emphasis on "praxis" – the combining of theory and practice – social medicine and collective health provide models of intellectual and practical work that envision a transition to a healthy life, recently called *buen vivir*, "to live well" (we discuss this concept further in Chapter 10).

> ## SOCIAL MEDICINE AND COLLECTIVE HEALTH IN THE TIME OF COVID-19
>
> The two main international organizations for social medicine and collective health in Latin America are the Latin American Association of Social Medicine (Asociación Latinomericana de Medicina Social, ALAMES) and the Brazilian Association of Collective Health (Associação Brasileira de Saúde Coletiva, ABRASCO). For more information about meetings and teleconferences, publications, teaching, research, service activities, and activism, please see their websites: http://www.alames.org, https://www.abrasco.org.br/site/. Both sites contain extensive information about COVID-19, racial capitalism, and activism in the global South. For the comprehensive statement by ALAMES on COVID-19, which expands on the perspectives of this book, see "ALAMES Against the Pandemic COVID 19," http://www.alames.org/index.php/documentos/articulos-de-prensa/146-eng-alames-against-the-pandemic-covid-19/file.

The accomplishments of this field remain relatively unknown outside Latin America, as major publications have not been translated from Spanish and Portuguese. A lack of attention also reflects an erroneous assumption that the intellectual and scientific productivity of countries in the global South[2] reflects a less relevant and rigorous approach to the important questions of our age. In this chapter, we describe the challenges and dangers of working in LASM, which show the links between health and praxis that the future will require.

Productivity and Danger

Many people who have worked in LASM have lived through dramatic personal experiences. These experiences show how the very nature of their work – because it reveals the social origins of health problems – can be seen as dangerous to the sectors of society that control wealth and power.[3]

★ ★ ★

> The social medicine expert is about to be tortured. The form of torture: electric shock applied to his testicles. His crimes have been simply to teach medical and other health science students in a community clinic, one of the major public health teaching sites for the University of Chile. A graduate of the Harvard School of Public Health, he is also accused of conducting research on the relationships between poverty and health outcomes in local communities. He knows that several of his colleagues have already been executed for similar crimes. In his interrogation, he has been asked to provide information about his friends and other colleagues, but so far he has refused.
>
> The torturer is a clean-cut and matter-of-fact person whose military affiliation isn't quite clear. He orders the social medicine expert to pull down his pants. The social medicine expert has no choice but to comply, looking at the electrodes in the torturer's right hand. Just then, the torturer glances at the watch on his right wrist. "Okay," the torturer says, "it's five-o'-clock. Time to go home." He leaves the room. The social medicine expert pulls his pants back up and waits for the guard to take him back to his cell.
>
> Recalling this experience in an interview, he mentions Max Weber's work on the sociology of bureaucracy: "bureaucratized torture."[4]

★ ★ ★

> The chief of surgery at a public hospital in a working-class neighborhood of Santiago, Chile, sits in his dimly lit office. His tall frame is bent over a notebook computer. He had trained on the surgical services at Massachusetts General Hospital. After completing his training, Salvador

Allende chose him as minister of health for the Unidad Popular (Popular Unity) government. Known as an outstanding surgeon and medical educator, he convened a "council of elders" from the University of Chile's School of Public Health to advise the Ministry of Health.

On September 11, 1973, he was the last person in the line of government officials who walked down the stairs to the first floor of La Moneda, the presidential palace, which was on fire after the air force's precision bombing, to surrender to the military victors of the coup d'état. As the last person to see Allende alive, he notes simply that Allende was not killed but instead committed suicide, in the tradition of José Manuel Balmaceda, the reformist president of Chile who killed himself in 1891 rather than surrender to a military coup.

After his own arrest, the surgeon and former minister of health was tortured and sent to prison for a year on frigid Dawson Island near Antarctica. Later, he worked in exile for fourteen years as a professor of surgery in Caracas, Venezuela. Following the Chilean election in 1988 that led to a new government, he returned as chief of surgery to the same public university hospital where he worked before the coup.

He writes mainly for the clinical journal that health professionals and workers at his hospital have produced intermittently since 1953. Currently, he is working on a series of articles that he has introduced with a quote from Alice in Wonderland: "Could you tell me please what road I should take?" These articles describe the deterioration of Chile's public health system under both the dictatorship and the country's subsequent civilian regime, whose polices call for further privatization of public industries, housing, education, and health programs.

★ ★ ★

The former dean of the medical school of the University of Buenos Aires explains why, at age seventy-three, he lives hand-to-mouth on small teaching and consulting fees and royalties, without a pension or other regular income. Before the dictatorship took control in Argentina during 1976, he had enjoyed a prominent career, applying the social sciences to medicine and public health administration. His articles and books in health planning had achieved international recognition. He frequently was asked to consult with the World Health Organization and the Pan American Health Organization and to give presentations at universities and professional organizations throughout the Americas.

When the military took control, he and his family happened to be outside Argentina. He was not able to return for more than ten years. His neighbors told him that they watched helplessly as soldiers knocked down the doors of his home and proceeded to ransack and burn his library. The burning of books and journals in this case and many others makes the Argentine intellectual productivity of the 1960s through

1980s difficult to locate, except in rare book collections. Sometimes books were handed over voluntarily by the owners of the publication for fear that the military would find them and use them as evidence of subversion – justifying imprisonment, torture, and death. The former dean points proudly to the bookshelf that contains his own publications, many of which were given as gifts after his return to his homeland, by friends who had bravely hidden them for many years.

★ ★ ★

During various periods in the history of LASM, the work of its leaders has proven threatening to those who governed their societies. The risks of working in this field have reflected a critique of the existing social order, a focus on the health problems of oppressed peoples, and a vision of a healthier and more just future.

Historical Roots of Latin American Social Medicine

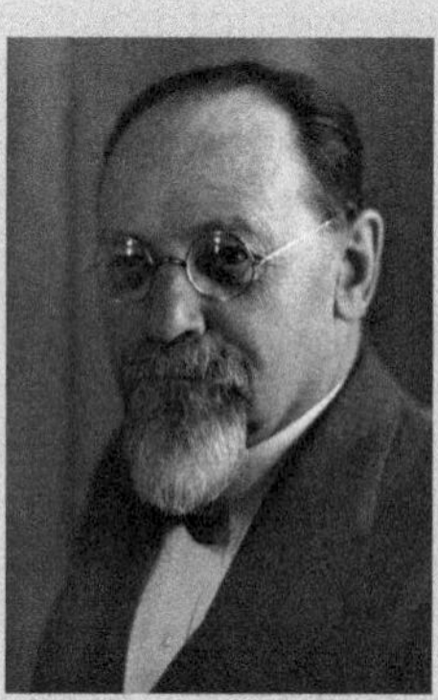

Figure 8.1 Max Westenhöfer, a student of Virchow, who later as a pathologist influenced social medicine in Chile.

To understand LASM's importance for the present and future, it helps to examine its origins during the nineteenth century, its flowering during the 1930s and again during the 1960s, its relation to empire during the late twentieth century, and its growing influence during the twenty-first century. Most Latin American accounts of social medicine's history refer to its sources in Europe, frequently citing the work of Rudolf Virchow in Germany (although indigenous sources also have influenced LASM more recently through concepts like *buen vivir*, as discussed Chapter 10).[5] Through his political activism in the reform movements that culminated in the revolutions of 1848, Virchow initiated a series of groundbreaking

MAX WESTENHÖFER: THE PATHOLOGIST WHO CONNECTED VIRCHOW AND CHILE

Adherents of Rudolf Virchow's vision about the social determinants of mortality and morbidity immigrated to Latin America near the turn of investigations concerning the effects of social conditions on illness and mortality. Presenting pathologic observations and statistical data, he argued that the solution to these problems required fundamental social change, rather than specific medical interventions. Virchow defined the new field of social medicine as a "social science" that focused on illness-generating social conditions.[6] (For more on Virchow, see Chapter 2.)

Followers of Virchow's vision immigrated to Latin America near the turn of the twentieth century. These supporters helped establish departments of pathology in medical schools and initiated courses in social medicine. Max Westenhöfer (Figure 8.1), a prominent German pathologist, teacher, and practitioner of social medicine, directed the department of pathology at the medical school of the University of Chile for some years and influenced a generation of students and practitioners. Among them was Salvador Allende, a medical student activist, pathologist, and future president of Chile.[7]

The "Golden Age" of Social Medicine in Chile and the Role of Salvador Allende

The roots of Chilean social medicine date back to the early twentieth century. In 1907, thousands of saltpeter workers and their families converged in the northern desert city of Iquique, calling for improved living and working conditions.[8] The Chilean army, led by General Roberto Silva Renard, told the strikers that they had to disband within the hour. When the deadline passed, the army opened fire on the crowds of men, women, and children. The number of victims remains unknown.

Despite the massacre, Chilean workers continued to fight for their health and safety. Sustained activism began after the nationwide strikes of 1918. During that year, saltpeter workers in the northern desert encouraged work stoppages in other industries with the goal of improving wages, benefits, and working conditions. A charismatic organizer – Luis Emilio Recabarren (pictured in our online document) – emphasized the destructive effects of malnutrition, infectious diseases, and other health problems with social roots that caused workers' illnesses and premature mortality. During the next three decades, Recabarren and his allies sought economic reforms to improve the social conditions that affected illness and mortality among the poor. In the 1920s and 1930s, social medicine flourished in Chile, partly as a response to the demands of the labor movement.

Within this so-called golden age of Chilean social medicine emerged Salvador Allende. Allende's experiences as a physician and a pathologist shaped much of his later career in politics. Acknowledging debts to others who studied the social roots of illness, Allende created a model of medical problems in the context of underdevelopment. Although parallel activities in social medicine were occurring during the same time period in both North America and Europe, these developments apparently did not influence Allende's work directly.

As discussed in Chapter 2, Allende served as minister of health for a newly elected popular-front government in 1939 and presented his analysis of the relationships among social structure, disease, and suffering in his classic book, *La Realidad Médico-Social Chilena (The Chilean Medico-Social Reality)*.[9] This book conceptualized illness as a disturbance of the individual, fostered by deprived social conditions. Allende specifically described the working class's living conditions that generated illness. He emphasized the social conditions of underdevelopment and international dependency, as well as the effects of foreign debt and the work process. Allende also focused on several specific health problems, including maternal and infant mortality, tuberculosis, sexually transmitted and other communicable diseases, emotional disturbances, and occupational illnesses. Describing public health problems that had not been studied previously, he analyzed illegal abortion, the responsiveness of tuberculosis to economic advances rather than innovations in treatment, housing density in the causation of infectious diseases, and the differences between generic and brand-name pricing in the pharmaceutical industry.

La Realidad Médico-Social Chilena took a unique direction by advocating social rather than medical solutions to health problems. In the book's conclusion, Allende proposed income redistribution, state regulation of food and clothing supplies, a national housing program, and industrial reforms to address occupational health problems. Rather than seeing improved health care services as a means toward a more productive labor force, Allende valued the population's health as an end in itself and advocated social changes that went far beyond the medical realm.

As an elected senator in the early 1950s, Allende introduced the legislation that created the Chilean National Health Service, the first national program in the Americas that aimed to guarantee universal access to health services.[10] He linked this reform to other efforts that tried to achieve more equitable income distribution, job security, improved housing and nutrition, and a less dominant role for multinational corporations within Chile. Similarly, as an elected senator during the 1960s and president between 1970 and 1973, Allende sought reforms in the National Health Service and other institutions that would have achieved structural changes throughout society. Allende's analytical position in *La Realidad Médico-Social Chilena* lay behind much of his political work until his death in 1973, during the military coup d'état.

Social Medicine versus Public Health Elsewhere in Latin America

Both historically and currently, leaders in Latin America have distinguished social medicine from traditional public health. From this perspective, as noted in Chapter 3, public health tends to define a population as a sum of individuals. Specific characteristics, such as sex, age, education, income, and race or ethnicity, permit the classification of these individuals into groups. In traditional epidemiology, rates for a population are calculated arithmetically from the characteristics of individuals who compose the population. By contrast, much work in social medicine envisions populations, as well as social institutions, as totalities whose characteristics transcend those of individuals.[11] Social medicine, therefore, defines problems and seeks solutions with social rather than "reductionist" individual units of analysis. In this way, the population can be analyzed through such categories as social class, economic production, social reproduction of the labor force mainly by women, and culture and not simply the characteristics of individuals.[12]

Another distinction between social medicine and traditional public health concerns the static versus dynamic nature of health versus illness, as well as the effect of social context. Social medicine conceptualizes "health–illness" as a singular, natural, and dialectical process rather than a dichotomous category. Social epidemiologists have studied disease processes in this contextualized model, considering the changing effects of social conditions over time.[13] Indeed, the epidemiologic profile of a society or a group within a society requires a multilevel analysis of how social conditions, such as economic production, social reproduction, culture, marginalization, and political participation, affect the dynamic process of health–illness. Meanwhile, statistical methods, such as logistic regression models with disease as a dependent variable, considered as either present or absent, obscure health–illness as a dialectical process rather than a yes–no condition of being.[14]

In line with this social medicine theme, a group in Argentina led by Juan B. Justo in the 1920s tried to go beyond the "public health" initiatives of the time. Known as hygienic interventions (*higienismo*), such initiatives emphasized infection control, sanitation, nutrition, and similar efforts to improve population health.[15] *Higienismo* usually aimed to improve labor force productivity in the interest of national development and international investment. Justo, a surgeon, became the founding leader of the Socialist Party in Argentina and provided an early Spanish translation of

Marx's *Capital*. Like Allende, Justo called attention to the pervasive effects of social class on health services and outcomes.[16] This work led to regional and national organizing efforts that sought broad social change as the basis for improved health. However, *higienismo* gained dominance, and Justo's remained a minority position.

Another line of work in social medicine that grew from Argentine roots was that of Ernesto "Che" Guevara (Figure 8.2). Guevara's childhood asthma, as well as role models in his family, led him to enter medical school and eventually to specialize in allergic diseases. After medical school, he toured South America, Central America, and Mexico by motorcycle. Through experiences of poverty and suffering during his trip, Guevara developed his views about the need for revolution as a prerequisite for improving health conditions (Figure 8.2).[17]

In his speeches and writings on "revolutionary medicine," Guevara called for a corps of physicians and other health workers who understood the social origins of illness and the need for social change to improve health conditions.[18] Guevara's work profoundly influenced LASM. Perhaps because of this, one might assume that Guevara was influenced by Allende, Justo, and others who came before him. However, this is not the case. Sources close to Guevara, including an uncle who served as a role model in medicine, reported that throughout his medical training and career, Guevara remained unexposed to earlier works in LASM and that he developed his analysis linking health outcomes with social conditions independently, largely through experiences from his motorcycle trip.[19]

Meanwhile, in Ecuador, leaders in social medicine trace their local roots back nearly 200 years. During the early nineteenth century, the physician

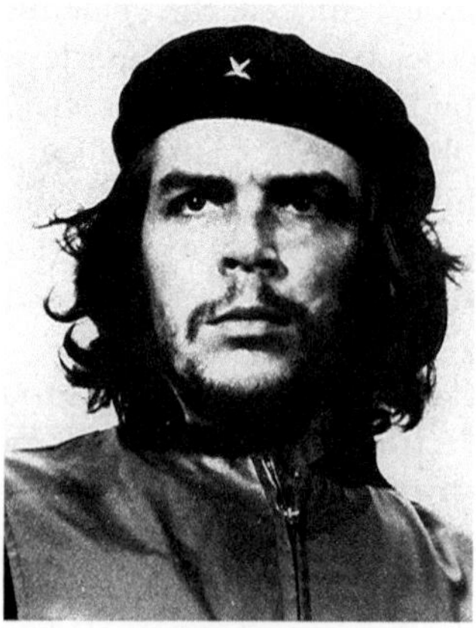

Figure 8.2 Ernesto (Che) Guevera, a physician whose views influenced social medicine in Cuba and other countries.

Eugenio Espejo linked his work as a physician from an indigenous family background to the revolutionary struggles against Spain.[20] In his efforts to control epidemics, Espejo became convinced – as Virchow later would be in Germany – that poverty, inadequate housing and sanitation, and insufficient nutrition fostered such outbreaks. Subsequently, in the early twentieth-century movement toward social security, Pablo Arturo Suárez's book on "the situation of the working class" provided epidemiologic data on adverse health outcomes.[21] During the 1930s, the physician Ricardo Paredes studied occupational lung diseases and accidents among Ecuadoran miners working at a U.S.-owned mining company.[22] In addition to legislation that improved working conditions, Paredes's efforts led to a broad consciousness in Ecuador of the effects on health of "economic imperialism" by multinational corporations during empire.

The early work in Chile, Argentina, and Ecuador influenced LASM, although there also were substantial efforts in Brazil, Colombia, Cuba, and Mexico. However, uncritical and reductionist public health efforts throughout Latin America, clarified by several investigations,[23] have provided a background to which contemporary practitioners of social medicine have reacted. For instance, leaders of social medicine in many Latin American countries responded critically to the Rockefeller Foundation's public health initiatives, which emphasized the productivity of labor in enhancing the ventures of U.S.-based multinational corporations (for more about Rockefeller, see Chapter 6).[24]

The 1960s and Later

Among the dramatic changes that occurred worldwide during the 1960s, the Cuban Revolution emerged as one of the most important for social medicine. Cuba's improved public health system flowered as part of a social revolution, where accomplishments in health occurred as an integral part of broad structural changes in the society as a whole.[25] The social transformations underlying Cuba's achievements in primary care, public health, medical education, planning and administration, and epidemiological surveillance inspired activists and scholars around the world.

If Cuba provided a positive model for LASM, Chile's policies created ambivalence. Social medicine groups took a keen interest when Allende and the Unidad Popular alliance won the presidential election in 1970, and many people in social medicine came to Chile to work with the new government. Allende had proposed a peaceful transition to socialism through electoral rather than military means – the first such transition in history. The government moved toward a "unified" national health program, in which the contradictions of coexisting private and public sectors would be reduced. Allende's plan for socialized medicine crumbled after the violent coup d'état of 1973, when repression of the population and especially of health care workers reached unprecedented levels of violence.[26] The failure of the peaceful road to socialism served as a reminder about the dangers of pursuing social medicine.

Nicaragua's revolution in 1979 also inspired social medicine activists, although many worried about the Sandinista government's social policies linked to health. Leaders of social medicine from several countries contributed to the new Nicaraguan government's health reforms, including extensive programs that dealt with infectious diseases and maternal and child health.[27] These leaders' concerns, not emphasized publicly, focused on the contradictions of the Nicaraguan revolution that, for instance, permitted a continuing major role for private practice, even for those health professionals who worked full time in the National Health Service. Government representatives argued that such policies, enhancing the private sector of the economy, would prevent an exodus of health professionals similar to the one that had occurred in Cuba. Owing to such contradictions, some social medicine leaders eventually reduced their support activities, especially after the Sandinistas' electoral losses.

Liberation theology became a source of inspiration for many of social medicine's activists. Priests such as Frei Betto in Brazil advocated participation in "base communities," which fused religious piety with struggles for social justice.[28] These struggles included efforts to improve health and public health services. Certain leaders of liberation theology grew skeptical about nonviolent processes in base communities, coming to believe that violence sometimes was needed to overcome the opposition of wealthy elites. Influenced by Camilo Torres, a priest who joined the revolutionary movement in Colombia, some social medicine activists entered armed struggle in several countries and later returned to the practice of social medicine.[29]

Another important influence on social medicine stemmed from the educational innovations of Paulo Freire and his co-workers in Brazil. Through adult literacy campaigns, Freire encouraged people in poor communities to approach education as a process of empowerment. In the efforts that led to his classic book, *Pedagogy of the Oppressed*, Freire fostered the organization of small educational "circles" by which local residents could link their studies to the solution of concrete problems in their communities.[30] Activists later began to extend this approach to public health education and organizing for improved health services.[31] Freire himself became more interested in applications of empowerment strategies to health.[32] While Freire's orientation also has influenced public health in the United States, the impact proved even greater in LASM.[33]

During the 1970s, a leader emerged who profoundly affected the course of LASM from a base in Washington, D.C. Trained as a physician in Argentina and a sociologist in Chile, Juan César García served as research coordinator within the Pan American Health Organization (PAHO) from 1966 until his death in 1984. García (Figure 8.3) produced seminal works

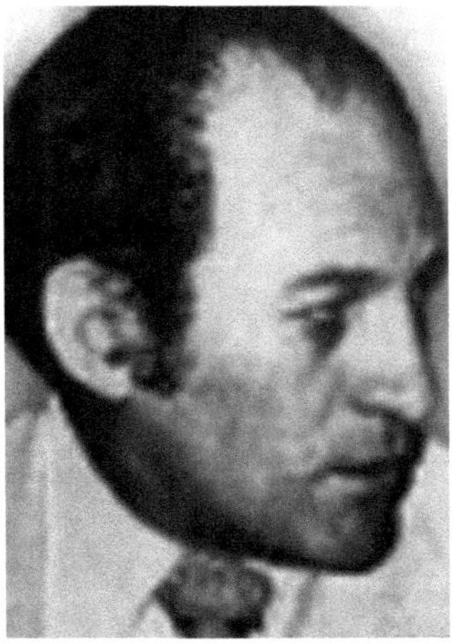

Figure 8.3 Juan César García, who helped support the growth of Latin American social medicine from a base at the Pan American Health Organization in Washington, DC.

on medical education, the social sciences, social class determinants of health outcomes, and the ideological bases of discrimination against Latinos.[34] Although his Marxist social philosophy manifested itself in several works published under his own name while he was working for PAHO, he also published more explicitly political articles under pseudonyms.

García also fostered LASM through the financial and socioeconomic support that he provided through PAHO. With his colleague María Isabel Rodríguez (Figure 8.4), who was living in exile after serving as dean of the school of medicine at the University of El Salvador, García orchestrated grants, contracts, and fellowships that proved critical for social medicine groups throughout Latin America. PAHO funding helped establish the first influential training program in LASM, at the Autonomous Metropolitan University – Xochimilco, in Mexico City, which attracted students from throughout Latin America. Current leaders consistently refer to García's initiative and tenacity, despite the opposition that he increasingly received within PAHO.

In advocating social medicine, García helped distribute Spanish-language translations of work by Vicente Navarro, a professor of public health at Johns Hopkins University who for many years resisted the dictatorship of Francisco Franco in his native Spain. Navarro's works have influenced LASM regarding the effects of capitalism, imperialism, and maldistribution of economic resources on health services and outcomes. The *International Journal of Health Services*, edited by Navarro, has provided an English-language forum for Latin American authors.[35]

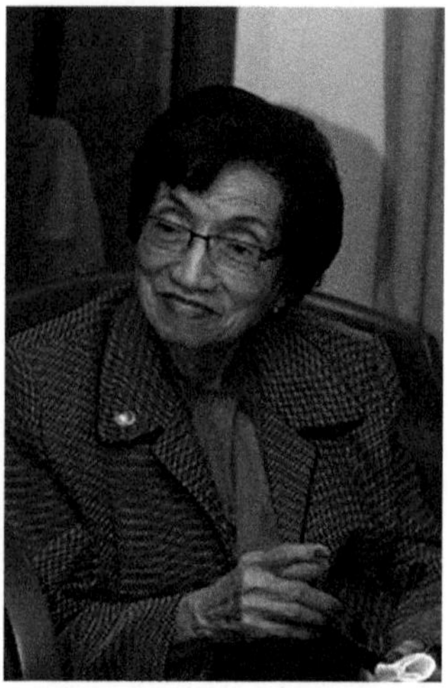

Figure 8.4 María Isabel Rodríguez, who became Minister of Health in El Salvador after spending years in exile while working for the Pan American Health Organization in Washington, DC.

Political Repression and Work Challenges

In a study that included in-depth interviews with 24 leaders of social medicine in Latin America, only four respondents denied having suffered some form of political repression.[36] Respondents had experienced repression because of their work in Chile's Unidad Popular government, their activity in human rights, or their role as health care activists. The forms of repression included torture, imprisonment in concentration camps, exile, exclusion from government jobs, loss of economic security and work stability, loss of professional prestige, and restriction of political activity.

Even after the dictatorships in Latin America, the work process of social medicine varies widely, depending on political and economic conditions. From Chile and Argentina, most leaders of social medicine took refuge in other countries. These refugees from South America's southern cone made major contributions to the diffusion of social medicine while they were living and working abroad. If people remained within their homelands, they usually supported themselves through clinical laboratory work, market research, or retail sales. Since the fall of the dictatorships, people in social medicine have faced great difficulties in attempts to reintegrate themselves into universities or medical schools. Many hold multiple jobs, usually in clinical or administrative work, and pursue social medicine as largely unpaid activities.

In countries without dictatorships, or where dictatorships proved somewhat less brutal – like Brazil – fewer people needed to emigrate and more remained at work in universities or teaching hospitals. In Colombia, owing to a tradition of violence, prominent leaders of social medicine have perished or entered exile despite the presence of elected governments. In other countries, such as Mexico, Ecuador, and Cuba, participants in social medicine have been able to maintain relatively stable academic positions. In general, the most favorable institutional conditions for social medicine have existed in Mexico, Ecuador, Brazil, and Cuba. Since conditions in Argentina, Chile, and Colombia remain more adverse, participants in social medicine struggle to achieve high levels of productivity.

Theory, Method, and Debate

LASM has developed into a rich and diverse field rather than a single, homogeneous tradition. Intense debates have focused on theory, method, and strategies for change.[37] For instance, theoretical debates have questioned the usefulness of traditional Marxist analysis as opposed to more recent theories. Theoretical differences have also focused on the primacy of economic forces versus other issues such as gender, race, and ethnicity. Methodological debates have considered the balance between quantitative and qualitative methodologies in research, as well as individuals versus groups as units of analysis. Strategically, practitioners of social medicine have differed widely in their willingness to collaborate with international health organizations and international financial institutions.

If there is one commonality that distinguishes the field, however, it is an emphasis on theory. Practitioners of social medicine have argued that a lack of explicitly stated theory in North American medicine and public health does not signify an absence of theory. Instead, an a-theoretic or anti-theoretic stance means that the underlying theory remains implicit. Latin American critics have used this prism to interpret the North American tendency to focus on the biological rather than the social components of such problems as cancer, hypertension, and occupational illnesses. From this perspective, the biological focus reduces the unit of analysis to the individual and, thus, obscures the social causes amenable to societal-level interventions.[38]

Referring to the linkage between theory and practice, practitioners of social medicine frequently use the term "praxis." Influenced by Gramsci's work in Italy, Latin American leaders have emphasized theory that both informs and takes inspiration from efforts toward social change.[39] Research and teaching activities often take place in collaboration with labor unions, women's groups, indigenous coalitions, and community organizations.

Although Marxist theory has stimulated social medicine, conceptual work has focused on the strengths and limitations of traditional Marxism in the Latin American context. Adverse experiences in socialist countries like the Soviet Union also have revealed the limited capability of traditional Marxist theory.[40] Certain components, however, have continued to ground conceptual work and research.

First, social medicine has emphasized social class, as defined by the relations of economic production. In Marxist theory, the most important characteristic of social class involves ownership and control of the means of production.[41] Practitioners of social medicine have argued that the exploitation of labor remains an inherent condition of economic production, especially in less developed countries. As a result, they have maintained a vision of social class rooted in economic production rather than in such demographic characteristics as income, education, and occupational prestige. This theoretical position concerning economic production has led to the choice of research questions that focus on the labor process itself, in both industrial and agricultural settings. The social medicine groups in Mexico, Chile, Ecuador, and Brazil have initiated studies of work hierarchies, the production process in factories, and the impact of work conditions on health and mental health outcomes.

A second focus, in addition to social class, involves the reproduction of economic production. Marxist theory questions how the capitalist system can reproduce the inherently exploitative relations of production across generations. Among the supporting institutions that accomplish this reproduction, the family figures most prominently, especially through the patterning of gender roles. Marx and Engels argued, for instance, that the exploitation of workers was inherently linked to the exploitation of women, since economic reproduction required the reproduction of the labor force mainly through the activities of women within families.[42] In contemporary societies, women often bear the "triple burden" of wage labor, housework, and child rearing. For that reason, social medicine groups in several countries have collaborated in research that focuses on women workers and the effects of their roles in economic production and reproduction.[43]

Ideology, a third theoretical focus, comprises the distinctive ideas and doctrines of a social group. A "hegemonic" ideology tends to justify the interests of the class that dominates a society during a specific historical period. Demystification of this dominant ideology then becomes a task for theoretical and political work.[44] The social medicine groups in Latin America have accepted this task of demystification as a priority. During earlier years, the work of demystification focused on "developmentalist" policies, fostered by North American and European governments. More recently, demystification efforts have emphasized the health policies of the World Bank and other international financial institutions. These agencies have encouraged increasing indebtedness, privatization, and cutbacks in public services, based on macroeconomic, market-based principles.

Contemporary European theory also influenced LASM. For instance, theoretical efforts in Italy on the work process have shaped the conceptual approach taken by the Mexican group in collaboration with industrial unions.[45] French psychoanalysis and institutional analysis have influenced the efforts of Argentine and Brazilian investigators in their studies of health services.[46] Philosophical advances in France, partly developed by Argentinians in exile, have informed the critique of ideologies in health policies and proposals for change.[47]

As noted already, the theory of health–illness as a dialectic process, developed initially by Asa Cristina Laurell and colleagues in Mexico, has generated criticisms of prior approaches to defining health and understanding its causes.[48] At a basic level, social medicine practitioners in Latin America have criticized mono-causal explanations of disease. Taking a perspective similar to Virchow's, they maintain that simplistic explanations by which a specific agent causes a specific disease do not adequately consider the social conditions that increase the likelihood of disease. However, even multi-causal models, such as those that consider the interactions among agent, host, and environment, still define disease in a relatively static fashion. Critiques from the standpoint of social medicine have argued that by dichotomizing the presence or absence of a disease, traditional multi-causal models do not adequately consider the dynamic linkages by which social conditions affect the dialectic process of health–illness. These analyses have suggested a more complex approach to causality, in which social and historical conditions receive more explicit emphasis.

Anticipating methodological trends in the United States and elsewhere, leaders in LASM have – since the mid-1970s – called for a multi-method approach that "triangulates" contemporary methods at both individual and societal levels of analysis. Even in early research, Mexican and Ecuadoran researchers combined quantitative, multivariate analyses with qualitative, in-depth interviews that they often conducted in group situations (so-called collective interviews).[49] Recent approaches to multilevel research have included quantitative techniques, such as structural equation modeling, combined with qualitative techniques, such as focus groups and computerized thematic analysis.[50]

Emerging Themes

Social medicine groups throughout Latin America have emphasized the effects on health of international policies under empire. Historically, this work has analyzed the extraction of raw materials and the exploitation of inexpensive labor. More recently, social medicine groups have focused on international macroeconomic policies, as well as the political power of multinational corporations and international financial institutions. The burden of foreign debt in the global South has emerged as a key concern. Public sector cutbacks, privatization of public services, and the opening of markets in health care to multinational corporations have received critical attention by social medicine groups in several countries. As one example, an assessment of managed care as a privatization initiative by multinational corporations and international financial institutions has emphasized the detrimental effects on access to services as the public sector "safety net" deteriorates and has demystified claims that market-oriented practices improve conditions for the poor.[51]

The social medicine groups have linked policy research with organizing efforts aimed at achieving progressive change in political systems. These actions aim to expand public debate and to redirect reform initiatives toward meeting the needs of vulnerable populations. For instance, social medicine groups have collaborated with the opposition Party of the Democratic Revolution, later the Movement for National Regeneration (Movimiento Regeneración Nacional, MORENA), and the Zapatista Army of National Liberation in Mexico; the coalition of indigenous and labor organizations in Ecuador; the Workers' Party in Brazil; and the Central Organization of Argentine Trade Unions.

Several groups have pioneered research on social and cultural determination of health–illness. Researchers in Ecuador have focused on urban ecology, economic changes stemming from petroleum production, and the relationship between gender and the work process in explaining morbidity and mortality patterns.[52] The Ecuadoran group has pioneered the use of multivariate, quantitative techniques to conduct multilevel research on social determinants, using data at the individual, social, and cultural units of analysis. Brazilian researchers have used multilevel and multi-method approaches – including anthropological, nonquantitative methods in epidemiology – to clarify mechanisms at the community, family, and biological levels that mediate the impact of social inequalities.[53]

This work emerges from a theoretical emphasis on economic production and reproduction, as well as a recognition that problems in these arenas represent some of the chief threats to health in countries of the global South. Mexican researchers have worked with industrial unions and local communities to clarify health and mental health problems that derive from the work process and environment. In this effort, the investigators have pioneered such methods as the collective interview mentioned earlier.[54] The Ecuadoran group has emphasized the differing health outcomes that women experience in industrial and agricultural work environments.[55] In Chile, the social medicine group has carried out research that links gender, work, and environmental conditions.[56] Research on the work process in Brazilian health institutions has informed the policy efforts of the national Workers' Party.[57]

Partly reflecting the violent conditions that practitioners of social medicine themselves have confronted, research on violence and trauma has received priority in several countries. In Colombia, the social tradition of violence – previously linked to poverty and cycles of rebellion, but more recently reflecting narcotics traffic and paramilitary operations – has generated research on the effects of violence on health outcomes.[58] Chilean investigators have studied families whose members experienced torture, exile, or death during the dictatorship.[59] Influenced by psychological studies of violence in El Salvador by Ignacio Martín-Baró, a U.S.-trained psychologist who himself was assassinated by paramilitary forces, researchers in Argentina have focused on the survivors among the more than 30,000 individuals who "disappeared" during the Argentine dictatorship.[60]

The Future of Latin American Social Medicine

While social medicine groups have achieved varying levels of influence on medical practice, public health programs, and medical education in their respective countries, they have pioneered a praxis that offers a standard for the future. For the most part, their work has not attained publication in English and remains little known outside Latin America. Wider knowledge of this work would prove helpful, not the least due to the courage of the individuals and groups that have continued their efforts under dangerous working conditions.

Practitioners of LASM have used theories and methods that distinguish their efforts from those of traditional public health. In particular, a focus on the social and historical contexts of health problems, an emphasis on economic production and social causation, and the linkage of research and education to political practice have provided innovative approaches to some of the most pressing problems of our age. Despite the challenges of struggling against the stream of dominant paradigms, the themes and findings of LASM have much to offer as medicine and public health throughout the world enter a period of profound transformation.

Indeed, the praxis of LASM provides a guide for an alternative future, especially in efforts of mutual aid and international solidarity.[61] Struggles oriented to social medicine show the contours of social reconstruction that increasingly will occur worldwide. As the exploitations of global capitalism and empire transform, along with ideas that have justified these exploitations, a new vision of medicine and public health is emerging, a vision based on solidarity and mutual support rather than exploitation and profit making.

Notes

1 Howard Waitzkin, *Medicine and Public Health at the End of Empire* (New York: Routledge, 2011), chapter 13, regarding praxis and other components of LASM in relation to empire. The following article explores the distinction between social medicine and collective health and devotes more attention to collective health in Brazil: Howard Waitzkin, Celia Iriart, Alfredo Estrada,

and Silvia Lamadrid, "Social Medicine in Latin America: Productivity and Dangers Facing the Major National Groups," *Lancet* 358 (2001): 315–23. For another helpful overview of LASM in the context of global heath, see Anne-Emanuelle Birn, Yogan Pillay, and Timothy H. Holtz, *Textbook of Global Health* (New York: Oxford University Press, 2017), chapters 3, 4, and 13. A trilingual collection of structured abstracts from LASM appears in the Latin American Social Medicine Collections, University of New Mexico, https://digitalrepository.unm.edu/lasm/; Howard Waitzkin, Celia Iriart, Holly Buchanan, Francisco Mercado, Jon Tregear, and Jonathan Eldredge, "The Latin American Social Medicine Database: a Resource for Epidemiology," *International Journal of Epidemiology* 37 (2008): 724–28.

2 For the distinction between global South and global North, we feel deeply indebted to the work of Samir Amin, who has illuminated the historical and contemporary importance of the exploited peripheries in the South and exploiting centers in the North. For instance, we try to extend Amin's recently expressed vision: "In the countries of the South, most people are victims of the system, whereas in the North, the majority are its beneficiaries.... The possible, but difficult, conjunction between the struggles of peoples in the South with those of peoples in the North is the only way to overcome the limitations of both." See Samir Amin, "Revolution from North to South," *Monthly Review* 69, no. 3 (July–August 2017): 113–27.

3 Waitzkin, *Medicine and Public Health at the End of Empire*, chapter 13.

4 Max Weber, *Max Weber on Capitalism, Bureaucracy, and Religion*, Stanislav Andreski, ed. (Boston: Allen & Unwin, 1983).

5 Saúl Franco and Everardo D. Nunes, "Presentación," in Saúl Franco, Everardo Nunes, Jaime Breilh, and Cristina Laurell, eds., *Debates en Medicina Social* (Quito: Organización Panamericana de la Salud, 1991), pp. 7–16.

6 Rudolf Virchow, *Gesammelte Abhandlungen aus dem Gebiet der Oeffentlichen Medicin und der Seuchenlehre* (Berlin: Hirschwald, 1879); *Letters to His Parents, 1839 to 1864* (Canton, MA: Science History Publications, 1990).

7 Howard Waitzkin, "Medicine and Social Change: Lessons from Chile and Cuba," in *The Second Sickness: Contradictions of Capitalist Health Care*, 2nd ed. (Lanham, MD: Rowman & Littlefield; 2000), chapter 7; María Angélica Illanes, *"En el Nombre del Pueblo, del Estado y de la Ciencia,...": Historia Social de la Salud Pública, Chile 1880–1973* (Santiago: Colectivo de Atención Primaria, 1993).

8 Daniela Estrada, "RIGHTS-CHILE: Workers' Massacre More Relevant Than Ever 100 Years On," Inter Press Service, December 8, 2007, http://www.ipsnews.net/2007/12/rights-chile-workersrsquo-massacre-more-relevant-than-ever-100-years-on/.

9 Salvador Allende, *La Realidad Médico-Social Chilena* (Santiago: Ministerio de Salubridad, 1939).

10 Howard Waitzkin and Hilary Modell, "Medicine, Socialism, and Totalitarianism: Lessons from Chile," *New England Journal of Medicine* 291 (1974): 171–77; Thomas J. Bossert and Thomas Leisewitz, "Innovation and Change in the Chilean Health System," *New England Journal of Medicine* 374 (2016): 1–5.

11 Franco and Nunes, "Presentación."

12 Wim Dierckxsens, *Capitalismo y Población: La Reproducción de la Fuerza de Trabajo Bajo el Capital* (San José: Editorial Universitaria Centroamericana, 1979); Raúl Rojas Soriano, *Capitalismo y Enfermedad* (Mexico City: Folios Ediciones, 1982), and *Sociología Médica* (Mexico City: Folios Ediciones, 1983).

13 Friedrich Engels, *Dialectics of Nature* (New York: International, 1940); Richard Levins and Richard Lewontin, *The Dialectical Biologist* (Cambridge, MA: Harvard University Press, 1985).

14 Jaime Breilh, "Componente de Metodología: La Construcción del Pensamiento en Medicina Social," in Saúl Franco, Everardo Nunes, Jaime Breilh, and Cristina Laurell, eds., *Debates en Medicina Social* (Quito: Organización Panamericana de la Salud, 1991).
15 Marcos Buchbinder, "Rol de lo Social en la Interpretación de los Fenómenos de Salud y Enfermedad en la Argentina," *Salud, Problema y Debate* (Buenos Aires, Argentina) 2, no. 4 (1990): 37–50.
16 Juan B. Justo, *Teoría y Práctica de la Historia* (Buenos Aires, Argentina: La Vanguardia, 1933).
17 Ernesto Che Guevara, "The Dilemma of What To Dedicate Myself To," in John Gerassi, ed., *Venceremos! The Speeches and Writings of Ernesto Che Guevara* (London: Weidenfeld & Nicholson, 1968).
18 Ernesto Che Guevara, "The Revolutionary Doctor," in John Gerassi, ed., *Venceremos! The Speeches and Writings of Ernesto Che Guevara* (London: Weidenfeld & Nicholson, 1968); Gordon Harper, "Ernesto Guevara, M.D.: Physician – Revolutionary Physician – Revolutionary," *New England Journal of Medicine* 281 (1969): 1285–89.
19 Francisco Lynch Guevara, personal communication, Buenos Aires, Argentina, 1995.
20 Eugenio Espejo, *Voto de un Ministro Togado de la Audiencia de Quito* (Quito: Comisión Nacional de Conmemoraciones Cívicas, 1994).
21 Pablo Arturo Suárez, *Contribución al Estudio de las Realidades entre las Clases Obreras y Campesinas* (Quito: Imprenta Fernández, 1934).
22 Ricardo Paredes, *Oro y Sangre en Portocavelo* (Quito: Editorial Artes Gráficas, 1938).
23 Mirta Z. Lobato and Adriana Álvarez, *Política, Médicos y Enfermedades: Lecturas de la Historia de la Salud en la Argentina* (Buenos Aires, Argentina: Editorial Biblos, 1996); Marcos Cueto, ed., *Salud, Cultura y Sociedad en América Latina* (Washington, DC: Organización Panamericana de la Salud – Instituto de Estudios Peruanos, 1996); Gilberto Hochman, *Aprendizado e Difusão na Constituição de Políticas: A Previdência Social e seus Técnicos* (Rio de Janeiro, Brazil: Instituto Universitário de Pesquisas do Rio de Janeiro, 1987); Eduardo Estrella, Antonio Crespo, and Doris Herrera, *Desarrollo Histórico de las Políticas de Salud en el Ecuador, 1967–1995* (Quito: Proyecto Análisis y Promoción de Políticas de Salud, 1997); Marcos Cueto, *El Regreso de las Epidemias: Salud y Sociedad en el Perú del Siglo XX* (Lima: Instituto de Estudios Peruanos, 1997); Anne-Emanuelle Birn, "Skirting the Issue: Women and International Health in Historical Perspective," *American Journal of Public Health* 89 (1999): 399–407.
24 Anne-Emanuelle Birn and Armando Solórzano, "Public Health Policy Paradoxes: Science and Politics in the Rockefeller Foundation's Hookworm Campaign in Mexico in the 1920s," *Social Science & Medicine* 49 (1999): 1197–213; E. Richard Brown, *Rockefeller Medicine Men* (Berkeley: University of California Press, 1979); Marcos Cueto, ed., *Missionaries of Science: The Rockefeller Foundation and Latin America* (Bloomington, IN: Indiana University Press, 1994); Saúl Franco-Agudelo, "The Rockefeller Foundation's Antimalarial Program in Latin America: Donating or Dominating?" *International Journal of Health Services* 13 (1983): 51–67.
25 Julie M. Feinsilver, *Healing the Masses: Cuban Health Politics at Home and Abroad*, (Berkeley: University of California Press, 1993); Howard Waitzkin, Karen Wald, Romina Kee, Ross Danielson, and Lisa Robinson, "Primary Care in Cuba: Low- and High-Technology Developments Pertinent to Family Medicine," *Journal of Family Practice* 45 (1997): 250–58; Waitzkin, "Medicine and

Social Change: Lessons from Chile and Cuba"; Don Fitz, *Cuban Health Care: The Ongoing Revolution* (New York: Monthly Review Press, 2020).
26 Waitzkin and Modell, "Medicine, Socialism, and Totalitarianism: Lessons from Chile"; Paul B. Cornely, et al., "Report of the APHA Task Force on Chile," *American Journal of Public Health* 67 (1977): 71–73.
27 Richard Garfield, *Health Care in Nicaragua: Primary Care under Changing Regimes* (New York: Oxford University Press, 1992); Richard M. Garfield, Thomas Frieden, Sten H. Vermund, "Health-Related Outcomes of War in Nicaragua," *American Journal of Public Health* 77 (1987): 615–18.
28 Frei Betto and Fidel Castro, *Fidel and Religion: Castro Talks on Revolution and Religion with Frei Betto* (New York: Simon and Schuster, 1987).
29 Camilo Torres, *Revolutionary Priest: The Complete Writings and Messages* (New York: Random House, 1971).
30 Paulo Freire, *Pedagogy of the Oppressed* (New York: Herder and Herder, 1970).
31 Nilson do Rosario Costa, "Transición y Movimientos Sociales: Contribuciones al Debate de la Reforma Sanitaria," *Cuadernos Médico Sociales* (Rosario, Argentina) 44 (1988): 51–61.
32 Paulo Freire, *Pedagogy of Freedom: Ethics, Democracy, and Civic Courage* (Lanham, MD: Rowman and Littlefield, 1998).
33 Nina Wallerstein and Edward Bernstein, "Empowerment Education: Freire's Ideas Adapted to Health Education," *Health Education Quarterly* 15 (1988): 379–94; Raúl Magaña, et al., "Una Pedagogia de Concientización para la Prevención del VIH/SIDA," *Revista Latino Americana de Psicología* 24, no. 1–2 (1992): 97–108.
34 Juan César García, *La Educación Médica en la América* (Washington, DC: Organización Panamericana de la Salud, 1972); *La Investigación en el Campo de la Salud en Once Países de la América Latina* (Washington, DC: Organización Panamericana de la Salud, 1982); *La Mortalidad de la Niñez Temprana Según Clases Sociales* (Medellín, Colombia: Universidad Pontífica Bolivariana, 1979); "The Laziness Disease," *History and Philosophy of the Life Sciences* 3, no. 1 (1981): 31–59.
35 Vicente Navarro, *Medicine under Capitalism* (New York: Prodist, 1977); *Dangerous to Your Health: Capitalism in Health Care* (New York: Monthly Review Press, 1993); "A Celebration of a Half a Century's Dedication to Relevance and Scholarship. A Note from the Founder and Editor-in-Chief, Professor Vicente Navarro," *International Journal of Health Services* 50, no. 1 (2020): 5–6.
36 Waitzkin, Iriart, Estrada, and Lamadrid, "Social Medicine in Latin America: Productivity and Dangers Facing the Major National Groups"; and "Social Medicine Then and Now: Lessons from Latin America," *American Journal of Public Health* 91 (2001): 1592–601; Waitzkin, Iriart, Buchanan, Mercado, Tregear, and Eldredge, "The Latin American Social Medicine Database." See also Debora Tajer, "Latin American Social Medicine: Roots, Development during the 1990s, and Current Challenges," *American Journal of Public Health* 93 (2003): 2023–27; Waitzkin, *Medicine and Public Health at the End of Empire*, chapter 13.
37 Saúl Franco, Everardo Nunes, Jaime Breilh, and Cristina Laurell, eds., *Debates en Medicina Social* (Quito: Organización Panamericana de la Salud, 1991).
38 Asa Cristina Laurell, "Social Analysis of Collective Health in Latin America," *Social Science & Medicine* 28 (1989): 1183–91.
39 Antonio Gramsci, *The Prison Notebooks* (New York: International, 1971); Saúl Franco, "Tendencias de la Medicina Social en América Latina," in Jaime Sepúlveda et al., eds., *Actualización en Medicina Social* (Santiago, Chile: GICAMS, 1989).

40 José Carlos Escudero, "Salud–Ecología– Política," *Salud y Cambio* 2, no. 3 (1991): 8–20.
41 Asa Cristina Laurell, "Trabajo y Salud: Estado del Conocimiento," in Saúl Franco, Everardo Nunes, Jaime Breilh, and Cristina Laurell, eds., *Debates en Medicina Social* (Quito: Organización Panamericana de la Salud, 1991).
42 Jaime Breilh, *Epidemiología: Economía, Medicina y Política* (Mexico City: Fontamara, 1989); Jaime Breilh, *Género, Poder y Salud* (Quito: Centro de Estudios y Asesoría en Salud, 1993); Jaime Breilh and Edmundo Granda, "La Epidemiología en la Forja de una Contrahegemonía," *Salud Problema* (Mexico City) 11 (1986): 25–40; Jaime Breilh and Edmundo Granda, "Epidemiología y Contrahegemonía," *Social Science & Medicine* 28 (1989): 1121–27.
43 Asa Cristina Laurell, "Mortality and Working Conditions in Agriculture in Underdeveloped Countries," *International Journal of Health Services* 11 (1981): 3–20; Asa Cristina Laurell, Mariano Noriega, Oliva López, and Victor Ríos, La Experiencia Obrera Como Fuente de Conocimiento: Confrontación de Resultados de la Encuesta Colectiva e Individual," *Cuadernos Medico-Sociales* 51 (1990): 5–26.
44 Mario Testa, *Saber en Salud: La Construcción del Conocimiento* (Buenos Aires, Argentina: Lugar Editorial, 1997); Emerson Merhy and Rosana Onocko, eds., *Agir em Saúde* (São Paulo, Brazil: Hucitec, 1997).
45 Asa Cristina Laurell, "La Salud-Enfermedad Como Proceso Social," *Revista Latinoamericana de Salud* 2 (1982): 7–25; Mario Testa, *Pensar en Salud* (Buenos Aires, Argentina: Lugar Editorial, 1993).
46 Testa, *Saber en Salud*; Merhy and Onocko, eds., *Agir em Saúde*.
47 Miguel Benasayag and Edith Charlton, *Esta Dulce Certidumbre de Lo Peor* (Buenos Aires: Nueva Visión, 1994).
48 Juan Samaja, "La Triangulación Metodológica: Pasos para una Comprensión Dialéctica de la Combinación de Métodos," in Francisco Rojas Ochoa y Miguel Márquez, eds., *ALAMES en la Memoria*: Selección de Lecturas (Havana: ALAMES, Cuba, and Editorial Caminos, 2009); Asa Cristina Laurell, "Lasting Lessons from Social Ideas and Movements of the Sixties on Latin American Public Health," *American Journal of Public Health* 108 (2018): 730–31.
49 Asa Cristina Laurell, et al., "Disease and Rural Development: A Sociological Analysis of Morbidity in Two Mexican Villages," *International Journal of Health Services* 7 (1977): 401–23; Jaime Breilh, Edmundo Granda, Arturo Campaña, and Oscar Betancourt, *Ciudad y Muerte Infantil* (Quito: Ediciones CEAS, 1983).
50 Jaime Breilh, *Nuevos Conceptos y Técnicas de Investigación* (Quito: Centro de Estudios y Asesoría en Salud, 1995); Alexis J. Handal, et al., "Occupational Exposure to Pesticides during Pregnancy and Neurobehavioral Development of Infants and Toddlers," *Epidemiology* 19 (2008): 851–59. For an update on Breilh's pathbreaking work in social epidemiology, see: Jaime Breilh, *Critical Epidemiology and the People's Health* (New York: Oxford University Press, 2020, in press).
51 Karen Stocker, Howard Waitzkin, and Celia Iriart, "The Exportation of Managed Care to Latin America," *New England Journal of Medicine* 340 (1999): 1131–36; Celia Iriart, Emerson Merhy, and Howard Waitzkin, "Managed Care in Latin America: the New Common Sense in Health Policy Reform," *Social Science & Medicine* 52 (2001): 1243–53; Celia Iriart, "La Reforma del Sector Salud en Argentina: De la Salud como Derecho Social a Bien Público a Responsabilidad Individual y Bien de Mercado," in Centro de Estudios y Asesoría en Salud, *Reforma en Salud: Lo Privado o lo Solidario* (Quito: CEAS, 1997); Jaime Breilh, "Reforma: Democracia Profunda, No Retroceso Neoliberal," in Centro de Estudios y Asesoría en Salud, *Reforma en Salud: Lo Privado o lo Solidario* (Quito:

CEAS, 1997); Emerson Merhy, Celia Iriart, and Howard Waitzkin, "Atenção Gerenciada: Da Micro-Decisão Corporativa à Micro-Decisão Administrativa, um Caminho Igualmente Privatizante?" in Haino Bursmester, ed., *Managed Care: Alternativas de Gestão em Saúde* (São Paulo, Brazil: Editora PROAHSA/ Editora Fundação Getulio Vargas, 1998); Asa Cristina Laurell and María Elena Ortega, "The Free Trade Agreement and the Mexican Health Sector," *International Journal of Health Services* 22 (1992): 331–37; Asa Cristina Laurell, "Three Decades of Neoliberalism in Mexico: The Destruction of Society," *International Journal of Health Services* 45 (2015): 246–64.

52 Colectivo CEAS, *Mujer, Trabajo y Salud*, (Quito: Ediciones CEAS, 1994); Oscar Betancourt, *La Salud y el Trabajo* (Quito: Centro de Estudios y Asesoría en Salud y Organización Panamericana de la Salud, 1995); Handal, "Occupational Exposure to Pesticides during Pregnancy and Neurobehavioral Development of Infants and Toddlers."

53 Naomar de Almeida Filho, *Epidemiología sin Números* (Washington, DC: Organización Panamericana de la Salud, 1992).

54 Asa Cristina Laurell, "The Role of Union Democracy in the Struggle for Workers' Health in Mexico," *International Journal of Health Services* 19 (1989): 279–93; Laurell, et al., "Disease and Rural Development."

55 Colectivo CEAS, *Mujer, Trabajo y Salud;* Betancourt, *La Salud y el Trabajo.*

56 Sonia Montecino, "Madres Niñas, Madresolas, Continuidad o Cambio Cultural?" *Salud y Cambio* (Santiago, Chile), 4, no. 11 (1993): 6–8.

57 Túlio Franco, Wanderlei Silva Bueno, and Emerson Merhy, "O Acolhimento e os Processos de Trabalho em Saúde: O Caso de Betim, Minas Gerais, Brasil," *Cadernos de Saúde Pública* (Rio de Janeiro) 15, no. 2 (1999): 345–53.

58 Saúl Franco, "International Dimensions of Colombian Violence," *International Journal of Health Serv*ice 30 (2000): 163–85; "A Social-Medical Approach to Violence in Colombia," *American Journal of Public Health* 93 (2003): 2032–36.

59 Alfredo Estrada, Mónica Hering, and Andrés Donoso, *Familia, Género y Terapia: Una Experiencia de Terapia Familiar Sistémica* (Santiago, Chile: Ediciones CODEPU, 1997).

60 Ignacio Martín-Baró, *Writings for a Liberation Psychology* (Cambridge, MA: Harvard University Press, 1994); "La Violencia en Centroamérica: Una Visión Psicosocial," *Salud, Problema y Debate* (Buenos Aires, Argentina) 2, no. 4 (1990): 53–66; Alicia Stolkiner, "Tiempos "Posmodernos": Ajuste y Salud Mental," in Hugo Cohen, et al., eds., *Políticas en Salud Mental* (Buenos Aires, Argentina: Lugar Editorial, 1994); Alicia Stolkiner, "Human Rights and the Right to Health in Latin America: The Two Faces of One Powerful Idea," *Social Medicine* 5 (2010): 58–63.

61 Anne-Emanuelle Birn and Carles Muntaner, "Latin American Social Medicine across Borders: South-South Cooperation and the Making of Health Solidarity," *Global Public Health* 14 (2019): 817–34, doi:10.1080/17441692.2018.1439517.

Chapter 9

Social Medicine and the Micro-politics of Medical Encounters

How Society Impinges on the Medical Encounter

During the Great Depression in 1935, the playwright Clifford Odets captured some key themes that still apply nearly nine decades later. In *Waiting for Lefty*, Dr. Benjamin – a medical resident in a large urban hospital – tries to diagnose and treat his patients supportively.[1] Through his work, he finds that broader social problems limit his relationship with his patients. Due to financial deficits, the hospital's board of directors decides to close yet another charity ward, where low-income patients previously could receive urgent services at a reduced cost. "Benj" soon learns that financial considerations govern the policies that affect not only the hospital but also the larger health care system of which he is a part.

As he becomes more dispirited about the possibilities for humane relationships with his patients, Benj reads about what appear to be more favorable possibilities under socialized medicine in the Soviet Union. He fantasizes that, there, his capabilities as a healer could be fulfilled with less social impediment. In the end, though, Benj opts to struggle within the United States. He enters political work in his minimal free time. Although he commits himself to the struggle, he also recognizes his own apprehension about the difficulties and uncertainties involved: "No! Our work's here – America! I'm scared... What future's ahead, I don't know."

Even today, as we will see in this chapter, those who work at the front lines of medicine cope with the same kinds of challenges, which during recent years have emerged as an important part of social medicine.

The Human Experience of Access Barriers

Barriers to health care access have become ever more pervasive in the United States, even after the enactment of the Affordable Care Act (ACA, Obamacare) in 2010. These barriers prevent patients from receiving needed services but also impose fundamental ethical problems for doctors and other health workers who find themselves unable to solve problems that sometimes lead to patients' deaths or continuing disabilities. Medical professionals have to deal with these barriers throughout their careers. As practitioners, the authors have shared with patients, students, and colleagues the anguish of not being able to receive or to provide needed services, due to the lack of suitable public policies. To put a human face to the troubling statistic data on access barriers, we give you the following stories. These are experiences of patients who have seen Howard Waitzkin personally in the practice of primary care and social medicine, or who have been seen by faculty members, residents, and students with whom he has worked.[2]

Medicaid is a national program in the United States that aims to ensure access to care for eligible, low-income people. The Medicaid program covers individuals with dependent children, those who are disabled, and many people in nursing homes. To be eligible, a person must earn a monthly income that falls below the level of poverty as determined by the state and federal governments.[3] However, U.S. citizens suffer from cutbacks and increased co-payments under Medicaid.

- *A 31-year-old diabetic and legally blind man began to experience severe unilateral headaches but could not afford a computerized tomographic (CT) scan of the head because his monthly deductible under Medicaid (which he was required to pay out of pocket each month) increased from $50 to $250. He was later brought – delirious – to the emergency room (ER), where an emergency CT scan revealed a brain tumor with poor prognosis. At his death, his physicians felt the tumor may have been resected successfully if he had received attention earlier, when his severe headaches first began.*

Some patients do not meet eligibility for Medicaid but have an income below the state-defined poverty limit. The Medically Indigent Adult (MIA) program helps to cover these adults. To help reduce costs, state governments decentralized the MIA programs to the county level during the early 1980s. States and counties vary widely in services provided and in co-payments, and there are many restrictions. Under Obamacare, some states expanded their Medicaid programs to cover more MIA patients, but other states did not.

- *A 63-year-old man with hypertension, renal insufficiency, and prostate enlargement causing urinary obstruction could not gain approval from the county's MIA program for a prostatectomy because it was considered an elective procedure. His urinary obstruction and renal function gradually worsened. When he finally required dialysis, he became eligible for federal Medicare benefits. The massive cost of dialysis (more than $100,000 per year) probably would have been avoided if he had received the prostatectomy.*

- *A 44-year-old man had malignant melanoma, confirmed by limited biopsy with incomplete excision. Outpatient surgery for wider resection was delayed for more than three months by MIA eligibility procedures, again because the procedure was considered elective. By the time that the biopsy was performed, the melanoma had metastasized widely, and the patient subsequently died.*

If patients have private insurance, many establish relationships with physicians who have followed them for many years. Yet, a patient can lose health insurance for many different reasons: losing a job that provides health insurance, having an employer who decides not to provide insurance, divorce or death of a spouse whose job provided insurance, geographic relocation, or other such changes in circumstance. When a patient loses insurance, his or her provider may decide to stop seeing the patient, because of concern about getting paid. "Abandonment" is the legal principle by which a doctor cannot refuse to see a previous patient, unless a suitable substitute is arranged and the patient agrees to the change.[4] However, neither governmental agencies nor professional organizations enforce these principles if a doctor refuses to see a previous patient due to loss of insurance.

- *A 44-year-old unemployed woman was followed by her physician for about eight years because of complex regional pain syndrome, a very painful condition of her legs and feet that periodically required low doses of a narcotic and a tranquilizer for symptomatic relief. When the patient went through a divorce, she lost her husband's insurance coverage. Shortly thereafter, her long-term physician informed her that he could no longer see her because she lacked insurance. Several months passed, during which she could not receive the needed treatment, until she could find a new physician to see her.*

One of the most troubling effects of access barriers in the United States involves premature deaths that could have been avoided if people could obtain the care that they needed. In our experience, such tragedies arise most commonly when patients cannot find appropriate services for the diagnosis and treatment of cancer. When symptoms of cancer arise, such patients experience critical delays, with disastrous effects on the eventual outcome of their disease. As mentioned earlier, problems in services can arise for patients despite coverage by public insurance. Barriers become especially grim, however, when patients lack insurance altogether.

- *A 48-year-old Japanese American woman ran her own small landscape-gardening business. Due to the high cost of individual health insurance policies, she decided to remain uninsured. After noticing a breast lump, she delayed seeking care. She did not have a regular doctor, was worried about the expense, and was hopeful that the mass would just disappear. When*

> the mass continued to grow after three months, she began to seek care from private physicians but was denied services because she was uninsured. After six months, she eventually found care at a community clinic. Evaluation for metastatic disease was arranged by special request with a nuclear medicine facility at a university hospital – without the personal intervention of her physicians and the donation of specialty services, the appropriate scan would not have been done. The scan revealed extensive metastatic cancer. Her chemotherapy was also delayed because of access barriers. Within six months, the patient died.

Another barrier to access involves homelessness. Homeless patients often are not able to obtain treatment for serious medical problems, including infectious diseases like tuberculosis that threaten the health of the general community. Despite their poverty, homeless people experience difficulty in getting needed care under public, government-run insurance programs. For example, many programs require an address to ensure that the expenses of care are assigned to the correct county or other governmental unit. Because they cannot provide an address, homeless people frequently cannot obtain public coverage.

- *A 38-year-old uninsured, homeless man was admitted to a university hospital from the ER because of active pulmonary tuberculosis. He had come to the ER because he was coughing up blood. During a week of hospitalization, he was treated with three antibiotics until his sputum was free of infectious organisms. Due to financial problems, the hospital recently had initiated a policy that outpatient prescriptions would not be filled unless they were paid for directly by the patient or were chargeable to public or private insurance. For this reason, the patient was asked to travel after discharge to the county health department for his outpatient prescriptions to continue the necessary treatment. However, the patient did not find transportation and, consequently, did not receive his medication. Four weeks later, he again developed bloody sputum and was re-admitted for tuberculosis. This time, his treatment became more complicated since he had developed medication-resistant organisms due to the interruption in antibiotic treatment.*

Similarly, undocumented immigrants often struggle to find adequate care because they do not have a government-issued identification. Furthermore, they are often not covered by most public programs. Undocumented immigrants contribute substantially to the economic productivity of the United States, especially in the West and Southwest regions, and pay much more in taxes than they receive in public benefits.[5] Although they tend to be healthier and to utilize health care services less than age-matched U.S. citizens, they have few options for care when illness strikes and are specifically excluded from Obamacare.[6]

- *A 31-year-old undocumented man from Mexico presented with carpal tunnel syndrome of his right hand that interfered with his work as a tailor. The patient and his family had noticed that his hands, feet, and facial features had been growing in size over several years. He had worked and had taxes deducted from his pay at a local clothing factory for the past 18 years. After a medical resident coordinated an in-depth evaluation, acromegaly associated with a pituitary tumor was diagnosed. But the needed treatment of radiation therapy or neurosurgery could not be arranged because of financial impediments. After waiting nearly three months, the patient was lost to follow-up when he returned to Mexico.*

The following two patients show the special problems of working people who lose their insurance because of job loss. They also illustrate psychosocial issues that practitioners and patients find especially challenging.

- *A 55-year-old man who served as an office worker in a small horticultural company lost his job after 25 years with the same firm. One month later, he lost his health insurance, which had been provided as a fringe benefit of employment. After another month, he suddenly passed out and was taken to a county hospital because his private physician refused to see him without insurance. Upper gastrointestinal hemorrhage from a bleeding duodenal ulcer, with resulting loss of consciousness, was diagnosed. After treatment with transfusions and medications, the patient slowly recovered. Nearly one year after losing his job, the patient found employment again as an office worker, received insurance coverage, and returned to his former physician for care.*
- *A 53-year-old receptionist and clerical worker was not working partly because of symptoms of pain and limited mobility that were associated with osteoarthritis and premature osteoporosis. She relied on the insurance coverage of her husband, the patient in the last case summary. About three months after he lost his job, she fell and fractured her forearm and wrist. Her private physician would not see her, due to lack of insurance coverage. She was taken to a county hospital, where resident physicians who did not receive supervision tried to realign the fractures, but she was left with a deformity.*

These last two patients deeply influenced one of the authors' commitments in primary care and social medicine: They were Howard Waitzkin's own parents. They experienced these problems just as he was completing residency training in internal medicine. They were proud people, who worked hard throughout their lives and were very reluctant to accept public welfare or insurance programs. They did not want help in contacting their physicians or the hospital staff where they were taken, since they viewed their problems as their own responsibility. At various times, they expressed the view that they somehow deserved the misfortunes that had befallen them, because they had not found a way to attend college during and after the Great Depression.

These and the earlier patients' experiences illustrate two central themes of social medicine regarding barriers to health care access in the United States and some other countries. First, these barriers involve fundamental issues of personal dignity. The difficulties in obtaining access to care degrade the individuals and families involved, at a time when they are most in need. Personal dignity requires more from social policy than yet has been achieved in the United States.

Second, such problems can happen to anyone, largely as a matter of luck. Severe illness can strike people who have lived their lives in accord with the mainstream standards of their communities. When misfortune arises, the United States does not provide a "safety net" that assures access to basic medical services. Further, these problems do not only affect poor people and members of minority groups, although their impact is particularly severe for such individuals and families. Instead, barriers to access can exert unpredictable and devastating effects for a large part of the U.S. population, including a substantial part of the middle class.

Patient–Doctor Relationships in the Era of Managed Care

As managed care has expanded, it has transformed the patient–doctor relationship. This transformation has occurred rapidly, with little preparation for either clinicians or patients. From the standpoint of social medicine, an assessment of managed care's impact should consider effects on the patient–doctor relationship.

Managed care is difficult to define, since it encompasses diverse organizational structures. However, it generally refers to administrative control over the organization and practice of health services through large corporations. Historically, managed care has included such prepaid approaches as health maintenance organizations (HMOs), preferred provider organizations (PPOs), and proposals for national programs such as the ACA.[7] Managed care assumes that quality is assured through administrative control and through competition in the marketplace. Although problems in patient–doctor relationships preceded the growth of managed care, the characteristics of managed care both worsen old problems and create new ones. The characteristics of managed care organizations (MCOs) differ, but in general their structural features introduce strain in the patient–doctor relationship.

Advocates of managed care often claim that this method of organizing services can and should improve the patient–doctor relationship. For instance, the MCOs generally assign patients to a single primary care physician, who presumably can provide continuity of care and help improve the coordination of services. The primary care provider can communicate about preventive services and screenings and can encourage their utilization. Since managed care services are mostly paid in advance through monthly capitation payments, the predictability of co-payments required for each outpatient visit may also reduce financial barriers to access for some patients.

Not a single research project, however, has conclusively demonstrated improved patient–doctor communication processes or patient satisfaction in managed care systems. The limited studies comparing communication and satisfaction in the managed care and fee-for-service sectors have found no difference or observations not favorable to managed care.[8] Meanwhile, the adverse impacts of managed care on communication processes and the patient–doctor relationship have received wide attention in influential editorials, position papers, and the public media.[9] Further, the claimed advantages of managed care in the arenas of communication and interpersonal relationships have not been assessed in detail for subgroups of enrollees, including minorities, the poor, non-English speakers, the elderly, and the chronically ill.

Managed care refers to primary care practitioners as "gatekeepers."[10] That is, such physicians tend the gate – keeping it closed for expensive procedures, referrals to specialists, or emergency visits and opening it only when absolutely necessary for preservation of life or limb. In carefully tending the gate, physicians and their bosses in for-profit MCOs keep or invest in global financial markets enough of the patients' capitation payments to generate large profits and accumulation of capital unprecedented in health care.[11]

Since the 1980s, from the social medicine perspective, the medical profession has become "proletarianized," which involves a sharp change in a doctor's previous social class position.[12] Proletarianization refers to a loss of professional autonomy and a conversion of health professionals into workers who no longer control the conditions of medical practice. Until the 1980s, doctors for the most part owned and/or controlled their means of production and conditions of practice. Although their work often was challenging, they could decide their hours of work, the staff members who worked with them, how much time to spend with patients, what to write about their visits in medical records, and how much to charge for their services.

Now, the corporations for which doctors work as employees usually control those decisions. Loss of control over the conditions of work has caused much unhappiness and burnout in the profession. Early on, an esteemed clinician and mentor described medical proletarianization when it was first emerging as "working on the factory floor."[13] Most doctors, about 70 percent, have become employees of MCOs or health system corporations that have adopted the same approach as MCOs to management practices.[14] Forty to fifty percent of doctors report feeling burned out due to the stresses of their work as employees, and the proportion is higher among women physicians than among men.[15] Burnout has worsened since the COVID-19 pandemic, when the risks to health and financial stability have increased even more the day-to-day stress of frontline health professionals.[16]

Due to the mystique of professionalism and relatively high salaries, doctors often do not realize that their discontent reflects in large part their changing social class position. Through the proletarianization and deprofessionalization of health care workers, "alienation" arises in the work process of clinical care. Here we refer to Marx's concept of alienation, which involves the separation of the worker from the control over work conditions and the product of his or her labor. The medical clinician now must learn what it means to become an employee. In the words of Marx: "The object which labor produces – labor's product – confronts it as *something alien*, as a *power independent* of the producer."[17]

Changes in the medical record contribute to professionals' alienation and deeply affect communication between patients and doctors. During the 1990s, work was advancing in the United States toward the creation of a unified national electronic medical record (EMR) system, which would have been not-for-profit and in the public sector. The national health programs of several European countries had adopted the not-for-profit, public sector approach for their EMR systems.

However, in the United States, the George W. Bush administration initiated a large federal initiative to promote the use of health technology and, specifically, EMRs created by for-profit corporations. Another member of the Bush family, Jonathan Bush, was a prime mover in fostering EMRs as a major new source of private profit making; he later became a multibillionaire as the chief executive officer of Athena, one of the largest EMR corporations. This initiative received further impetus during the first year of the Obama administration, when medical practices were given incentives to purchase EMR systems under the American Recovery and Reinvestment Act, the 2009 stimulus package.[18] EMRs became a new, federally subsidized profit center, and dozens of for-profit vendors came forth to sell their EMR software to clinicians. The result, ironically, is that health information in the United States has become even more fragmented. Now practitioners experience a bewildering variety of EMR systems, none of which talks to each other; within individual institutions, there are often several different types of EMRs, sold in the for-profit marketplace.

EHR* STATE OF MIND

http://zdoggmd.com/ehr-state-of-mind/

This popular video, featuring internist and hospitalist Zubin Damania, MD (also known as ZDoggMD), captures doctors' and patients' frustrations with the EMR. Ironically, AthenaHealth – the corporation that produced one of the most profitable EMRs under the leadership of Jonathan Bush – sponsored the video as a public relations and advertising tactic.

* "EHR" stands for electronic health record, which means the same as "EMR."

Troubling features of EMRs impact patient–doctor communication. Most EMR systems were designed to capture billing and quality information, not to facilitate clinical care. As a result, clinicians, rather than looking at their patients, sit hunched over their computers, clicking little boxes to summarize what happens in the medical encounter or to document discussion of preventive measures, such as whether they have advised their patients to get a colonoscopy or not to smoke. The transformation of medical records from a narrative about patients' experiences to a standardized process that involves clicking boxes has become a process that worsens even further the alienated labor of health professionals. As one of Matt Anderson's frustrated patients told him: "I used to talk to my doctor; now I just see the back of his head."[19] There is no particular reason behind the flow of the clinical interview, since it now follows computer-generated prompts that guide a doctor to work one's way through the required screens with the required answers. Not only is the voice of the doctor gone in many EMRs, but, more crucially, so is the voice of the patient. In a menu-driven EMR, clinical histories are reduced to a collection of facts taken out of context: *left abdominal pain/quality: crampy/duration: 2–4 days/relieved by: defecation*. Electronic standardization transforms the essential task of understanding the patient's experience, to assist in diagnosis and treatment.

"Double agent" has become another compelling way in social medicine to think about physicians' role under managed care, as pointed out by Marcia Angell, a former editor of the *New England Journal of Medicine*, and others.[20] While physicians continue to present themselves as advocates for patients, they in actuality work as double agents – for both patients and MCOs. The MCOs hold interests that are often very different from those of patients.

However, referring to doctors as double agents in the context of managed care does not adequately convey the conflict. For example, in one of many similar incidents, Howard Waitzkin as a primary care physician spent nearly a day advocating for a single patient, a 58-year-old psychologist with a displaced fracture of her elbow, to various bureaucrats working in a major MCO. The goal was to convince them that she really did need an orthopedic appointment today rather than in three weeks and also really needed surgery within three days rather than the indefinite future. Yet, the passion that leads some clinicians to struggle on behalf of patients appears to be burning out, since such time-consuming tasks generate little apparent benefit for either the patient or the physician. Because the struggle to obtain services for patients is so inconvenient, an incentive arises not to pursue the matter vigorously; this constraint decreases the probability that the patient will receive services, even when they are needed.

Physicians participating in managed care rarely, if ever, explain to patients that their own financial earnings under a capitation arrangement often improve when they limit services such as diagnostic tests, expensive treatments, and specialty consultations. MCOs also do not communicate this conflict of interest to patients whom they seek to enroll. Some MCOs have even required their physician employees to follow "gag rules." These rules explicitly have prohibited physicians under contract from disclosing a range of diagnostic or treatment options to patients when the administrators of the organization do not approve. In other words, under managed care, physicians' income may be related to how little they do. This structural condition is in direct conflict with physicians' responsibilities under the Hippocratic Oath and other ethical norms, which call for prioritization of the patient's welfare above all other concerns.

Seen from the patients' viewpoint, contracts that forbid a physician to reveal the full range of treatment options or diagnostic techniques violate patients' rights, particularly the right to informed consent. The legal doctrine of informed consent requires physicians to explain to their patient all the choices available, the risks and benefits of the proposed treatment, and any alternatives. Because a patient's access to this information is restricted as a result of managed care rules, informed consent is not achieved and the patient is put at risk. Disturbingly, patients are often unaware that such rules even exist and, therefore, falsely assume that they are receiving all the relevant information to give informed consent for a procedure. Indeed, informed consent could not be obtained because the patient is not given all the necessary information to make a consensual decision. In addition, the consent is obtained under false pretenses: Patients believe that they are given all the information because it is the physician's responsibility to do so.

These constraints have led to a strange and ethically difficult situation in which patients remain naive about the financial motivations that underlie many clinical decisions.[21] In some ways, this naiveté has become reminiscent of the ignorance and lack of information that physicians formerly maintained for patients who developed cancer or other fatal illnesses. Physicians used to assume that revealing a professional inability to cure would prove deleterious to patients' morale, and so patients often remained in the dark even when they strongly wanted to know.[22] This norm has changed over recent decades, partly in response to the demands of the consumer movement and parallel struggles for full information within the women's and civil rights movements.[23]

In recognition of ethical dilemmas that gag rules impose, consumer rights organizations have advocated their abolition. As a response, the federal government eventually banned explicit gag rules for MCOs participating in the national Medicare and Medicaid programs. In addition, patients' rights laws in many but not all states have extended this ban to private managed care plans. However, even when formal gag clauses are eliminated from physicians' contracts with MCOs, the financial motivations that MCOs frequently impose on physicians to limit their services maintain a subtle pressure that restricts the communication of diagnostic and therapeutic options.[24] Under these circumstances, although formal gag clauses appear less frequently, the financial conditions that encourage less than full communication have persisted.

Many clinicians feel uncomfortable with this moral anomaly and become frustrated with MCOs influencing their clinical decisions, even when they may benefit from their role as a gatekeeper. After all, MCOs dictate what services, procedures, and medications a patient can obtain even when a physician's recommendations may differ. Beyond that, MCOs may limit when a patient can seek the care that is needed. The following encounters illustrate some generic issues that manifest themselves under managed care.

- *A 58-year-old male physics professor, insured by his university's new self-insured managed care program, developed severe substernal chest pain at 1 a.m. during a Thanksgiving holiday weekend. The patient called the on-call primary care internist to approve a visit to the ER, as he had been instructed to do so when he signed up for the plan. The on-call physician had covered more than 30 patients on the inpatient wards, in the intensive care units, and by phone that day for his colleagues. He had just managed to catch some much-needed sleep when the patient called. As he was also hard of hearing, he did not wake up until a half hour after the patient called, when the answering service again tried to reach him. By that time, the patient had left for the ER because of continuing pain. When the patient arrived, his electrocardiogram (EKG) revealed a large myocardial infarction. If the patient had waited for the approval as he was supposed to do, he would have arrived too late for treatment with the medication streptokinase that helped break up the clot in his coronary arteries.*
- *A 25-year-old Spanish-speaking woman who was a hospital custodial worker obtained the cheapest MCO coverage that was possible through her job. She went to the ER during her shift at 3:00 a.m., on the same night as the previous case, with a sore throat and a fever of 101 degrees. Because she had not realized that she was supposed to call the on-call physician for permission, the ER staff called the same physician, again, waking him up. The physician was mad at being awoken solely for this bureaucratic reason and asked to speak with the patient (fortunately, the physician could speak Spanish). He realized the problem could wait until daytime, so he did not approve the ER visit. The patient complained that it would be difficult to come during the day because of child care responsibilities, but she could not persuade the physician to approve the visit, since he had been instructed not to approve such visits for minor outpatient problems.*

The two patients in the above case summaries, based on Howard Waitzkin's clinical practice in primary care and social medicine, show the limitations that managed care imposes on individual discretion. In the first case, the patient – though knowledgeable about the rule that ER visits must be preapproved – overrode that constraint through a judgment decision about the urgency of his symptoms. As it later became clear, his background as a scientist and educator contributed to his choice to take action without the gatekeeper's permission, a decision that may have saved his life. The second patient acted from a position of ignorance about the structural constraints of a plan in which she enrolled and could not provide a convincing-enough argument to accomplish her own preferences to be seen sooner rather than later. In neither case did the constraints imposed by managed care's gatekeeping principles conform with a close and trusting patient–doctor encounter, in which the patient's preferences should guide the course of care in a predictable way.

Social Context and Patient–Doctor Communication

The social context of the medical encounter raises important issues for social medicine, especially in the setting of managed care. The following encounter, recorded in a study of patient–doctor communication in primary care, conveys an elderly woman's loss of home, community, and autonomy.

- *An elderly woman visited her physician for follow-up of her heart disease. During the encounter, she expressed concern about her decreased vision, her ability to continue driving, lack of stamina and strength, weight loss and diet, and financial problems. She discussed her recent move to a new home and her relationships with family and friends. Her physician assured her that her health was improving; he recommended that she continue her current medical regimen and that she see an ophthalmologist.*

    From the questionnaires that the patient and the physician completed after their interaction, some pertinent information was available: The patient was an 81-year-old high-school graduate. She was Protestant, Scottish American, and widowed. She had five living children whose ages ranged from 45 to 59, and she described herself as a "homemaker." She recently moved from the home that she had lived in for 59 years. The reasons for giving up her home remained unclear, but they seemed to involve a combination of financial factors and difficulties in maintaining it.

    The physician is a 44-year-old male who is a general internist. The physician had known the patient for about one year and believed that her primary diagnoses were atherosclerotic heart disease and prior congestive heart failure. The encounter took place in a suburban private practice near Boston.

During silent periods in the physical examination of the patient's heart and lungs, the patient spontaneously mentioned more details about the loss of possessions and relationships with previous neighbors, along with satisfaction about certain conveniences of her new living situation. As the patient spoke, the physician asked clarifying questions about the move and gave several pleasant fillers, before he cut off this discussion by helping the patient from the examination table.

PATIENT: *I sold a lot of my stuff.*
DOCTOR: *Yeah, how did the moving go?*
PATIENT: *And y'know, take forty-ni... fifty-nine years' accumulation. Boy, and I've got cartons in my closet it'll take me till doomsday to... ouch!*
DOCTOR: *Gotcha!*
PATIENT: *But I've been kept out of mischief by doing it. But I've got a lot to do, I sold my rugs cause they wouldn't fit where I am. I just got a piece of plain cloth at home.*
DOCTOR: *Mmhmm.*
PATIENT: *Sometimes I think I'm foolish at eighty-one. I don't know how long I'll live. Isn't much point in putting money into stuff, and then, why not enjoy a little bit of life? And I've got to have draperies made.*
DOCTOR: *Now then, you're...*
PATIENT: *But that'll come. I'm not worrying. I got an awfully cute place. It's very, very comfortable. All electric kitchen. It's got a better bathroom than I ever had in my life.*
DOCTOR: *Great! Met any of your neighbors there yet?*
PATIENT: *Oh, I met two or three. And my... some of my neighbors from Belmont here, there's Mrs. F – and her two sisters are up to see me, spent the afternoon with me day before yesterday. And all my neighbors, um, holler down the hall. They're comin', so they say. So I'm hopin' they will. I hated to move, cause I loved, um, I liked my neighbors very much.*
DOCTOR: *Now, we'll get you down. You watch your step.*
PATIENT: *You're not gonna let me, uh, disrobe today?*
DOCTOR: *Don't have to, I think.*
PATIENT: *Well!*
DOCTOR: *Your heart sounds good.*
PATIENT: *It does?*
DOCTOR: *Yep.*

After the physician mentioned briefly that the patient's heart "sounds good," he and the patient moved on to other topics. Probably unintentionally, the physician's cutoff and return to a technical assessment of cardiac function marginalized the patient's loss of home and community.

From the patient's perspective, the move held several meanings. First, her new living situation, an apartment (she mentioned a hallway), contained several physical features that she viewed as more convenient, or at least "cute." On the other hand, she apparently has sold many of her possessions, which carried the memories of 59 years in the same house.

Further, she felt the need to decorate her new home but doubted the wisdom of investing financial resources in such items as rugs and draperies at her advanced age.

Aside from physical objects, the patient confronted a loss of community. In response to the physician's question about meeting new neighbors, the patient said that she has met "two or three." Yet, she "hated to move" because of the affection she held for her prior neighbors. Describing her attachment, she first mentioned that she "loved" them and then modified her feelings by saying that she "liked" them "very much." Whatever pain this loss has created, the full impact remained unexplored, as the physician cut off the line of discussion by terminating the physical exam and returning to a technical comment about her heart.

Throughout these passages, the physician supportively listened. He offered no specific suggestions to help the patient, nor did he guide the dialogue toward a deeper exploration of her feelings. Despite his supportive demeanor, the physician here functioned within the traditional constraints of the medical role. When tension mounted with the patient mourning a much-loved community, the physician returned to the realm of medical technique.

Even before managed care made its way into clinical practice, many practitioners felt reluctant to get involved in helping improve the social problems that patients faced, no matter how important such problems may have been. Physicians rationalized: There was not time. Or, exploring social problems went beyond the medical role. The answers have never been simple, but the productivity expectations and the financial structure of managed care have discouraged efforts to deal with such problems even further.

To what extent *should* physicians intervene in the social context? The answer to this important question in social medicine depends partly on clarification of the practitioner's role, especially the degree to which intervention in the social context comes to be seen as appropriate and desirable. Practitioners may reasonably respond by referring to the time constraints of current practice arrangements, the need to deal with challenging technical problems, and the lack of support facilities and personnel to improve social conditions. How physicians should involve themselves in contextual difficulties, without increasing professional control in areas where physicians claim no special expertise, therefore, takes on a certain complexity.

On the other hand, the presence of social problems in medical encounters warrants more critical attention. Based on research about patient–doctor communication, recommendations have emerged that encourage physicians to let patients tell their narrative in an open-ended way, with far fewer interruptions, cutoffs, or returns to technical matters. According to these recommendations, when patients refer to personal troubles as the result of social issues, physicians should at least acknowledge the patient's concerns; preferably, the provider should point the patient in the right direction to seek out additional resources. These are some criteria that could prove helpful for physicians in deciding when and under what circumstances they should initiate, extend, or limit discussions about social issues.[25]

Managed care has created troubling contradictions in patient–doctor encounters and relationships. Under the constraints of managed care, practitioners' role as double agents and the financial structures that limit open communication have changed the nature of the patient–doctor interaction, including the ability to address the problems of social context that affect many patients' lives. While the era that predated managed care was not free of problems, the conflicts of interest and mixed loyalties inherent in managed care arrangements have clouded the picture even further: Managed care has created enduring legal and ethical dilemmas that warrant attention in social medicine.

Trauma, Militarism, Mental Health, and Physical Symptoms

Access barriers and managed care, of course, are not the only characteristics of society that impinge on the medical encounter. Militarism also exerts profound effects, not only for peoples in invaded countries but also for those who carry out military policy. Military campaigns figure as an important part of imperialism, whose adverse effects on health have received attention in social medicine, as we have described in prior chapters. For example, recent combat operations in Iraq, Afghanistan, and elsewhere around the world have taken the lives of military personnel and have damaged the physical and mental health of many who survived. Despite military officials' publicly stated intention to implement high-quality military health care, reports originating both inside and outside the military have called attention to the unmet medical and psychological needs of service personnel.[26] Physical and emotional injuries sustained by U.S. soldiers and their families have become a public health epidemic that continues to stress the country's already overextended health and mental health systems. And, of course, such injuries and deaths happen alongside the devastation inflicted by war on civilian populations.

Several challenges interfere with access to medical and mental health services for active duty military personnel. During recent wars, soldiers have experienced a command and medical care system where illness and injury were viewed as obstacles to the military mission, inconveniences to local commands, or malingering.[27] As a result, some soldiers have faced deployment to active combat zones before full evaluation of physical illness. Those with mental health problems such as depression or post-traumatic stress disorder (PTSD) often have entered a combat zone despite being newly diagnosed or just beginning a medication such as a tranquilizer, antidepressant, or antipsychotic drug. Such prescriptions of psychotropic medications have continued even though the medications may increase the risks of severe depression and suicide when used in young adults.[28]

We previously have discussed the "double agent" health professional in the managed care context: one that is serving both the patient and the managed care business model that rewards the physician for being "the gatekeeper." There is also the problem of "double agency" interwoven in the provision of health and mental health services in the military. In this case, double agency refers to the dual allegiances of military health and mental health professionals that inevitably arise in their relationship with patients. Personnel shortages and the pressure to deploy and redeploy troops rapidly to the Middle East, for instance, have put increasing pressure on military physicians, psychiatrists, and psychologists. As they encounter soldiers with health and mental health problems, military health professionals by necessity must consider the goals of maintaining the numbers and readiness of combat forces.[29] This dual role of military health professionals raises inherent tensions that reduce the likelihood that soldiers receive suitable care and increase the likelihood of their seeking care outside the military.

These tensions led to the creation of networks, inspired by principles of social medicine and involving civilian professionals who try to meet the medical and mental health needs of soldiers, without the burden of double agency. The networks provide services that parallel those of the military that have failed to deliver effective care. One organization in particular shows the challenges of addressing the physical and psychological injuries that military personnel sustain.

CIVILIAN MEDICAL RESOURCES NETWORK

This website gives more information about the purposes and activities of this volunteer network to deal with the unmet medical and mental health needs of active duty military personnel: http://civilianmedicalresources.net.

The Civilian Medical Resources Network (CMRN) has worked as a small national network of professionals established to offer soldiers an alternative to the military health and mental health care system.[30] Through the network, primary care providers, psychiatrists, psychologists, social workers, and public health workers try to address the needs of active duty U.S. military personnel when they seek medical and psychological care in the civilian sector. Because other resources at least partly address the needs of veterans, the network has focused on active duty personnel.

Recruitment of clinicians for the network occurred initially through personal outreach to professional colleagues. In addition, two national organizations oriented toward social medicine – Physicians for Social Responsibility and Physicians for a National Health Program – announced the program to their members. Approximately 100 professionals have participated, mostly primary care and mental health practitioners, based in all regions of the United States.

Referrals to the network have come from the GI Rights Hotline (GIRH), a national effort maintained by 25 religious and peace organizations, as well as the Military Law Task Force of the National Lawyers Guild.[31] Legal professionals provide advice to the network and assist clinicians with documentation of soldiers' medical and mental health problems, as needed, to support their requests for discharge or reassignment. At its height, the hotline has received approximately 3000 calls per month from active duty soldiers and their families. When a soldier or family member calls the hotline and describes unmet needs for physical or mental health services, a counselor may contact the network to set up a referral to one or more participating professionals.

Because soldiers generally do not have financial resources or insurance coverage to pay for civilian services, network professionals provide care for free or at a greatly reduced cost. When possible, soldiers visit network professionals in person. If a face-to-face visit is unfeasible due to geographical distance, network professionals assist soldiers through telephone and e-mail consultations. In addition to communication with soldiers based in the United States, professionals conduct assessments and treatment interventions with soldiers deployed to the Middle East, Afghanistan, Europe, or Korea, some of whom decompensate emotionally with suicidal or sometimes homicidal intentions. Volunteers conduct the referral procedures and coordinate with the GIRH and the Military Law Task Force.

For less acute situations, soldiers seek independent second opinions of diagnoses made by military medics or physicians or advice about treatment options and the impact of military service on their illnesses or injuries. Other soldiers request independent evaluations for their own peace of mind or independent treatment because of concerns about the adequacy of services in military clinics. Furthermore, the actions of civilian professionals help soldiers gain access to specialized military physicians. This work also reduces the likelihood that commanding personnel block or oppose visits to medical personnel.

Several recurrent themes pertinent to social medicine have emerged from encounters with military clients. First is the concept of the "economic draft." Many soldiers report that they enlisted because of financial challenges or lack of employment opportunities. In addition to experiencing low-income financial conditions, soldiers in the U.S. armed forces often come from ethnic or racial minority backgrounds or grew up in less developed countries, especially in Latin America. Second, psychological problems among soldiers often involve perceived deception during the recruiting process: Clients report that they received inaccurate assurances about deployments, combat requirements, salaries and benefits, and support for families. Longer and more frequent deployments than promised become a source of major distress.

Beyond the problems associated with the recruitment process, emotional problems emerge from the ethical conflict and "moral injury" of witnessing or perpetrating violence without a sense that the violence led to progress in meeting military, political, or social goals.[32] Many soldiers were not briefed about the military's goals, so they do not understand the purpose of military involvement in Afghanistan, Iraq, or other countries. Violent acts perpetrated against civilians, especially children, generate guilt, depression, and PTSD.

As previously mentioned, another theme involves the existing barriers to care built into the military system. Soldiers who stay with their units experience barriers when they attempt to contact the GIRH and receive evaluations through the CMRN. Scheduling problems due to work demands inhibit appointments with civilian professionals. Clients report difficulties that they or their families experience in obtaining privatized services from MCOs that contract with the military. Inconvenience in obtaining services and managed care practitioners' diminishing the importance of clinical problems motivate soldiers and their families to seek services from CMRN professionals.

Although most soldiers using the CMRN network did not engage in torture or other forms of abuse, they express awareness of these practices as part of military operations. In their training, soldiers learn that such practices contradict rules of war, such as the Geneva Convention, as well as specific regulations that govern actions by U.S. military forces. In practice, however, many soldiers also learn that officers tolerate and sometimes encourage the use of torture and similar abuses.[33] This contradiction causes stress, stigma, and shame about unethical actions perpetrated by military colleagues. Professionals working with soldiers in the network note high levels of shame, a situation that inhibits them from seeking help.

Such problems speak to the larger social issues of an all-volunteer military force in an increasingly militarized society. During the Vietnam War, a military draft led to the induction of young people from a broad range of social positions. A volunteer army of the present, however, depends on men and women predominantly from low-income and minority backgrounds. Services for GIs and veterans periodically enter public consciousness, especially after scandals, and there is no shortage of scandals in the military. For example, the substandard conditions at Walter Reed Army Medical Center came to light in a series of documentaries in 2007.[34] There have also been instances of military personnel acting violently against their military superiors or colleagues. In 2009, a stressed military psychiatrist opened fire at Fort Hood, Texas, and was sentenced to death.[35]

More recently, in January 2017 a former soldier opened fire at a crowded Florida airport.[36] However, the predominantly working-class origins of those serving in war — as opposed to the more privileged class position of officials in government and industry who make the key decisions about initiating and expanding war — limit the attention that the injuries of war among front-line warriors receive from policy makers. During the wars in Iraq and Afghanistan, only a handful of legislators in the U.S. Congress have had children in the military.

Due to a new cluster of ethical conflicts related to changing military operations in the service of empire, mental health problems predominate among those participating or anticipating participation in combat. Soldiers report suicidal ideation that goes unrecognized or unacknowledged when they seek care in the military system. Within a report published in *Military Medicine* about 233 of their clients, a team from CMRN found very high rates of mental health disorders and suicidality: Almost half, 48 percent, reported suicidal thoughts. Seventy-two percent of clients met criteria for major depression, 62 percent PTSD, 20 percent generalized anxiety disorder, 25 percent panic disorder, and 27 percent alcohol use disorder.[37]

Military statistics indicate rapid increases in suicide, suicide attempts, and self-injuries among active duty soldiers. An average of more than one active duty GI and more than 20 veterans commit suicide each day. More U.S. soldiers currently die from suicide than from combat. In one calendar year, the U.S. Army reported approximately 2,100 suicide attempts and self-injuries, a rate of more than five per day, much increased from prior years. The probability of suicide increases with the number of deployments and time spent in Afghanistan or Iraq. Suicides committed outside combat zones remain underreported.[38] Even though suicide rates have increased markedly in the United States during recent years, the rates among active duty military personnel and among veterans remain higher.[39]

The epidemic of mental health problems in the military coincides with the unprecedented privatization of medical and mental health services for active duty soldiers and their families. Although the military previously offered such services within its own facilities, private corporations later received substantial contracts from the military to provide these services. This policy change reflects the same neoliberal principle that favored privatization of services previously provided by public hospitals and clinics for underserved populations. As a result of privatizing military health and mental health services, the chief executive officer who benefited most, financially, from the Iraq War did not head a corporation traditionally considered part of the military–industrial complex, but rather a large MCO (Health Net), whose contractor (ValueOptions) provided mental health services for soldiers and their families.[40]

During this same time period, for soldiers who sought help within the military sector for PTSD, depression, and other mental health problems stemming from military service, military psychologists increasingly diagnosed personality disorders. Since military policy considers personality disorders as preexisting conditions that antedate military service, soldiers who receive these diagnoses lose financial and health benefits after discharge.[41] This policy applies even though military officials did not diagnose personality disorder during soldiers' mental health evaluation when inducted into the armed forces.

During current wars, military leaders implement strategies that involve less combat engagement with identified combatants and more violence against civilians.[42] In a context where both torture and systematic human rights abuse occur, soldiers suffer from high levels of psychological distress. Resistance to war, thus, becomes increasing medicalized. With accumulated injuries, both physical and psychological, soldiers turn to professionals in the civilian sector as a route to less dangerous assignments or to discharge.

Except in social medicine, efforts to deal with the physical and mental health damage caused by war rarely address the linkages among empire, militarism, and health. As recurrent financial crises devastate less economically developed countries and eventually begin to plague dominant nations as well, war increasingly becomes one of the few remaining methods to stimulate a failing global economy. The physical and emotional suffering of soldiers, who over time occupy an ever more marginalized position in dominant societies, apparently seems an acceptable price for economically driven war. For those who might otherwise call a halt to militarism without a clear narrative to justify it, the symbolism of terrorism and security provides a justification.

Characteristics of society impinge on the medical encounter in many ways. In this chapter we have considered only a few: social causes of barriers to access for needed services; the growth of managed care and the closely associated processes of corporatization, proletarianization, and alienation of health professionals from their work; how patients and health professionals process the social context of medical encounters; and the effects of militarism and endless war. Proposals to improve patient–doctor communication, while helpful to a limited extent, usually do not address the more fundamental distortions of clinical services that derive from the economic and political structures of our societies. As the founders of social medicine such as Engels, Virchow, and Allende argued, health care and health itself depend much more on our confronting these root causes of illness, suffering, and early death. Studying and practicing in medicine and other health professions will continue to generate illusion and disappointment until we address those "fundamental causes" much more directly.[43] That is the daunting but worthy goal to which we turn now.

Notes

1 Clifford Odets, *Waiting for Lefty* (New York: Dramatists Play Service, 1962).
2 Adapted and updated from Howard Waitzkin, *At the Front Lines of Medicine: How the Health Care System Alienates Doctors and Mistreats Patients… and What We Can Do about It* (Lanham, MD: Rowman & Littlefield, 2001), chapter 1.
3 Centers for Medicare & Medicaid Services, "Eligibility," www.medicaid.gov/medicaid/eligibility/index.html.
4 "Medical Abandonment Law and Legal Definition," Legal Definitions, USLegal Inc., https://definitions.uslegal.com/m/medical-abandonment/.
5 Alexia Fernández Campbell, "The Truth about Undocumented Immigrants and Taxes," *The Atlantic*, September 12, 2016, www.theatlantic.com/business/archive/2016/09/undocumented-immigrants-and-taxes/499604 ; Institute on Taxation and Economic Policy (ITEP), "Undocumented Immigrants' State & Local Tax Contributions," March 2, 2017, https://itep.org/immigration/.
6 A. Taylor Kelley and Renuka Tipirneni, "Care for Undocumented Immigrants – Rethinking State Flexibility in Medicaid Waivers," *New England Journal of Medicine* 378 (2018): 1661–63; Michael S. Cohen and William L. Schpero, "Household Immigration Status Had Differential Impact on Medicaid Enrollment in Expansion and Nonexpansion States," *Health Affairs* 37, no. 3 (March 2018): 394–402, https://www.healthaffairs.org/doi/abs/10.1377/hlthaff.2017.0978; Altaf Saadi, Sameer Ahmed, and Mitchell Katz, "Making a Case for Sanctuary Hospitals," *JAMA* 318 (2017): 2079–80; Jens Hainmueller, Duncan Lawrence, Linna Martén, et al., "Protecting Unauthorized Immigrant Mothers Improves Their Children's Mental Health," *Science* 357 (2017): 1041–44.
7 Howard Waitzkin and Ida Hellander, "Obamacare: The Neoliberal Model Comes Homes to Roost in the United States – If We Let It," in Howard Waitzkin and the Working Group on Health Beyond Capitalism, *Health Care Under the Knife: Moving Beyond Capitalism for Our Health* (New York: Monthly Review Press, 2018); Adam Gaffney, David Himmelstein, and Steffie Woolhandler, "The Failure of Obamacare and a Revision of the Single-Payer Proposal after a Quarter-Century of Struggle," in Howard Waitzkin and the Working Group on Health Beyond Capitalism, *Health Care Under the Knife: Moving Beyond Capitalism for Our Health* (New York: Monthly Review Press, 2018).
8 Gaffney, Himmelstein, and Woolhandler, "The Failure of Obamacare and a Revision of the Single-Payer Proposal after a Quarter-Century of Struggle"; Katherine Baicker and Jacob A. Robbins, "Medicare Payments and System-Level Healthcare Use: The Spillover Effects of Medicare Managed Care," *American Journal of Health Economics* 1 (2015): 399–431; Theodore Marmor and Jonathan Oberlander, "From HMOs to ACOs: The Quest for the Holy Grail in US Health Policy," *Journal of General Internal Medicine* 27 (2012): 1215–18.
9 Marcia Angell, "The Doctor as Double Agent," *Kennedy Institute of Ethics Journal* 3 (1993): 279–286; Waitzkin, *At the Front Lines of Medicine*, chapter 4; Gordon Schiff and Sarah Winch, "The Degradation of Medical Labor and the Meaning of Quality in Health Care," in Howard Waitzkin and the Working Group on Health Beyond Capitalism, *Health Care Under the Knife: Moving Beyond Capitalism for Our Health* (New York: Monthly Review Press, 2018).

10 Waitzkin, *At the Front Lines of Medicine*, chapter 4; Christopher B. Forrest, "Primary Care Gatekeeping and Referrals: Effective Filter or Failed Experiment?" *British Medical Journal* 326 (2003): 692–95; Gaffney, Himmelstein, and Woolhandler, "The Failure of Obamacare and a Revision of the Single-Payer Proposal after a Quarter-Century of Struggle"; Howard Waitzkin and the Working Group on Health Beyond Capitalism, *Health Care Under the Knife: Moving Beyond Capitalism for Our Health* (New York: Monthly Review Press, 2018), Part 1.

11 Matt Anderson and Robb Burlage, "The Transformation of the Medical Industrial Complex: Financialization, the Corporate Sector, and Monopoly Capital," in Howard Waitzkin and the Working Group on Health Beyond Capitalism, *Health Care Under the Knife: Moving Beyond Capitalism for Our Health* (New York: Monthly Review Press, 2018).

12 Waitzkin and the Working Group, *Health Care Under the Knife*, Part 1.

13 John D. Stoeckle, "Working on the Factory Floor," *Annals of Internal Medicine* 107, no. 2 (1987): 250–51.

14 Leslie Kane, "Medscape Physician Compensation Report 2018," *Medscape*, April 11, 2018, www.medscape.com/slideshow/2018-compensation-overview-6009667#13.

15 Carol Peckham, "Medscape National Physician Burnout & Depression Report 2018," *Medscape*, January 17, 2018, www.medscape.com/slideshow/2018-lifestyle-burnout-depression-6009235#3.

16 Jianbo Lai, Simeng Ma, Ying Wang, et al., "Factors Associated With Mental Health Outcomes Among Health Care Workers Exposed to Coronavirus Disease 2019," *JAMA Network Open* 3, no. 3 (2020): e203976, doi:10.1001/jamanetworkopen.2020.3976; Charlene Dewey, Susan Hingle, Elizabeth Goelz, and Mark Linzer, "Supporting Clinicians During the COVID-19 Pandemic," *Annals of Internal Medicine*, June 2, 2020, https://doi.org/10.7326/M20-1033; Marwa Saleh, "A Double Whammy: The COVID-19 Pandemic and Burnout in Medical Professionals," *Harvard Medical School Lean Forward*, April 9, 2020, https://leanforward.hms.harvard.edu/2020/04/09/a-double-whammy-the-covid-19-pandemic-and-burnout-in-medical-professionals/.

17 Karl Marx, "Estranged Labor," in *Economic and Philosophical Manuscripts of 1844*, www.marxists.org/archive/marx/works/1844/manuscripts/labour.htm.

18 Catherine M. DesRoches et al., "Electronic Health Records' Limited Successes Suggest More Targeted Uses," *Health Affairs* 29 (2010): 639–46.

19 See also: Pamela Hartzband and Jerome Groopman, "Off the Record: Avoiding the Pitfalls of Going Electronic," *New England Journal of Medicine* 358 (2008): 1656–58.

20 Angell, "The Doctor as Double Agent."

21 Marc A. Rodwin, "Conflicts of Interest, Institutional Corruption, and Pharma: An Agenda for Reform," *Journal of Law, Medicine and Ethics* 40 (2012): 511–22.

22 Howard Waitzkin and John D. Stoeckle, "The Communication of Information about Illness: Clinical, Sociological, and Methodological Considerations," *Advances in Psychosomatic Medicine* 8 (1972): 180–215.

23 Waitzkin, *At the Front Lines of Medicine*, chapter 4.

24 Ibid.

25 Howard Waitzkin, "Culture, Communication, and Somatization in Health Care," in Dale E. Brashers and Daena Goldsmith, eds., *Communicating to Manage Health and Illness* (New York: Routledge, 2009).

26 Howard Waitzkin, Mario Cruz, Bryant Shuey, Daniel Smithers II, Laura Muncy, and Marylou Noble, "Military Personnel Who Seek Health and Mental Health Services Outside the Military," *Military Medicine*, 183 (2018): e232–e240, doi:10.1093/milmed/usx051; Defense Health Board: *Ethical Guidelines and Practices for U.S. Military Medical Professionals* (Falls Church, VA: Office of the Assistant Secretary of Defense Health Affairs, 2015), https://health.mil/search-results?query=Ethical+Guidelines+and+Practices; Leonard S. Rubenstein, Scott A. Allen, and Phyllis A. Guze, "Advancing Medical Professionalism in US Military Detainee Treatment." *PLOS Medicine* 13 (2016): e1001930, doi:10.1371/journal.pmed.1001930; Amy B. Adler, Amanda L. Adrian, Marla Hemphill, Nicole H. Scaro, Maurice L. Sipos, and Jeffrey L. Thomas, "Professional Stress and Burnout in U.S. Military Medical Personnel Deployed to Afghanistan," *Military Medicine* 182 (2017): e1669–e1676, doi:10.7205/MILMED-D-16-00154.

27 Joseph Lieberman and Barbara Boxer, "Make Mental Health a Priority: When Service Members Go Untreated, the Entire Military Suffers," *Army Times* 68, no. 3 (2007): 42; Waitzkin et al., "Military Personnel Who Seek Health and Mental Health Services Outside the Military."

28 National Institute of Mental Health, "Antidepressant Use in Children, Adolescents, and Adults," www.nimh.nih.gov/health/topics/child-and-adolescent-mental-health/antidepressant-medications-for-children-and-adolescents-information-for-parents-and-caregivers.shtml (under revision, 2020); Gregory Simon, "Effect of antidepressants on suicide risk in adults," *UpToDate*, May 28, 2019, https://www.uptodate.com/contents/effect-of-antidepressants-on-suicide-risk-in-adults?search=antidepressants%20suicide&source=search_result&selectedTitle=1~150&usage_type=default&display_rank=1#H16005424; U.S. Food and Drug Administration, "Suicidality in Children and Adolescents Being Treated With Antidepressant Medications," February 5, 2018, https://www.fda.gov/drugs/postmarket-drug-safety-information-patients-and-providers/suicidality-children-and-adolescents-being-treated-antidepressant-medications; Glen I. Spielmans, Tess Spence-Sing, and Peter Parry, "Duty to Warn: Antidepressant Black Box Suicidality Warning Is Empirically Justified," *Frontiers in Psychiatry*, February 13, 2020, https://www.frontiersin.org/articles/10.3389/fpsyt.2020.00018/full.

29 Victor W. Sidel and Barry S. Levy, "The Roles and Ethics of Military Medical Care Workers," in Barry S. Levy and Victor W. Sidel, eds., *War and Public Health* (New York: Oxford University Press, 2008); Waitzkin et al., "Military Personnel Who Seek Health and Mental Health Services Outside the Military"; W. Brad Johnson, Roderick Bacho, Mark Heim, and John Ralph, "Multiple-Role Dilemmas for Military Mental Health Care Providers," *Military Medicine* 171 (2006): 311–15.

30 Waitzkin et al., "Military Personnel Who Seek Health and Mental Health Services Outside the Military"; Howard Waitzkin, *Medicine and Public Health at the End of Empire* (Boulder, CO: Paradigm Publishers, 2011), chapter 12; Waitzkin, Howard and Marylou Noble, "Caring for Active Duty Military Personnel in the Civilian Sector," *Social Medicine* 4 (2009): 56–69, www.socialmedicine.info/index.php/socialmedicine/article/view/295.

31 GI Rights Hotline, https://girightshotline.org; Military Law Task Force of the National Lawyers Guild, http://nlgmltf.org.

32 Anthony Nazarov et al., "Role of Morality in the Experience of Guilt and Shame within the Armed Forces," *Acta Psychiatrica Scandinavica* 132 (2015): 4–19; William P. Nash, Teresa L. Marino Carper, Mary Alice Mills, Teresa

Au, Abigail Goldsmith, and Brett T. Litz, "Psychometric Evaluation of the Moral Injury Events Scale," *Military Medicine* 178 (2013): 646–52.

33 Steven F. Miles, *Oath Betrayed: America's Torture Doctors* (Berkeley, CA: University of California Press, 2009); Jonathan H. Marks and Mark G. Bloche, "The Ethics of Interrogation – The U.S. Military's Ongoing Use of Psychiatrists," *New England Journal of Medicine* 359 (2008): 1090–92; George G. Annas, "Military Medical Ethics – Physician First, Last, Always," *New England Journal of Medicine* 359 (2008): 1087–90.

34 Tom Bowman, "Walter Reed Was the Army's Wake-Up Call in 2007," *NPR*, August 31, 2011, www.npr.org/2011/08/31/139641856/in-2007-walter-reed-was-the-armys-wakeup-call.

35 Billy Kenbar, "Nidal Hasan Sentenced to Death for Fort Hood Shooting Rampage," *Washington Post*, August 28, 2013, www.washingtonpost.com/world/national-security/nidal-hasan-sentenced-to-death-for-fort-hood-shooting-rampage/2013/08/28/aad28de2-0ffa-11e3-bdf6-e4fc677d94a1_story.html?noredirect=on.

36 Lizette Alvarez, Frances Robles, and Richard Pérez-Peña, "In Year Before Florida Shooting, Suspect's Problems Multiplied," *New York Times*, January 7, 2017, www.nytimes.com/2017/01/07/us/esteban-santiago-fort-lauderdale-airport-shooting-.html.

37 Waitzkin et al., "Military Personnel Who Seek Health and Mental Health Services Outside the Military."

38 Office of Suicide Prevention, U.S. Department of Veterans Affairs, "Suicide Among Veterans and Other Americans 2001–2014," August 2017, www.mentalhealth.va.gov/docs/2016suicidedatareport.pdf; Robert J. Ursano, Lisa J. Colpe, Steven G. Heeringa, et al., "Army Study to Assess Risk and Resilience in Servicemembers Collaborators: Suicide Attempts in the US Army during the Wars in Afghanistan and Iraq, 2004 to 2009," *JAMA Psychiatry* 72 (2015): 917–26; Robert J. Ursano, Ronald C. Kessler, James A. Naifeh, et al., "Associations of Time-Related Deployment Variables With Risk of Suicide Attempt Among Soldiers: Results from the Army Study to Assess Risk and Resilience in Servicemembers (Army STARRS)," *JAMA Psychiatry* 75 (2018): 596–604; Mark A. Reger, Derek J. Smolenski, Nancy A. Skopp et al., "Risk of Suicide among US Military Service Members Following Operation Enduring Freedom or Operation Iraqi Freedom Deployment and Separation from the US Military," *JAMA Psychiatry* 72 (2015): 561–69; Patricia Kime, "Active-duty Suicides Up, Guard and Reserve Down in 2014," *Military Times*, February 8, 2016, www.militarytimes.com/story/military/2016/02/08/active-duty-suicides-up-guard-and-reserve-down-2014-military-suicide-attempts/80021990/; Waitzkin et al., "Military Personnel Who Seek Health and Mental Health Services Outside the Military."

39 Deborah M. Stone, Thomas R. Simon, Katherine A. Fowler, et al., "Trends in State Suicide Rates — United States, 1999–2016 and Circumstances Contributing to Suicide — 27 States, 2015," *MMWR Morbidity and Mortality Weekly Report* 67 (2018): 617–24. doi:10.15585/mmwr.mm6722a1.

40 Sarah Anderson, John Cavanagh, Chuck Collins, and Eric Benjamin, *Executive Excess 2006: 13th Annual CEO Compensation Survey* (Washington, DC, and Boston, MA: Institute for Policy Studies and United for a Fair Economy, 2007), pp. 8–9, https://ips-dc.org/wp-content/uploads/2006/08/Executive-Excess2006.pdf.

41 Joshua Kors, "How Specialist Town Lost His Benefits," *The Nation*, April 9, 2007, pp. 11–21; "Disposable Soldiers," *The Nation*, April 26, 2010), www.thenation.com/article/disposable-soldiers.
42 Winter Soldier, Iraq and Afghanistan, http://ivaw.org/wintersoldier.
43 Jo C. Phelan, Bruce G. Link, and Parisa Tehranifar, "Social Conditions as Fundamental Causes of Health Inequalities: Theory, Evidence, and Policy Implications," *Journal of Health and Social Behavior* 51 (2010): S28–S40; Waitzkin, *Medicine and Public Health at the End of Empire*, chapters 13–14.

Chapter 10

Health Praxis, Reform, and Sociomedical Activism

Praxis, as we have said before, is the uniting of theory and practice, study and action.[1] In social medicine, as in life more generally, there is an obvious difference between knowledge about social conditions and changing those conditions. Understanding the problems of medicine and society are not enough.

Knowledge alone will not solve the difficulties we face. Research and analysis must be linked to action that changes the social conditions responsible for illness and early death. Also, for meaningful improvements in the health care systems of the United States and other countries, it is important not only to understand the social roots of illness and suffering, but also to confront the practicalities of activism (Figure 10.1).

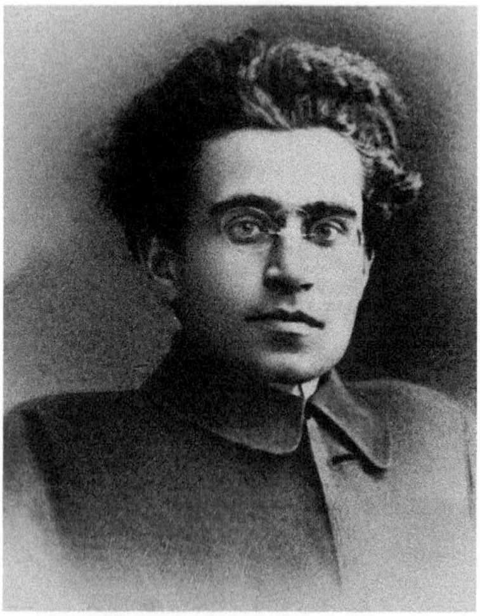

Figure 10.1 Antonio Gramsci, who interpreted praxis and hegemony during the ten years prior to his death in 1937 at the age of 46, while imprisoned by Italian fascism.

> Antonio Gramsci developed the understanding of praxis – the uniting of theory and practice – in his *Prison Notebooks*, while incarcerated for his activism in struggling against Italian fascism. Among his theoretical contributions, Gramsci analyzed "hegemony," the dominant ideologies of a society. He argued that fascist governments cannot obtain a population's acquiescence to domination by force alone. Instead, those who rule must communicate key ideas that justify their domination, and these ideas then become hegemonic in achieving a population's compliance with otherwise unacceptable policies. A major part of the praxis that Gramsci advocated involved theoretical understanding and then action to demystify those hegemonic ideas that helped preserve the wealth and power of society's ruling elite.
>
> Some have argued that Gramsci's physical disabilities influenced his own attempts to combine a theory about social conditions that generate illness and suffering, with political practice to change those conditions.

Throughout this book, we already have considered many examples of praxis: the theoretical studies of social class and inequality that guided the work of Engels, Virchow, and Allende as founders of social medicine (Chapter 2); the analyses of poverty and racism that informed the struggles of social medicine activists in the United States (Chapter 5); the understanding of imperialism and its impact on health that has motivated activists struggling to resist privatization and to strengthen public sector services in Latin America (Chapters 7 and 8); and the analysis of militarism and imperialism that has given direction to practitioners who try to address the unmet medical and mental health needs of military personnel (Chapter 9). In this final chapter, we look at some directions of progressive health care praxis in efforts to achieve national health programs (NHPs) and to bring about fundamental changes in the social determination of illness, suffering, and early death.[2]

Contradictions of Reform

Health care workers and activists concerned about the relationship between social change and health face difficult challenges in their daily work. People's problems often have roots in social conditions. For instance, consider those who cannot find a job or adequate housing; the elderly or disabled who need periodic medical certification to obtain welfare benefits that are barely adequate; prisoners who develop illnesses because of prison conditions; patients with cancer whose insurance does not cover treatment; and workers with high blood pressure or heart disease who need to choose among buying medications, purchasing food, and paying the rent. These problems are complex, and end up being "patched" rather than fixed. On the individual level, patching allows patients to continue functioning in the same social system that is often the source of the problem. However, even health workers who are highly critical of these societal conditions devote most of their clinical time to patching the system's victims. Frequently, this work has the paradoxical effect of preserving the system's overall stability.

The contradictions of "patching" have no simple resolution. One conclusion is that health work in itself is not sufficient. Instead, health workers should try to link their clinical activities to efforts aimed directly at basic sociopolitical change. The goal is to encourage health care praxis that points to progressive change in the social order. If health care workers do not address the social roots of medical problems, solutions will remain limited and unsatisfactory.

To achieve this goal, it is important to acknowledge the contradictions of reform, which can slide into reformism. That is, improved material circumstances may seem beneficial but can actually reinforce the status quo by reducing the potential for social conflict. Then political praxis seems no longer needed, and reform morphs into reformism. In other words, people fight for reform when conditions grow more oppressive. Therefore, in the realm of health and welfare, a repetitive pattern takes place: Reforms most often follow social protest, resulting in incremental improvements that do not change the overall patterns of oppression, and these limited improvements suffer cutbacks when protest recedes.[3] So, reform often proves unhelpful or temporary.

A distinction developed initially by French activist and journalist André Gorz helps clarify this problem.[4] "Reformist reforms" provide small material improvements while leaving current political and economic structures intact. These reforms may reduce discontent while helping to preserve the system in its present form. In contrast, "non-reformist reforms" achieve lasting changes in the present system's structures of power and finance. They do not simply modify material conditions. Instead, they provide the potential for massive political action. Rather than obscuring sources of exploitation by small incremental improvements, non-reformist reforms expose and highlight structural inequities. Such reforms ultimately increase frustration and political tension in a society, and they can contribute to revolutionary upheaval. According to Gorz, such reforms are dynamic phases in a progressive struggle, not stopping places.

In social medicine it is important to clarify which reform proposals are reformist and which are non-reformist, and to promote the latter. The distinction between reformist and non-reformist reforms is not easy, however, since few proposals address the underlying social causes of medical and public health problems. We believe it is essential to understand and to criticize piecemeal reformism. It is also necessary to examine carefully the much smaller number of health reforms and progressive directions of health activism that actually challenge broad social contradictions and that heighten the potential for basic social change. Without addressing these links among health, medicine, and social structure, both problems and solutions will continue to float in a haze of confusion and mystification. We now talk about some recent health reform proposals in the United States and try to distinguish which are reformist and which non-reformist, and why.

Struggles for National Health Programs

Obamacare and its predecessors. Since at least the 1920s, people in the United States have organized in support of an NHP that would provide universal access to comprehensive medical services. At that time, the "problem of sickness" became a major source of poverty if people became unemployed while sick: No work meant no pay.[5] Unions were starting to mobilize. Furthermore, universal health care was not a novel idea. Activists in European countries had been striving for health care reform since before 1883, when Germany became the first country in the world to establish an NHP.

In the United States, the most recent attempt to improve access to services involved former President Barack Obama's highly contested Patient Protection and Affordable Care Act (ACA), dubbed "Obamacare" by the press.[6] Early in his political career, Obama had supported a single-payer public sector program of universal health care. However, in his 2008 and 2012 presidential campaigns, he received the largest financial contributions in history from the insurance industry, more than the contributions received by his Republican adversaries, John McCain and Mitt Romney. Similarly, Obama became the first presidential candidate ever to turn down government funds for his campaign, based mostly on contributions from corporations in the financial sector linked to Wall Street and the health insurance industry.[7] So, it should come as no surprise that Obamacare called for the preservation and strengthening of the private insurance industry through vastly increased public payments to care for the uninsured, while leaving a substantial proportion of the population uninsured or underinsured. As an example of a reformist reform, Obamacare improved social conditions somewhat without changing the overall structure of the health care system or the broader society.

Obamacare followed the model of market-based reform proposals promoted since the era of neoliberalism began in the early 1980s, spearheaded by the governments of Ronald Reagan in the United States and Margaret Thatcher in the United Kingdom. Under neoliberalism, political and economic elites have supported capitalist, market-based reforms as a route to enhance investment opportunities and profitability for corporations selling private health insurance, medications, and equipment. The leadership of these corporations and international financial institutions, such as the World Bank, have advocated such market-based proposals utilizing public sector funds to subsidize private sector corporate expansion.

In the neoliberal model, private insurance corporations receive public funding from tax-generated government trust funds (Medicare, Medicaid, Social Security, etc.) as well as premiums and co-payments from employers and employees. The private insurance companies then pay for services delivered not only to privately insured patients but also to some but not all of the previously uninsured population. Due to the participation of private insurance corporations, there is much administrative waste. Specifically, the proportion of total health expenditures that goes for administration is usually around 25 percent, and the proportion of health experiences that pay for actual clinical services is about 75 percent.

In other words, under private insurance and under neoliberal national programs that include private insurance corporations, about one-quarter of every dollar spent on health care goes to administration. Many of these administrative expenditures pay for activities such as billing, denial of claims, supervision of co-payments and deductibles, pursuit of conditions that disqualify people from eligibility, and exorbitant salaries for executives. For example, in 2016, CEOs of the major U.S. insurance corporations earned annual salaries in the range of $20 million plus stock ownership options.[8]

Obamacare required that participating insurance companies maintain a "medical loss ratio" (MLR) of 80 percent, meaning that most insurance companies covering individuals and small businesses would spend at least 80 percent of their premium income on health care claims and quality improvement, with the remaining 20 percent going for administration, marketing, and profit. The MLR conveys the for-profit orientation of insurance corporations, who experience the requirement to provide medical care as a "loss" to their profit making. Research has shown that overall Obamacare did not achieve even this degree of control over administrative costs. In contrast, administrative costs within public sector programs that do not depend on private insurance companies for administration, such as traditional Medicare in the United States or Canada's single-payer NHP, comprise about 10 percent or less of expenditures, and the vast majority of funds get spent on clinical services for patients.[9]

> **EXTRA CREDIT ASSIGNMENT FOCUSING ON SCIENTIFIC CLAIMS ABOUT ECONOMIC PRINCIPLES REGARDING MARKETS AND COMPETITION**
>
> - Please find a single scientific research study that demonstrates the advantage of market competition for any health outcome.
>
> **More Extra Credit**
>
> - Please find a single scientific research study that demonstrates the advantage of market competition for any financial or other economic outcome.
>
> **Disclosure**
>
> One of the authors (Howard) has offered extra credit for this assignment during more than 20 years. No student has ever found such a study. If any reader does find such a study, please contact Howard, who will provide a prize that will make you happy.

The basic components of Obamacare resembled those of many health reform proposals favored by insurance corporations and international financial institutions. These proposals enhance corporations' access to public sector health and social security funds. The for-profit corporations justify these reforms through unproven claims about the efficiency of the private sector and about the enhanced quality of care under principles of competition and business management. Arguments in favor of neoliberal health policies usually present these claims as scientific truths, despite a lack of research findings supporting such claims.[10] (See box for another perspective on the lack of scientific evidence supporting the economic assumptions about market-based competition and managerial practices in health services.)

The so-called revolving door, by which corporate executives move into and out of government jobs directly related to their jobs in corporations, also helps determine how health policies favor corporate interests. For instance, the individual most responsible for drafting the 961-page bill known as the ACA was Liz Fowler, former Chief Counsel of the U.S. Senate Finance Committee.[11] Fowler previously had worked as vice president of Wellpoint, later Anthem, one of the largest for-profit insurance corporations. She also helped design Medicare Part D, the medication coverage supplement for Medicare. Part D favored the pharmaceutical industry by not allowing the government to negotiate prices of medications with drug companies or to require generic drug formularies that could reduce the high costs of brand-name drugs. In 2012, two years after the ACA went into law, Fowler left the Obama administration to become Director of Global Health Policy for Johnson & Johnson, focused on lobbying operations for this major pharmaceutical corporation. Fowler embodied the "revolving door" pattern, by which executives move between government and large corporations for personal and professional benefit, thus shaping legislation to favor corporate interests.

This process led to a "mixed" approach linking the public and private sectors. In the mixed model, private health insurance corporations receive public sector funds mostly from tax revenues. These funds subsidize partial insurance coverage, still with substantial co-payments and deductible payments, for a proportion of the previously uninsured population. Even at full implementation, Obamacare would leave about 23 million people still without coverage.[12] Private insurance companies continued to administer these policies, with continuing high administrative costs. Although the Obama administration also proposed a "public option" to be operated by the federal government, this proposal eventually was dropped due to opposition from the private insurance industry and industry supporters in Congress.[13]

Obama and his core staff members consistently argued that it was important to preserve the for-profit private insurance industry. As a result, under the ACA, families and individuals have bought insurance from private corporations. The ACA has assisted the poor through a means-tested approach that requires a large administrative overhead to determine eligibility based on limited income and assets. Prior state-run programs that involved a mixed private and public approach failed to achieve universal coverage and generated crippling cost overruns. Such was the example in Massachusetts, the first state to strive for universal coverage, under Governor Mitt Romney, and which later became a model for the ACA.[14] Similar problems arose in the health reform of 1994 in Colombia, which the World Bank spearheaded as the first neoliberal proposal to be implemented throughout a country. The proposal of Hillary and Bill Clinton in 1994, which failed to pass the U.S. Congress, also favored the private insurance industry and contained the same neoliberal approach that characterized the health reforms in Colombia and Massachusetts.[15]

Because it retained private insurance corporations as the main administrative entities, the ACA projected a high level of administrative costs. Because administrative waste would not decrease, the anticipated costs of the ACA predictably would become prohibitive, despite assurances to the contrary. Concern about these high costs became a key focus of debate in Congress and throughout the United States.

Indeed, administrative waste did increase even further under the ACA. Despite the Trump administration's attempts to repeal it, Obamacare survived, and the overall costs of the health system were projected to rise from 17.4 percent of the gross domestic product in 2013 to 19.6 percent in 2024. A conservative projection showed that premiums and out-of-pocket expenditures for the average family would equal the full average income by 2030. Regarding accessibility, many who obtained coverage under the ACA reported that the insurance remained mostly unusable due to the patient's required high share of cost.[16] At the time of this writing, about 30 million people in the United States were still uninsured and at least twice that number are underinsured. Due to loss of jobs and then loss of employment-based health insurance during the economic collapse in the United States that accompanied the COVID-19 pandemic, an estimated additional 7.3 million additional people would become uninsured.[17]

Other countries have implemented mixed private–public systems and have encountered their own challenges. Although some European systems have received critical attention,[18] several middle-income countries in Latin America have also tried to implement mixed systems. These initiatives resulted from requirements of international financial institutions like the World Bank and the International Monetary Fund, which demanded a reduction of public sector services and an expansion of private sector services as a condition for new or renegotiated loans.[19]

In these countries, neither the conversion of public to private sector insurance, nor the expansion of private insurance through enhanced public financing and participation by corporate entrepreneurs, succeeded in assuring access to needed services. Expansion of private insurance often generated additional co-payments. Privatization of social security and other public sector trust funds for health services generally favored private corporations by providing publicly subsidized insurance and by increasing the capital these corporations held. In addition, privatization led to higher administrative costs.

The impact of mixed private–public systems varies across countries. For Argentina, these policies led to increasing economic crises and major cutbacks of services, especially for the elderly and disabled. In Chile, where privatization occurred largely during the military dictatorship, private managed care organizations, subsidized by public tax funds, prospered as they covered relatively healthy groups in the population, while a constricted public sector continued to provide services to the uninsured.[20] Mexico faced pressures from the World Bank to privatize its social security system and public sector health services; as avenues opened to the participation of private corporations, public sector institutions encountered budget reductions that led to eroded services.[21]

In recent years the neoliberal approach has taken on the misleading name "universal health coverage (UHC)," referring to insurance coverage.[22] UHC does not mean "health care for all" (HFA) – a delivery system that provides equal services for the entire population regardless of an individual's or family's financial resources.[23] As leaders of Latin American social medicine have pointed out, the UHC orientation has become "hegemonic" in global health policy circles.[24] Those limited studies that have analyzed UHC's outcomes in countries such as Colombia, Chile, and Mexico based on data rather than assertion of success have not confirmed ideological claims favoring managed care, competition in markets, efficiency, cost reduction, or quality. Under UHC, access barriers remain or worsen as costs and corporate profits expand.[25]

There are also multiple examples of countries that have not accepted neoliberal health reforms but have constructed health systems based on the goal of HCA. These countries struggle to achieve universal access to care but without tiers of differing benefit packages for the rich and the poor. Canada, for instance, prohibits private insurance for services provided in its NHP. Wealthy people in Canada must participate in the publicly funded system, and the presence of the entire population in a unitary system assures a high-quality national program.[26] Countries trying to advance the HCA model in Latin America during recent years have included Bolivia, Brazil, Cuba, Ecuador, Uruguay, and Venezuela.

The single-payer approach. Like many NHPs around the world, a single-payer program in the United States would basically extend an improved version of Medicare to the entire population. Although Medicare is not without problems, most people over 65 years of age have supported the system and expressed satisfaction with it. Under traditional Medicare, the government actually occupies a very small role: collecting payments from workers, employers, and Medicare recipients for services received and distributing funds to health care providers. Medicare's administrative costs have averaged between 2 and 5 percent of expenditures, compared with private insurance companies' approximately 25 percent. This small percentage indicates that the vast majority of Medicare's expenditures pay for clinical services instead of administrative costs.

Because the single-payer approach will drastically reduce the role of private insurance corporations and will greatly restrict the role of other corporations, including the pharmaceutical industry, a single-payer NHP will become a non-reformist reform. Its progressive financing also will make a single-payer NHP a non-reformist reform, because the rich pay proportionally more than the poor. That is, the single-payer NHP would create meaningful structural changes in health care and also would redistribute wealth through its financing. Predictably, the political struggle that will precede and follow implementation of a single-payer NHP will generate conflict and continuing activism that focus on the social contradictions of a single-payer NHP within an overall capitalist economy, as has happened in essentially every country that has implemented a single-payer system.

The following features of a single-payer option come from the proposals of Physicians for a National Health Program (PNHP), which includes more than 22,000 members spanning all specialties, states, age groups, and practice settings.[27] According to the PNHP proposals, coverage would be universal for all needed services, including medications and long-term care. There would be no out-of-pocket premiums, co-payments, or deductibles. Costs would be controlled by "monopsony" financing from a single, public source. The NHP would not permit competing private insurance and would eliminate multiple tiers of care for different income groups. Practitioners and clinics would be paid predetermined fees for services without any need for costly billing procedures. Hospitals would negotiate an annual global budget for all operating costs. For-profit, investor-owned facilities would be prohibited from participation. Most nonprofit hospitals would remain privately owned. To reduce overlapping and duplicative facilities, capital purchases and expansion would be budgeted separately, based on regional health planning goals.

Funding sources would include current federal spending for Medicare and Medicaid, a payroll tax on private businesses less than what businesses currently pay for coverage, and an income tax on households, with a surtax on high incomes and capital gains. A small tax on stock transactions would be implemented, while state and local taxes for health care would be eliminated.[28] Under this financing plan, 95 percent of families would pay less for health care than they previously paid in insurance premiums, deductibles, co-payments, other out-of-pocket spending, and reduced wages.

From the corporate viewpoint, the insurance and financial sectors would lose a major source of capital accumulation. Other large and small businesses would experience a stabilization or reduction in health care costs. Companies that do not currently provide health insurance would pay more, but far less than the cost of buying private coverage.

A single-payer NHP would achieve universal access to care by drastically reducing administrative waste. National polls consistently have shown that about two-thirds of people in the United States favor the single-payer approach,[29] despite a lack of support by the Obama and Trump administrations and Congressional representatives who receive extensive financial support from the insurance industry. However, 122 members of Congress, led formerly by Representative John Conyers and more recently Representatives Keith Ellison, Pramila Jayapal, and Debbie Dingell, and 17 members of the Senate, led by Senator Bernie Sanders, have co-sponsored single-payer legislation.[30]

Moving Beyond Single Payer. The coming failure of Obamacare will mark a moment of transformation in the United States. For that moment, those struggling for a just and accessible health system will need to address some profound changes that have occurred during the era of neoliberalism. These transformations pertain to the shifting social and class position of health professionals and to the increasing oligopolistic and financialized character of the health insurance industry.

First, as already discussed in Chapter 9, the class position of physicians and other health professionals has changed drastically. Previously, most physicians worked in individual or group practices. Although some were employees receiving relatively high salaries and benefits, most were small entrepreneurs. In the "fee-for-service" system, they seldom accumulated capital on the scale of industrialists or financiers, but they still saw themselves and others saw them as members of an "upper class." Some Marxian theorists viewed them as members of a "professional managerial class."[31]

Physicians increasingly have become employees of hospitals or practices at least partially owned by large health systems. In a large 2017 survey, 69 percent of all physicians reported being employed, including 72 percent of women physicians.[32] These changes mainly reflect the increased costs of owning a private practice, due to billing and other administrative requirements. In the average practice, annual overhead costs have reached about $83,000 per physician in the United States, compared with $22,000 in Canada.[33] As a result, doctors mostly have become employees of hospital and health system corporations, where relatively high salaries tend to mask the reality of their employee status.

Before neoliberalism, physicians for the most part owned or controlled their own means of production and conditions of practice. Although their work was often challenging, they could decide their own hours, staff members, how much time to spend with patients, what to record about their visits in medical records, and how much to charge for their services. Today, the corporations for which physicians work control all of these decisions. This loss of control over the conditions of work has eroded doctors' professional well-being and satisfaction.

With loss of control over the work process and a reduced ability to generate very high incomes, the medical profession has become proletarianized.[34] In a way, doctors have joined that highest stratum of workers that Lenin and others referred to as the "aristocracy of labor."[35] From Samir Amin's perspective, the current wave of "generalized proletarianization" has engulfed the medical profession: "A rapidly growing proportion of workers are no more than sellers of their labor power to capital…a reality that should not be obscured by the apparent autonomy conferred on them by their legal status."[36]

Beyond the changing class position of health professionals, the transition as Obamacare fails will need to address the "oligopolistic" character of the insurance industry, with dominance by a small number of very large insurance corporations that do not achieve meaningful levels of competition among themselves. These corporations receive prepaid, capitated payments from publicly supported programs like Obamacare and then invest much of the funds in global financial markets. As a result, the health insurance industry increasingly overlaps with banks, investment corporations, hedge funds, and real estate companies – referred to as the FIRE sector of the global capitalist economy (*f*inancialization, *i*nsurance, and *r*eal *e*state), which accumulates capital by financial transactions and investments rather than the production of goods and services.[37] Due to these interrelationships, health insurance premiums largely reflect gains and losses in insurance corporations' financial investments, more than patients' utilization of health services. Obamacare has increased the flow of capitated public and private funds into the insurance industry, and, thus, has extended the overall financialization of the global economy. In addition to the marked enlargement and concentration of insurance corporations, a parallel set of large and oligopolistic for-profit corporations employ doctors and other health professionals to deliver health services under tight managerial control. Consolidation of large health systems has paralleled consolidation of large insurance corporations.[38]

In this context, it is important to consider the distinction between national health insurance (NHI) and a national health service (NHS). NHI involves socialization of payments for health services but usually leaves intact private ownership at the level of infrastructure. Except for a small proportion of institutions like public hospitals and clinics, under NHI, the means of production in health care remain privately owned. Canada is the best-known model of NHI. The PNHP single-payer proposal, as well as the Congressional legislation that embodies the singer-payer approach, is based on the Canadian model of NHI.

An NHS, by comparison, involves socialization of both payment for health services and the infrastructure through which services are provided. Under an NHS, the state generally owns and operates hospitals, clinics, and other health institutions, which become part of the public sector rather than remaining under private control. In the capitalist world, Scotland and Sweden provide examples of NHSs, where most health infrastructure exists within the public sector and most health professionals are employees of the state. For such countries, the state apparatus includes elements that provide "welfare state" services, including health care, while still ultimately protecting the capitalist system. In the socialist world, Cuba offers the clearest remaining model of an NHS where a private sector does not exist. In the United States, a legislative proposal introduced during the 1970s and 1980s by Representative Ronald Dellums explicitly adopted the goal of an NHS.[39]

The PNHP single-payer proposal emerged from a retreat in New Hampshire during 1986, where activists struggled with these distinctions. Although most participants at the retreat had worked hard for the Dellums NHS proposal, they reached a consensus – albeit with some ambivalence – to shift their work to an NHI proposal based on Canada. The rationale for this shift involved two main considerations. First, Canada's proximity and cultural similarity to the United States would make NHI more palatable for the U.S. population and, especially, for its Congressional representatives.

Second, a Canadian-style NHI proposal could be "doctor-friendly." Under the PNHP proposal, physicians could continue to work in private practice, clinics, or hospitals. The main difference for physicians is that payments would be socialized, so that they would not have to worry about billing and collecting their fees for services provided.[40]

While PNHP has achieved great success in its research and policy work, these efforts, and those of many other organizations supporting single payer, have not yet generated a broad social movement supporting a Canadian-style NHI. Meanwhile, the neoliberal model, with all its benefits for the ruling class and drawbacks for everyone else, has solidified its hegemony. Partly as a result, physicians and other health professionals are becoming proletarianized employees of an increasingly consolidated, profit-driven, financialized health care system. And under Obamacare, the state has continued to prioritize protection of the interests of capital, in this case by overseeing huge public subsidies for private insurance and pharmaceutical corporations.

Under these circumstances, it is no longer evident that socialization of payments for health services under a single-payer NHI is the only goal of progressive health praxis. PNHP calls for the removal of for-profit corporations from U.S. health care. But that change will not occur within the context of capitalism as we know it. As neoliberalism draws to a close and as Obamacare fails, a much more fundamental transformation is needed to reshape not just health care, but also the capitalist state and capitalist society, within which health care is situated.

Struggles to Address the Social Determination of Health and Illness

Priorities of non-reformist praxis. While the United States spends more on health care than any other country – over $3.5 trillion each year – the country continues to fall behind other advanced countries in health outcomes such as life expectancy and infant mortality.[41] As we have mentioned earlier, especially in Chapter 4, health care is one determinant of health outcomes, but overall is less important than other social conditions. Studies using meta-analysis, a technique that combines the results of many studies to allow stronger statistical conclusions, found that social determination of health includes components like socioeconomic status, racism and discrimination, education, neighborhood and physical environment, employment, and social support networks, as well as access to health care. The environment where a child grows up may exert health effects over several generations. Researchers determined that social conditions including racism and racial segregation, educational deficits, inadequate social supports, and poverty accounted for over a third of annual deaths in the United States. Studies have documented disturbing social class differences in life expectancy and deteriorating life expectancy among the middle-aged white population in the United States.[42] Addressing social determination of health is important for improving health and reducing long-standing inequalities in health and health care.

The range of non-reformist praxis reveals that several problems are especially urgent. So, what are the priorities? First, the recurrent economic crises of advanced capitalism present both dangers and opportunities. Stagnation and cutbacks in health care and other public services have heightened tensions throughout capitalist societies. For example, the far-right has emerged as a well-financed, politically powerful network of interest groups with a striking public presence and leadership style. Such organizations show an authoritarian fervor that borders on fascism. At the same time, openly racist groups have grown in size and public visibility. Under conditions of economic and political instability, polarization along class and racial lines deepens.

Such a social and political climate has emerged in the United States and some other countries. In the throes of the 2016 presidential election, racial tensions came to a head following several police shootings of young African American men and the inflammatory rhetoric of the Republican nominee, Donald Trump. While Trump never specifically endorsed the racist outcry taken up by some of his supporters, he also did not reject the support of Ku Klux Klan leader David Duke, among many others with similar views and actions. Partly in response to increasing racist attacks, antiracist activism has become a crucial priority in workplace and community organizing. On January 21, 2017 – the day after President Trump was inaugurated – millions of women and their supporters of various sexual orientations held protests in all 50 states and several other countries to express dissent at how the new president treated women and minority groups. The massive worldwide protests against racism and police brutality that arose after the killing of George Floyd in Minneapolis during the COVID-19 pandemic also reflect that growing resistance against the injustices and violence of racial capitalism. In health care and in our broader social systems, as we discussed in Chapter 4, racism, classism, and sexism remain as interrelated structures of oppression.

International work, especially in opposition to militarism, is a second priority. Medicine, capitalism, and imperialism historically have intertwined. As we describe in Chapter 6, medical and public health professionals have played an important role on behalf of imperialist expansion. Dominant nations frequently have tried to maintain their power through direct military intervention. At other times these efforts are subtler, as in the economic destabilization of new governments or covert military support for dictatorships. The availability of nuclear weapons vastly increases the stakes of political action against militarism. Warfare, if unchecked, will continue to create devastating effects on health and well-being throughout the world. Poignant examples of militarism's effects involve several countries of the Middle East, including Palestine, Afghanistan, Iraq, Syria, and Yemen. Endless war has emerged as an enduring characteristic of global capitalism, partly as a reliable route to capital accumulation by the military–industrial complex. "Disaster capitalism" has enhanced the fortunes enjoyed by a tiny proportion of the world's population. Victims of war increasingly include (as we have seen in the last chapter) military personnel. Meanwhile, war remains invisible to most people who live in the United States, even though approximately one-half of federal income taxes pay for present and past wars.[43]

Third, there is the inescapable problem of illness-generating conditions in the workplace and environment. As we have discussed in previous chapters, over the past two centuries the world has become a dumping ground for toxic wastes. While market-place ideology continues to push forward, health problems due to work and the environment worsen. The earth's surface temperatures between 2015 and 2019 were the five warmest since modern record keeping began in 1880.[44] Environmental exploitation has emerged as a damaging effect of capitalist development, but similar problems also have arisen in socialist countries. Epidemics of cancer and other chronic diseases have appeared among workers in a variety of industries. The hazards of nuclear power and stockpiled weapons threaten humanity and other species because of potential accidents as much as the intentional use of these technologies. In capitalist societies, as we have noted in Chapter 3, the structure of private profit consistently impedes efforts to deal systematically with occupational and environmental health problems. These medical consequences emerge from the very fabric of our society as currently organized. Changing the social roots of illness-generating conditions must be a major goal if we are to have a future at all.

READER ADVISORY: BEWARE OF WHAT FOLLOWS!

The following sections express information and viewpoints that may seem even more controversial or preposterous than others that we have expressed in this book. Some readers, though interested in social medicine, may become annoyed or worse because of what we have to say about moving beyond capitalism and how to do that. Based on our studies and experiences of activism, we do conclude that strategies to address the social determination of health without addressing the sources of illness-generating social determinants in global capitalism will not succeed. However, we do not claim to have a corner on the truth about how to get from A to B, and we individually hold somewhat different views about the following suggestions for praxis in social medicine. We expect that you will too. Because we respect your views, we actually welcome your feedback and constructively critical suggestions. You can reach us by email at waitzkin@unm.edu (Howard), alinaperez1190@gmail.com (Alina), and maanders@montefiore.org (Matt). We also would respect your decision to stop your encounter with social medicine here at this time, although we do hope you'll return in the future.

Moving beyond capitalism for our health. So, in capitalist societies, a central question for social medicine becomes: Are humane social conditions that foster health and a humane health care system possible in a capitalist society?[45] Previously, social medicine practitioners at least could point to some countries in Europe and elsewhere with mixed capitalist–socialist systems creating conditions that fostered good health and access to needed services. But all those countries have experienced attacks on their public sector NHPs, and inequality and racism have increased as causes of ill-health and early death. Non-reformist reforms aim to transform capitalist society and to move beyond the contradictions of capitalism that weaken NHPs and that create illness-generating social conditions. But how can that transition actually happen? How can we move beyond capitalism for our health?[46] These questions have emerged as crucial, especially for social medicine as we enter the coming transformation.

"It's easier to imagine the end of the world than the end of our economic system." This statement, attributed to Fredric Jameson,[47] conveys how simple it is to visualize scenarios leading to the end of humanity and other life forms (global warming with rising oceans and hot, uninhabitable land masses; nuclear Armageddon with radioactivity killing all animals and plants; etc.). The quote also conveys a vacuum of creative thinking that continues to stand in the way of moving beyond global capitalism, which each year benefits an ever tinier part of the world's population (now roughly 0.5 percent) at the expense of the rest of us. Yet, how to get from A to B, capitalism to postcapitalism, is the question that we need to answer during this critical period of history, when the destructive forces of the global capitalist system threaten the survival of us human beings and other living species.

Our current historical period contains tremendous dangers: nuclear war, global warming and other environmental catastrophes, and fascism – a world based on deepening exploitation of nature, inequality, repression, and suffering. But these dangers have generated worldwide resistance and social movements aiming to create societies based on harmony with nature, cooperative relationships of mutual aid, and decision-making by ordinary people about the directions that our lives and our children's and grandchildren's lives will take.

Because it is hard to imagine a viable path from capitalism to postcapitalism, most people who try to address our world's challenges assume that capitalism will continue to exist. So we engage in peculiar ways of struggling to improve our most important problems without confronting capitalism, even though we recognize that capitalism generates these problems and continues to make them worse (Figure 10.2). In concluding this book on social medicine, we argue for a shift in our approach, so that we struggle to improve our key problems by confronting and moving beyond capitalism itself through revolutionary transformation, even if that transformation involves actions and inactions on a day-to-day basis that may seem unglamorous and "rinky-dink," but also safe and feasible in every person's life (Figures 10.3 and 10.3.a; Figure 10.3.a. expands the bottom boxes about the rinky-dink revolution). We no longer can afford to wait by deferring this struggle for future generations to resolve.[48]

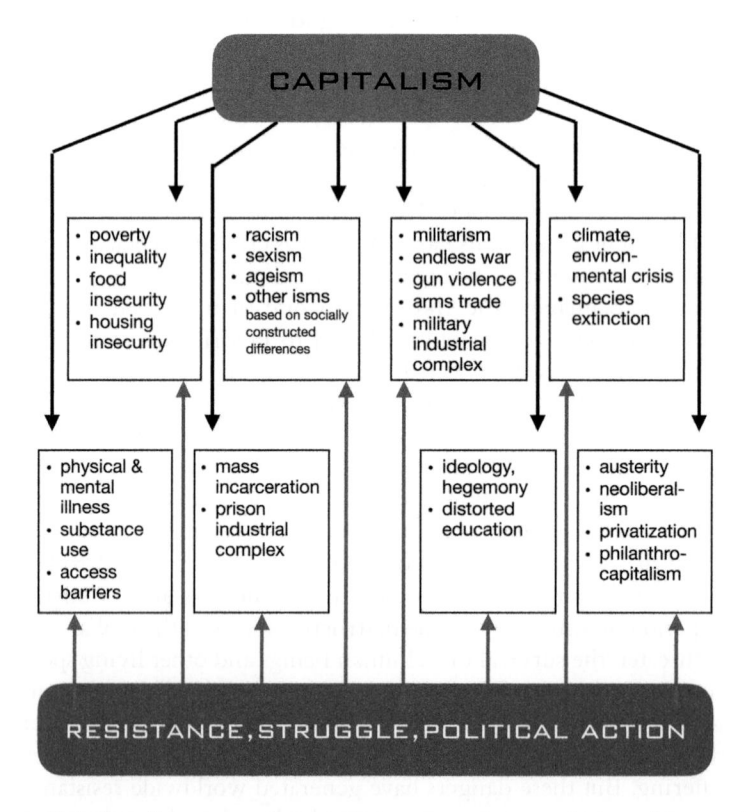

Figure 10.2 Peculiar ways of struggling to improve our key problems without confronting capitalism.

CAPITALISM

- poverty
- inequality
- food insecurity
- housing insecurity

- racism
- sexism
- ageism
- other isms
  based on socially constructed differences

- militarism
- endless war
- gun violence
- arms trade
- military industrial complex

- climate, environmental crisis
- species extinction

- physical & mental illness
- substance use
- access barriers

- mass incarceration
- prison industrial complex

- ideology, hegemony
- distorted education

- austerity
- neoliberalism
- privatization
- philanthrocapitalism

Creative *constructive* actions

- Solving the housing problem
- Solving the food problem
- Building the solidarity economy
- Taking part in limited electoral work to achieve "dual power"

Creative *destructive* actions

- Withholding consent to the global capitalist system
- Direct actions to block capitalism
  - Avoiding symbolic politics
- Tax resistance
- Redirection of investment into non-capitalist enterprises
- Demystification

RESISTANCE, STRUGGLE, POLITICAL ACTION

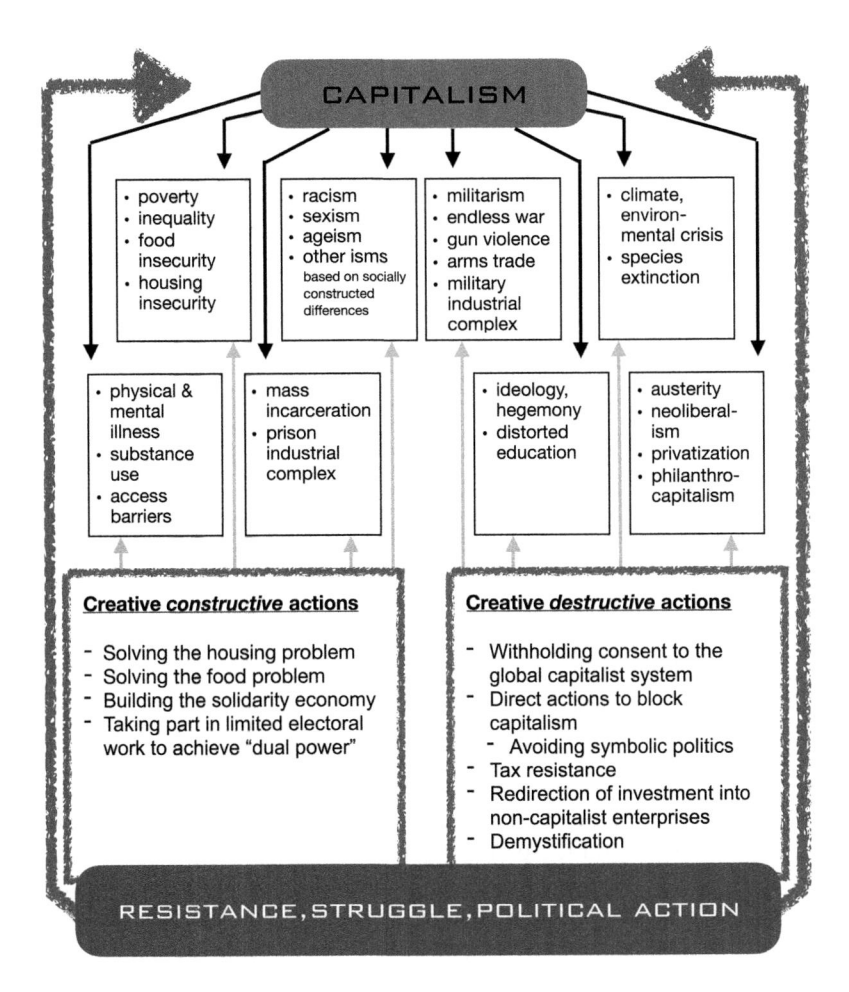

Figure 10.3 Rinky-dink revolution: struggling to improve our key problems by confronting and moving beyond capitalism.

As poverty, inequality, racism, sexism, food insecurity, job insecurity, climate change and environmental catastrophe, militarism, and the threat of nuclear war persist and worsen, millions of people throughout the world now realize that limited reforms in capitalism will not work. They/we – often with leadership from social medicine practitioners and activists – are ready to move ahead on the road beyond capitalism. For people who value social medicine, the road beyond capitalism involves clearly identifying the fundamental determination of illness and early death in the global capitalist system and struggling to change that determination through radical transformations leading to a postcapitalist economic system.

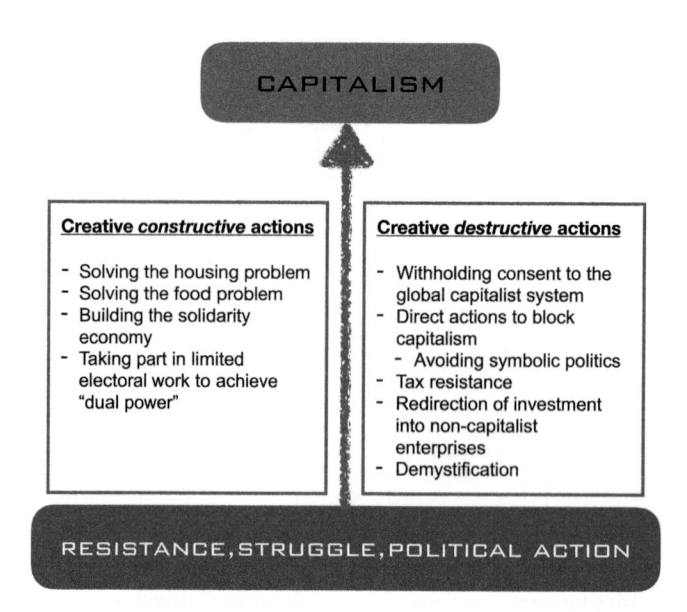

```
                    ┌─────────────────┐
                    │   CAPITALISM    │
                    └────────▲────────┘
                             │
    ┌────────────────────────┴─────────────────────────┐
    │ Creative constructive actions │ Creative destructive actions │
    │                               │                              │
    │ - Solving the housing problem │ - Withholding consent to the │
    │ - Solving the food problem    │   global capitalist system   │
    │ - Building the solidarity     │ - Direct actions to block    │
    │   economy                     │   capitalism                 │
    │ - Taking part in limited      │   - Avoiding symbolic politics│
    │   electoral work to achieve   │ - Tax resistance             │
    │   "dual power"                │ - Redirection of investment  │
    │                               │   into non-capitalist        │
    │                               │   enterprises                │
    │                               │ - Demystification            │
    └───────────────────────────────────────────────────┘
    
    ┌───────────────────────────────────────────────────┐
    │     RESISTANCE, STRUGGLE, POLITICAL ACTION        │
    └───────────────────────────────────────────────────┘
```

Figure 10.3.a Rinky-dink revolution: struggling to improve our key problems by confronting and moving beyond capitalism (expanded view).

How can that happen? Answering this question and then acting on the answers have emerged as the central challenges of praxis for thinkers and activists in social medicine and actually all others who are concerned about planet earth and the beings who live here. In conclusion, we indicate some reasons why electoral "democracy," which we are taught to see as the way to achieve needed changes in society (i.e., by electing leaders who will work toward those changes), will not actually achieve the fundamental changes in capitalism that will enhance health rather than illness and death. Then, we summarize an emerging field of analysis and struggle that focuses first on constructing a "solidarity economy" outside global capitalism and secondly on creative acts of resistance and nonparticipation in the global capitalist system. Here we provide a brief overview and some examples of efforts that move along a path toward transformation of the core social determination in capitalism that social medicine has identified throughout its history over the last two centuries.

Elections are not the point. Defects of the electoral process within what we usually consider as democracy manifest themselves often but arguably never more clearly than in the U.S. presidential election of 2016. This election clarified several glaring characteristics of electoral procedures that cast doubt on our ability to achieve meaningful change by voting:

- apathy, nonparticipation, intimidation, and exclusion of voters through complex voter registration requirements, insufficient polling places and staffing, and similar maneuvers that discourage voters from voting – leading in this case to Trump's so-called triumph when he received votes from less than 25 percent of eligible voters and less than one-sixth of all citizens, lost the popular vote, and faced no run-off election;
- scheduling election days on workdays rather than national holidays or Sundays;
- buying politicians through campaign contributions and other financial support; and
- creation of false consciousness through manipulation of the media.

Elections play a small role in the struggle to transform oppressive social conditions, and the role that elections do play is to clarify that much more fundamental revolutionary strategy is needed. As social medicine nurse and anarchist Emma Goldman pointed out long ago, elections are mostly symbolic actions that never in themselves bring fundamental change. In a quote attributed to her, she said, "If voting changed anything, they'd have made it illegal long ago."[49]

The understandable longing for humane government with responsive leaders chosen through elections probably belongs in the proverbial dustbin of history, because that desire has been realized rarely if ever. Since the origins of so-called democracy during the Greek empire, elections have remained the tool of rich and powerful elites. Capitalism has only magnified the inherent social class characteristics of electoral processes.

What Karl Marx and others call "bourgeois democracy" prevails throughout the world, with rare exceptions. Such democracy enacts a symbolic ritual of voting. As Tommy Douglas, the great left-wing Canadian politician and founder of the Canadian single-payer NHP, orated, mice vote for white cats or black cats, but never for mice.[50] So the problem we face now is not just presidents and other elected leaders who are neofascist, racist, sexist, and xenophobic, but rather a system that assures its elected leader will be, whether Republican or Democrat, a representative of the feline class. It is this system that must change, not the candidates who become the anthropomorphized symbols of the system. Years before Douglas, according to Vladimir Lenin, Marx described the process less metaphorically: "Every once in a while, the oppressed are allowed to decide which particular representatives of the oppressing class will represent them and oppress them."[51]

One reason why most of us rodents, sometimes depicted as the 99 percent, including many of us who work in social medicine, find it so hard to recognize the lunacy of our aspirations to elect good people to run good government involves our illusions about what government is and where it resides. The state in which elected government resides is the capitalist state; it is not a neutral state, let alone a state that aims to benefit people other than the small group of those at the top of the pyramid of wealth and power who control the state. Time and again, political economic realities have confirmed Marx and Engels's claim that the main role of the capitalist state is to protect the capitalist economic system, or, to use their metaphor, the state is the "executive committee of the bourgeoisie."[52]

Despite this understanding, we nevertheless cling to the illusion that the capitalist state can become a benevolent entity. NHPs, championed by activists and social medicine practitioners like the authors, are components of a benevolent welfare state. Other components include public education, housing, and transportation; livable wages; and adequate food supplies. Welfare states became fixtures of multiple European countries after the Great Depression of the 1930s, as Keynesian economic policies encouraged high levels of government spending. These welfare states also became models for development in some countries of the global South, such as Chile, Argentina, Costa Rica, and Mexico.

But welfare states within capitalist states suffer from inherent contradictions. First, the welfare components remain vulnerable to cutbacks and elimination during economic crises, as we have seen in the NHPs of essentially all European countries.[53] Important public programs of the welfare state constrict or disappear as that other key function of the capitalist state gears up to address the recurrent crises of the capitalist system.

Second, these welfare components contribute to a false consciousness and hegemonic beliefs about the state's beneficent potentialities. This ideological impact has been called the state's "legitimation function."[54] By providing helpful services, including health services through an NHP, the state legitimates the continuing inequalities and exploitations inherent in the capitalist system.[55]

Many of us, especially in the health professions and social medicine, respond to the suffering we encounter everywhere by advocating expansion or at least maintenance of the capitalist state's welfare components. We do this even though we understand that these welfare components remain perpetually vulnerable and legitimate a system that inherently causes exploitation, inequality, hunger, ill-health, and early death. And we persist in advocating for the welfare state although we know that the global capitalist system has become weaker and more vulnerable due to deepening crises, loss of legitimacy, and effects on the environment that threaten the survival of humanity and other life forms.

In the current period of world history, with all its dangers but also with its deep potential for transformation, the time has come to move beyond our illusions that electoral politics and reforms of the capitalist state can achieve the revolutionary changes that we know are necessary. So what is the nature of that revolution, and what is the eventual aim?

A solidarity economy. Many groups worldwide, including many who work in social medicine, are trying to achieve revolutionary change by creating a solidarity economy outside capitalism. In the United States, over 200 organizations currently are collaborating in constructing such a noncapitalist economy.[56] People in some of the poorest and most marginalized areas of the country (such as Jackson, Mississippi; the Rust Belt in the Midwest; and low-income neighborhoods of major cities) are pursuing this work, with some remarkable accomplishments.

Similar organizations are growing outside the United States in areas of the world most affected by imperialism and more recent austerity policies under neoliberalism, such as southern Europe and Latin America. These efforts often emphasize the social medicine goal of "living well" (*sumak kawsay* in Quechua, *buen vivir* in Spanish). Social medicine activists in Latin American countries such as Bolivia, Ecuador, Venezuela, and Nicaragua have advanced this goal as a key component of proposed national health policies. Living well usually implies community-based solidarity and sustainability through "mutual aid," moving away from the social conditions of capitalist society that worsen poverty, inequality, environmental pollution, and unacceptable health outcomes.[57]

Most of these efforts aim to free people from spending most of our lives as workers in precarious, proletarianized jobs, where we are unable to survive with healthy lives, let alone feel a sense of accomplishment in work and solidarity in community. One way of describing this struggle is to reduce the need to work as "wage slaves," without energy and time to create a new and different world. Moving into a postcapitalist world means finding solutions to some age-old problems.

First, groups trying to achieve a solidarity economy develop ways to solve the housing problem. For most people, paying for housing becomes the biggest expense, requiring us to labor for wages in the capitalist economy and also emerging as the main source of day-to-day insecurity. So the solidarity economy first of all finds ways to create cheap, small-scale, cooperative, pleasant, and comfortable housing units that require very little money, with collaborative solutions to avoid the exploitative conditions, such as rent, debt, burdensome taxes, and insurance, that capitalism imposes on people who need housing. Housing co-ops find inexpensive properties in cities or rural areas where housing can be rehabilitated or constructed with the increasingly sophisticated technologies that reduce the costs of labor and improve the environmental sustainability of housing materials.[58] The aim is about $150 per person per month of housing costs, which can be in dollars, local currency of a city or town, or nonmonetary time equivalents of donated work (called by such names as "Mutual Exchange of Work" units, or "MEOWs") (Figure 10.4).

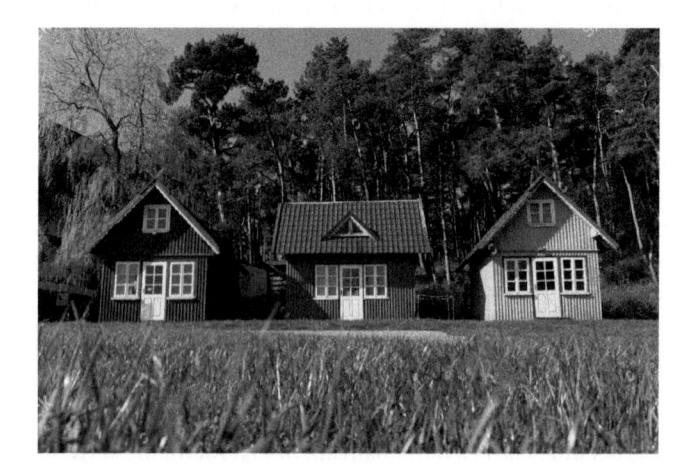

Figure 10.4 Examples of affordable housing within the solidarity economy.

Second, the path to achieving a solidarity economy includes solving the food problem. The goal is sustainable, local food production and consumption with a low carbon footprint (meaning minimum petroleum products used for fertilizers, pesticides, and, especially, transportation of food and its raw materials) and with a more favorable impact on the health of human beings, other living species, and mother earth.

Community gardens and food cooperatives figure as key components of achieving food autonomy, which people active in social medicine increasingly recognize as a critical goal. Gardening principles include cultivating plants that produce healthy nutrients such as nonanimal sources of proteins, with limited fats and carbohydrates. These principles recognize the worldwide epidemics of obesity and diabetes, which reflect a combination of food insecurity, "food deserts" (where healthy foods are unavailable or too expensive for purchase in many inner-city and rural areas), and overpromotion of sugar- and fat-rich foods by capitalist agricultural and food industries that produce and market processed food. Animals for products like meat, fish, eggs, and milk for human beings who opt for continuing nonvegetarian or nonvegan diets are locally raised, slaughtered, and packaged for local consumption.

An overall objective is independence from capitalist agriculture. Food independence means giving up consumption of food that requires access to seasonal production in distant places with carbon-based transportation over long distances, whose high financial costs and pollution contribute to climate change, depletion of fresh water supplies, and continuing exploitation of agricultural workers. For families of average size, the aim again is

$150 per person per month of food costs, which can be in dollars or time equivalent (MEOWs).[59]

While solving the housing and food problems both hold tremendous importance for health and "good living," several other key elements of constructing the solidarity economy beyond capitalism also deserve attention in social medicine. For instance, we must replace economic activities that are ecologically unsustainable. In addition to its inherent need to exploit human beings and animals in producing goods and services for sale, capitalism also requires a continuing "expropriation of nature" in order to accumulate capital for the tiny portion of humanity at the top of society's pyramid of wealth and power.[60] To survive and flourish through endless accumulation of capital, the capitalist economy depends on unending economic growth. The need for growth becomes an inherent contradiction within capitalism, because growth requires the endless exploitation of natural resources that actually are limited or whose use generates problems that threaten the survival of humanity and other species. Among many examples, fossil fuels cannot last forever, and their use meanwhile generates pollution and climate change, with dangerous effects on health and well-being.

So, constructing the solidarity economy outside capitalism requires not only less growth but actually degrowth, which means stopping the vicious cycle that inherently exploits humans, animals, and mother earth. These changes also require shifts in desires that capitalist markets have generated. As one of many examples, each roundtrip transcontinental airplane flight generates an impact on global warming that leads to the melting of 3 cubic meters of arctic ice.[61] So, those of us who care about social medicine need to let go of seeing so much of the world so much of the time. Simple changes in our patterns of economic consumption, which become massive changes if enough people act on them, will reverse the unhealthy habits of growth that capitalism inherently generates.

Day-to-day life in the solidarity economy means engaging in cooperative economic activities to meet one's own needs and wants, as well as meeting the needs and wants of others in one's community. The underlying principle of such economic activities involves mutual aid, by which people exchange goods and services without the exploitative structures and processes by which capitalism encourages a small proportion of the world's population to accumulate vast wealth while millions suffer from poverty, precarious jobs, housing insecurity, and hunger. Interestingly, one doesn't need money for many of these economic activities. Communities all over the world are discovering and implementing local economies that do not require much, if any, national currency, such as dollars. Instead, people are returning to simpler versions of economic exchange, where goods and services are produced and exchanged directly at the local level.

Several types of noncapitalist economic activities are emerging, with importance for social medicine. Through barter, people can directly exchange a good or service, satisfying what each person needs or wants; barter can include services provided by health and mental health professionals. With time banking, a person can do one hour of work anywhere in a specified community of participants; after one person provides one hour of work, he or she can request one hour of work from the time bank, which coordinates requests for services and keeps track of time worked. Health and mental health cooperatives within communities can operate within a time bank framework: Practitioners provide services they are trained to offer and, in return, receive goods and services that they need. Communities also can create their own local currencies, which people use to exchange goods and services, including services involving health and mental health.

By participating in the solidarity economy, community members enhance the local economy and also reduce dependency on expensive and carbon-producing transportation of products and workers to and from other parts of the world. Within many communities, people are deciding to share their infrastructure, including tools, kitchens, libraries, workspaces, equipment, communications including phone and internet, and buildings for housing, stores, clinics, hospitals, and other facilities that respond to common needs and wants. Such spaces become components of a "commons," which is available for everyone to share but does not generate profits that some people can enjoy at the expense of others.

What is the role of "electoral democracy" in the solidarity economy? Not much. Communities worldwide that are trying to construct economies not dependent on or dominated by the global capitalist system have developed a profound skepticism about the capitalist state, and this skepticism applies also to the feasibility of successful and enduring health care systems managed by the capitalist state. Rather than investing time, money, and energy in national electoral politics and politicians to advance goals like an NHP, activists have realized that noncapitalist NHPs cannot survive without social movements that transform the fundamental characteristics of capitalism itself.

As this understanding applies to elections, the focus moves from the national and state levels to the local level, usually the county or municipality. Activists take part in limited electoral work to achieve "dual power" at the local level. But they let go of illusions about elections and maintain clarity about the adverse effects of elections through history.

As implemented most clearly by Cooperation Jackson, dual power involves two elements of power. First, to summarize briefly, activists build a network of strong community-based organizations that focus on different components of the solidarity economy (such as housing, food, ecologically sustainable energy production and waste management, transportation, education, and health and mental health services) and that make decisions by direct participatory discussion and consensus within a "communal" structure. Adapting their model from revolutionary struggles in other countries and theories of transition beyond the capitalist state, local communes eventually assume the main responsibility for governance in a postcapitalist society and choose the regional and national leaders who implement policies shaped mostly from below.[62]

Second, during a transitional period, activists prioritize winning local elections, especially for mayor and municipal or county councils, as has occurred in Jackson. Local elections accomplish some narrow purposes. One key purpose involves the prevention of repression and brutality by police and other wings of "law enforcement" at various levels of government and by those outside government who take justice into their own hands through gun violence, paramilitary violence, and other forms of victimization. Another key purpose involves access to funds and labor based in the public sector to help provide housing, food, and needed services such as water, electricity, heat, sanitation, fire protection, public education, and health and mental health services that, in the short term, community residents cannot fully provide by themselves.

While efforts to build solidarity economies will constitute a fundamental part of praxis for social medicine in the future, this creative and often experimental work will not in itself lead to a full transformation of global capitalism and its pernicious effects on health and well-being. In addition to the positive construction of a new world, those who work in social medicine and many others can contribute to the peaceful and also creative destruction of our destructive economic system.

Creative acts of resistance and non-participation in the global capitalist economic system. Is there a military route to revolution in the United States and other powerful capitalist countries? With the exception of Cuba, most countries transitioning from capitalism through military means, such as the ex-Soviet Union, China, Vietnam, Nicaragua, Angola, and others, have wound up implementing systems involving strong elements of a capitalist economy. Cuba recently has been expanding opportunities for international investment and for people in Cuba to support themselves through private businesses and markets, without permitting multinational for-profit corporations to engage in the usual capitalist practices of exploiting workers for private capital accumulation. Some other countries that have carried out violent anti-capitalist revolutions (e.g., Nicaragua, China, Vietnam, and Angola), while permitting the intrusion of traditional corporate capitalism, have improved health outcomes, education, housing, and other quality of life indicators for large parts of their populations. Also, taking up arms as a defensive strategy is a crucial part of the U.S. experience.[63] For these and other reasons, a military wing of a revolutionary movement may happen, as it has in many countries of the global South and some in the global North.

Before turning to violence, the leaders of all those revolutions had agitated through political struggles that did not initially involve arms. But the brutality of the previous dictatorial regimes proved so great that no option other than armed struggle appeared viable. And those raising arms did so with the usual ambivalences about injuring and killing other beings, usually those conscripted or hired to fight on behalf of rulers who rarely risk making their bodies vulnerable in battle. Some leaders of social medicine have participated in armed revolutionary struggle, recognizing that revolutionary transformation of illness-generating social conditions could accomplish more than clinical interventions to treat illnesses that resulted from those social conditions. For instance, Doctor Ernesto (Che) Guevara (discussed in Chapter 8), who became a physician in his native Argentina, famously had to choose during the Cuban revolution between carrying his doctor's bag or carrying his rifle. He decided to carry his rifle because, as he later explained to a class of postrevolutionary Cuban medical students, he realized he could do more to improve health conditions through his rifle than through his doctor's bag. The human psyche usually justifies this kind of violence by invoking some variant of what Che called the revolutionary motivation of love.[64]

For most practitioners of social medicine, including the authors, who oppose violence or who cannot bring ourselves to injure or kill other human beings, the nonmilitary wing of revolutionary action opens up countless exciting possibilities. Surprisingly, fairly rigorous research shows that a small proportion of a country's population, estimated at 3.5–5 percent, can achieve revolutionary change through nonviolent resistance, even in countries with brutal dictatorships.[65] But these nonviolent actions move far beyond electoral politics to include direct action, whose conscious aim is to slow down and shut down the capitalist economic system and the state that protects that system.

Mass protests in the United States and many other countries often involve huge peaceful demonstrations, carried out with permits from the local police. Activists in social medicine tend to participate in such protests. The tremendous accomplishment of the women's marches on Washington, D.C., and other cities around the world on the day after Trump's inauguration, for instance, counts as probably the largest single protest action in the world's history. Coordinated marches against war taxes, for science, for the environment, and many other causes followed.[66]

Despite their importance, such actions do nothing to shut down the capitalist system. Neither did the smaller protests on inauguration day that destroyed some property and led to felony arrests that incapacitated key activists with legal proceedings and jail time for months or years afterward. And neither did most of the Occupy actions in which many subjected

Praxis, Reform, Sociomedical Activism 251

ourselves to police brutality in order to fill a public space for periods of time. These important nonviolent actions reverberate mostly in the realm of symbolic politics.

What kinds of actions actually do slow down or shut down the capitalist system, and why are they important for social medicine? The heroic struggle at Standing Rock to stop the Dakota Access Pipeline by indigenous communities is one such action. Here, the explicit purpose has not been just to demonstrate against a monstrous, last-ditch effort to accumulate massive profits by robbing indigenous lands, polluting water supplies, and worsening climate change by burning oil. As discussed throughout this book, all three of these goals – protecting indigenous land from the health-damaging effects of capitalism and imperialism, preserving accessibility of safe water supplies, and addressing the social and environmental determination of illness and early death – are fundamental goals of social medicine. However, one key purpose of the Standing Rock actions also has been to stop the pipeline's construction and to block transport of oil to refineries and eventually to "consumers"; in other words, to slow down and to stop this important component needed for the smooth functioning of the capitalist economic system. Similar heroic struggles by indigenous communities to block oil transport have happened in Canada and Latin American countries, including Bolivia and Ecuador (Figure 10.5).

So how might Latin American social medicine activists advise social medicine and other activists in the United States? Focusing on oil transportation, they would explain for starters that the Dakota Access Pipeline,

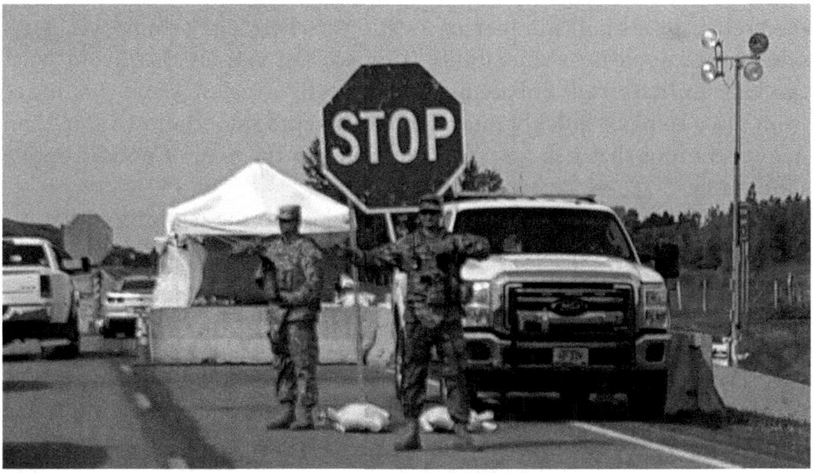

Figure 10.5 Protest in support of the struggle to block the Dakota Access Pipeline at Standing Rock.

as only one of many petroleum pipelines that traverse North America, lies four to five feet underground along 1,134 miles of geographically isolated territory in North Dakota, South Dakota, Iowa, and Illinois, vulnerable and largely unprotected from direct actions of many types. The pipeline originates in the Bakken shale oil fields in northwest North Dakota and terminates at the oil storage facility at Patoka Township in southern Illinois.[67]

Patoka probably would interest Latin American revolutionaries eager to shut down sectors of the capitalist economy and to block flow of fossil fuels. Google Maps, among other imaging sources, depict this quaint, sparsely populated agricultural area, where a highly concentrated collection of huge oil tanks contrasts with the surrounding farmlands, schools, shops, eateries, and pristine lakes used by folks who like to fish. The Dakota Access Pipeline and the BNSF rail yards where Bakken oil arrives by train are not the only interesting oil transport facilities that converge here. Patoka also is a main terminus for the Keystone and Keystone XL Pipelines, as well as the hub for existing pipelines used by Mobil Exxon, Marathon, and Shell. Energy Transfer Partners owns much of the storage infrastructure in Patoka, as well as pipelines carrying oil there and then to refineries mainly in Louisiana and Texas.[68]

In direct actions that target transport of fossil fuels, toxic chemicals, conventional and nuclear weapons, military equipment, precious metals, timber, and other items that keep the capitalist system afloat, social medicine and other activists may focus on pipelines, roads, waterways, air facilities, and so forth, many of them far from existing population centers and their associated security operations. The geographical distances and wide variety of potential targets means that activists need not restrict themselves to a small number of locations, where gatherings over periods of time increase vulnerability. Instead, fast actions that avoid what the U.S. military calls collateral damage to living beings and that move from place to place quickly interrupt the system's smooth flow more than demonstrations that risk arrest and injuries for the sake of nondisruptive symbolism.[69]

Tactically, experiences in Latin America lead to the realization that direct actions can disrupt business as usual, even if disrupters disperse when they receive warnings that they are about to be arrested. Despite efforts to restrict demonstrations in several states, U.S. legalities do require warnings by police and military forces before arrests or physical attacks begin. Latin American revolutionaries have shown that blocking a highway, railway, port, or airport for quite a long time does not necessarily imply the need to block it until arrest or injury. One misconception about nonviolent resistance involves the vision that one ethically needs to hang around until incarcerated, injured, or both.

Besides direct action, social medicine activists can change through our praxis what we do with our money, especially in the realms of taxes, investments, and local economic activities. Such changes can disrupt, undermine, and create space for further actions to transform illness-generating conditions fostered by global capitalism. Although some very rich doctors who identify with social medicine earn incomes or hold wealth that ranks them in the 1 percent at the top of capitalism's financial pyramid,[70] most of us in social medicine, even with comfortable lives, number in the 99 percent below the ultrarich. Nevertheless, we in the 99 percent persist as the main funders of the capitalist state, which passes our money on to corporations that exploit workers, destroy nature, raise the earth's temperature, and keep us in permanent war and perpetual inequality. We need to change our habits of giving up our money, and if enough of us do so, the capitalist state no longer will be able to prop up the capitalist economy for the benefit of the ultrarich.

Tax resistance can take several forms. For more than a century, pacifists in the United States have resisted taxes that pay for war, some eventually going to prison but the vast majority, like one of the authors, Howard, suffering no substantial harm as a result. If one honestly declares one's income, there is nothing illegal about claiming a war deduction of 50 percent, which is the approximate percentage of the federal budget that pays for past, present, and future wars. In addition to the destructive effects of war on health, longevity, and survival, of great interest to social medicine practitioners is that the portion of the federal budget that pays for war is about the same as the portion that pays for the combined total of health and mental health services, social security, public education, food and nutrition, housing and urban development, services for workers, children's services, and all other human resources.[71] For some of us, the realization that about half of our taxes support the war machine rather than the goals that we seek to achieve in social medicine makes the contradictions of our compliance with taxes too excruciating to accept any longer.

The problem with either explicit (openly claiming a war deduction) or implicit (using loopholes instead) tax resistance is that tax resisters number in the thousands rather than millions. "Death and taxes," the two inevitabilities as we are taught, seem hard to resist, but corporations and rich individuals understand very well that at least taxes actually are not inevitable. As a strategy to slow down or stop the usual function of the capitalist state to support the military industrial complex and perpetual war as a method of capital accumulation, tax resistance by social medicine and other activists could allow millions of us to stop functioning as the main financiers for the capitalist state.

Our investments also help corporations achieve the unhealthy goals we despise. What happens to the money we save in our little bank or retirement accounts and pay for our mortgages, car loans, and credit card bills? Off that money goes to big banks that give loans to corporations for the Dakota Access Pipeline, arms manufacturing, privatized prisons and schools, pharmaceutical and for-profit health insurance companies, and more. Even if we invest in "socially conscious" funds, that usually means substituting "clean" drug, insurance, and technology companies for "dirty" tobacco and oil companies in our portfolios.

The movement to get cities, universities, and other institutional investors to divest from banks that support pipelines, companies that sell fossil fuels, the Israeli military's repression of Palestinians, and a host of other destructive entities, while helpful, misses the point that we as millions of individuals and families are actually more important as aggregated investors than any of the institutional investors that we try to influence. Collectively, social medicine practitioners and others who want to change the world need to seize control and move our investments into organizations that protect our planet, support the health of our peoples, help our communities, and nurture noncapitalist economic enterprises. If we do so, we can move our money into locally controlled economies not linked to the global capitalist system. Local responses to neoliberal austerity policies in Latin America and southern Europe, including drastic cutbacks in previously accessible public sector health services, have led to a clear understanding that communities can produce and consume most of the goods and services that they need through noncapitalist forms of cooperative social organization. With solidarity economies, as discussed already, communities can develop markets, bartering procedures, cooperative health and mental health services, and even currency, while drastically reducing the flow of their earnings into the global capitalist economy. As many affected by austerity already have learned, we really do not need global capitalism – we can live and thrive without the 1 percent easier than they can without us.

Praxis and the Health and Mental Health of Social Medicine Practitioners

So what stands in our way? We ourselves stand in our way. Actions like these usually entail a very small risk of bodily harm and a somewhat larger risk of inconvenience such as arrest. Reasons for inaction include emotions like fear, especially when we feel a need to protect those who depend on us, including children. Comfort and our illusions also slow us down, especially when believe we can make a big difference by winning the next round of elections or by trying to create a single-payer NHP within the capitalist state or by protecting the environment, fighting militarism, and so forth, all the while preserving a system whose inherently exploitative structure makes inevitable the weakening or reversal of whatever we accomplish.

As usual, it is wonderful for two of the authors, Howard and Matt, to communicate about fear, comfort, and illusions with Latin American revolutionaries who practice social medicine. For these comrades, fears about physical safety give way to confidence in the nurturance they receive from others and the pride of a life worth living. Worries about revolution yield to pleasures of the moment – eating and drinking with friends who are also comrades, knowing that on a deep level "mi casa es tu casa" ("my home is your home") and dancing late into the night. And about illusions, they understand that a central characteristic of revolution involves counter-hegemonic struggle, in this case rejecting the crippling ideology that reforming small parts of a destructive system without changing the destructive system itself is somehow okay. Not acting to change the system generates despair about continuing to live on planet earth.

Revolutionary life in the solidarity economy actually can be healthy and a lot of fun, especially when compared with the lives of alienation, insecurity, and fear that many or most people live within the global capitalist system. This "good living" (*buen vivir*) is the essence of health that communities around the world are creating by constructing cooperative economic systems outside global capitalism. Growing evidence shows that people who engage in struggle to transform their societies enjoy better health and mental health than nonactivists, especially those who constantly fret about how capitalism ruins their lives but do little to change that.[72] Activism is an upper, and despite setbacks, it generates a high that comes from living life according to one's deepest values, with beloved friends and comrades who share "mutual aid."[73]

One criticism of social medicine is that it presents many problems with few solutions. Some useful directions of praxis, however, are clear. Social contradictions lie behind many medical problems; the social organization of medicine both reflects and fosters structures of oppression. These contradictions and oppressive structures are important targets of activism. Our future health care system, as well as the social order of which it will be a part, depends largely on the praxis we choose now.

Notes

1 Antonio Gramsci, *Selections from the Prison Notebooks* (New York: International, 1971), Part 3.
2 This presentation of praxis updates a discussion in Howard Waitzkin, *The Second Sickness: Contradictions of Capitalist Health Care*, revised edition (Lanham, MD: Rowman & Littlefield, 2000), chapter 8.

3 Frances Fox Piven and Richard A. Cloward, *Regulating the Poor* (New York: Vintage, 1971), pp. 3–79.
4 André Gorz, *Socialism and Revolution* (Garden City, NY: Anchor, 1973), pp. 135–77.
5 Beatrix Hoffman, "Health Care Reform and Social Movements in the United States," *American Journal of Public Health* 93 (2003): 75–85.
6 Daniel Béland, Philip Rocco, and Alex Waddan, *Obamacare Wars: Federalism, State Politics, and the Affordable Care Act* (Lawrence, KS: University of Kansas Press, 2016).
7 "Barack Obama on Single Payer in 2003," www.pnhp.org/news/2008/june/barack_obama_on_sing.php; Brad Jacobson, "Obama Received $20 Million from Healthcare Industry in 2008 Campaign," The Raw Story, http://rawstory.com/2010/01/obama-received-20-million-healthcare-industry-money-2008/; Center for Responsive Politics, "2012 Presidential Race," www.opensecrets.org/pres12/.
8 Paige Minemyer, "What the CEOs of the 8 Largest Insurers Earned in 2018," *FierceHealthcare*, https://www.fiercehealthcare.com/payer/health-insurance-ceos-took-home-a-hefty-pay-day-2018-how-does-compare-to-their-employees; Shelby Livingston, "Health Insurer CEOs Score Big Paychecks Despite Public Scrutiny," *Modern Healthcare*, April 22, 2019, https://www.modernhealthcare.com/insurance/health-insurer-ceos-score-big-paychecks-despite-public-scrutiny.
9 Howard Waitzkin and Ida Hellander, "Obamacare: The Neoliberal Model Comes Home to Roost in the United States – If We Let It," *Monthly Review* 68, no. 1 (2016): 1–18; "The History and Future of Neoliberal Health Reform," *International Journal of Health Services* 46 (2016): 747–66. For details about the Medical Loss Ratio under Obamacare, see: Kaiser Family Foundation, "Explaining Health Care Reform: Medical Loss Ratio (MLR)," February 29, 2012, https://www.kff.org/health-reform/fact-sheet/explaining-health-care-reform-medical-loss-ratio-mlr/; Benjamin Day, David U. Himmelstein, Michael Broder, and Steffie Woolhandler, "The Affordable Care Act and Medical Loss Ratios: No Impact in First Three Years," *International Journal of Health Services* 45, no. 1 (2015): 127–31, doi:10.2190/HS.45.1.i.; and Healthinsurance.org, "ACA's 2019 Medical Loss Ratio Rebates," April 20, 2020, https://www.healthinsurance.org/obamacare/acas-2019-medical-loss-ratio-rebates/.
10 Howard Waitzkin, *Medicine and Public Health at the End of Empire* (Boulder, CO: Paradigm, 2011), chapters 5 and 10; Howard Waitzkin and the Working Group on Health beyond Capitalism, *Health Care under the Knife: Moving beyond Capitalism for Our Health* (New York: Monthly Review Press, 2018), chapters 7, 8.
11 Physicians for a National Health Program, "Wellpoint 'Really Did' Write the Baucus Health Plan" [series of articles], www.pnhp.org/news/2009/september/wellpoint_really_di.php.
12 Rachel Nardin, Leah Zallman, Danny McCormick, Steffie Woolhandler, and David Himmelstein, "The Uninsured after Implementation of the Affordable Care Act: A Demographic and Geographic Analysis," *Health Affairs (Millwood) Blog*, June 6, 2013, http://healthaffairs.org/blog/2013/06/06/the-uninsured-after-implementation-of-the-affordable-care-act-a-demographic-and-geographic-analysis/.
13 John Geyman, *The Human Face of ObamaCare* (Friday Harbor, WA: Copernicus Healthcare, 2016). This source conveys the multiple gaps in coverage that remained under Obamacare. The public option also appeared in earlier

proposals by the World Bank for neoliberal health reform in countries of Latin America; see further below.
14 Steffie Woolhandler, Benjamin Day, and David U. Himmselstein, "State Health Reform Flatlines," *International Journal of Health Services* 38 (2008): 585–92.
15 Waitzkin and Hellander, "Obamacare"; Waitzkin and Hellander, "The History and Future of Neoliberal Health Reform."
16 Richard A. Young and Jennifer E. DeVoe, "Who Will Have Health Insurance in the Future? An Updated Projection," *Annals of Family Medicine* 10 (2012): 156–62; Timothy Jost, "Affordability: The Most Urgent Health Reform Issue for Ordinary Americans," *Health Affairs (Millwood) Blog*, February 29, 2016; Geyman, *The Human Face of ObamaCare*.
17 Robin A. Cohen, Emily P. Zammitti, and Michael E. Martinez, "Health Insurance Coverage: Early Release of Estimates from the National Health Interview Survey, 2017, National Center for Health Statistics, 2018, www.cdc.gov/nchs/data/nhis/earlyrelease/insur201805.pdf; Steffie Woolhandler and David U. Himmelstein, "Intersecting U.S. Epidemics: COVID-19 and Lack of Health Insurance," *Annals of Internal Medicine*, April 7, 2020, https://doi.org/10.7326/M20-1491.
18 Howard Waitzkin, Rebeca Jasso-Aguilar, and Celia Iriart. "Privatization of Health Services in Less Developed Countries: An Empirical Response to the Proposals of the World Bank and Wharton School," *International Journal of Health Services* 37 (2007): 205–27.
19 María Amparo Cruz Saco and Carmelo Mesa-Lago, "*Do Options Exist? The Reform of Pension and Health Care Systems in Latin America* (Pittsburg, PA: University of Pittsburg Press, 1998).
20 Julie Cupples, *Latin American Development* (London: Routledge, 2013).
21 Waitzkin, *Medicine and Public Health at the End of Empire*, chapter 9.
22 Julio Frenk, "Leading the Way towards Universal Health Coverage: A Call to Action," *Lancet* 385 (2015): 1352–58.
23 Howard Waitzkin, "Universal Health Coverage: The Strange Romance of *The Lancet*, MEDICC, and Cuba," *Social Medicine/Medicina Social* 9 (2015): 93–97, http://socialmedicine.info/index.php/socialmedicine/article/view/845/1607.
24 Nila Heredia, Asa Cristina Laurell, Oscar Feo, et al., "The Right to Health: What Model for Latin America?" *Lancet* 385 (2015): e34–e37. doi:10.1016/S0140-6736(14)61493-8. Epub October 15, 2014.
25 Waitzkin, *Medicine and Public Health at the End of Empire*, chapter 9; Asa Cristina Laurell, "Three Decades of Neoliberalism in Mexico," *International Journal of Health Services* 45, no. 2 (2015): 246–64; Amit Sengupta. "Universal Health Coverage: Beyond Rhetoric," Ottawa, Canada, International Development Research Centre, Occasional Paper No. 20, November 2013, www.municipalservicesproject.org/sites/municipalservicesproject.org/files/publications/OccasionalPaper20_Sengupta_Universal_Health_Coverage_Beyond_Rhetoric_Nov2013_0.pdf\; David Stuckler, Andrea B. Feigl, Sanjay Basu, and Martin McKee, "The Political Economy of Universal Health Coverage," Background Paper for the Global Symposium on Health Systems Research, Montreux, Switzerland, World Health Organization, November 16–19, 2010, www.pacifichealthsummit.org/downloads/UHC/the%20political%20economy%20of%20uhc.PDF.
26 Meena D. Thever, *Health Care for All: Is Canada's System a Model for America?* (Philadelphia, PA: Xlibris, 2005).
27 Adam Gaffney, Steffie Woolhandler, Marcia Angell, and David U. Himmelstein, "Moving Forward from the Affordable Care Act to a Single-Payer System,"

American Journal of Public Health 106 (2016): 987–88; Himmelstein, Woolhandler et al., "A National Health Program for the United States: A Physicians' Proposal"; Kevin Grumbach, Thomas Bodenheimer, David U. Himmelstein and Steffie Woolhandler, "Liberal Benefits, Conservative Spending: The Physicians for a National Health Program Proposal," *JAMA* 265 (1991): 2549–54; Charlene Harrington, Christine Cassel, Carroll L. Estes, et al., "A National Long-Term Care Program for the United States: A Caring Vision," *JAMA* 266 (1991): 3023–29.

28 Gerald Friedman, "Funding HR 676: The Expanded and Improved Medicare for All Act: How We Can Afford a National Single-Payer Health Plan," July 31, 2013, www.pnhp.org/sites/default/files/Funding%20HR%20676_Friedman_7.31.13_proofed.pdf; Robert Pollin, James Heintz, Peter Arno, Jeannette Wicks-Lim, and Michael Ash, "Economic Analysis of Medicare for All," Political Economy Research Institute, University of Massachusetts, Amherst, November 2018, https://www.peri.umass.edu/publication/item/1127-economic-analysis-of-medicare-for-all.

29 Yusra Murad, "As Coronavirus Surges, 'Medicare for All' Support Hits 9-Month High," April 1, 2020, https://morningconsult.com/2020/04/01/medicare-for-all-coronavirus-pandemic/; Lunna Lopes, Liz Hamel Follow @lizhamel on Twitter, Audrey Kearney Follow @audrey__kearney on Twitter, and Mollyann Brodie, "KFF Health Tracking Poll – January 2020: Medicare-for-all, Public Option, Health Care Legislation And Court Actions," January 30, 2020, https://www.kff.org/health-reform/poll-finding/kff-health-tracking-poll-january-2020/.

30 "The Medicare for All Act (H.R. 1384)," https://www.congress.gov/bill/116th-congress/house-bill/1384/text; "S.1129 - Medicare for All Act of 2019," https://www.congress.gov/bill/116th-congress/senate-bill/1129?q=%7B%22search%22%3A%5B%221129%22%5D%7D&r=7.

31 Barbara Ehrenreich and John Ehrenreich, "The Real Story behind the Crash and Burn of America's Managerial Class," *Alternet*, February 13, 2013, www.alternet.org/economy/barbara-and-john-ehrenreich-real-story-behind-crash-and-burn-americas-managerial-class?page=0%2C0; Ehrenreich Barbara and John Ehrenreich, "The Professional-Managerial Class," *Radical America* 11, no. 2 (March–April 1977): 7–31.

32 Sarah Grisham, "Medscape Physician Compensation Report 2017," www.medscape.com/slideshow/compensation-2017-overview-6008547; Elisabeth Rosenthal, "Apprehensive, Many Doctors Shift to Jobs with Salaries," *New York Times*, February 13, 2014, www.nytimes.com/2014/02/14/us/salaried-doctors-may-not-lead-to-cheaper-health-care.html?_r=0.

33 Dante Morra, Sean Nicholson, Wendy Levinson, David N. Gans, Terry Hammons, and Lawrence P. Casalino, "US Physician Practices Versus Canadians: Spending Nearly Four Times as Much Money Interacting with Payers," *Health Affairs*, August 2011, http://content.healthaffairs.org/content/early/2011/08/03/hlthaff.2010.0893.

34 John B. McKinlay and Joan Arches, "Towards the Proletarianization of Physicians," *International Journal of Health Services* 15 (1985): 161–95; Adam Reich, "Disciplined Doctors: The Electronic Medical Record and Physicians' Changing Relationship to Medical Knowledge," *Social Science & Medicine* 74 (2012): 1021–28.

35 Eric Hobsbawm, "Lenin and the 'Aristocracy of Labor'," *Monthly Review* 64, no. 7 (December 2012): 26–34.

36 Samir Amin, "Contra Hardt and Negri: Multitude or Generalized Proletarianization? *Monthly Review* 66, no. 6 (November 2014): 25–36.
37 Robb Burlage and Matthew Anderson, "The Transformation of the Medical-Industrial Complex: Financialization, the Corporate Sector, and Monopoly Capital," in Waitzkin and the Working Group on Health beyond Capitalism, *Health Care Under the Knife*, chapter 5.
38 These financial flows of health insurance cohere with Foster's comment about Marx's "general formula for capital": "At the more stratospheric level represented by contemporary finance, the general formula for capital, or M-C-M' [money-commodity-increased money], is being increasingly supplanted by the circuit of speculative capital, M-M', in which the production of use values disappears altogether and money simply begets more money." John Bellamy Foster, "The Epochal Crisis," *Monthly Review* 65, no. 6 (October 2013): 1–12, commenting on Karl Marx, "The General Formula of Capital," *Capital*, volume 1, part 2, chapter 4, www.marxists.org/archive/marx/works/1867-c1/ch04.htm.
39 Waitzkin and Hellander, "Obamacare"; Waitzkin and Hellander, "The History and Future of Neoliberal Health Reform"; David Matthews, "The Battle for the National Health Service: England, Wales, and the Socialist Vision," *Monthly Review* 68, no. 10 (March 2017): 25–35.
40 David Himmelstein and Steffie Woolhandler, "The Political Economy of Health Reform," in Waitzkin and the Working Group on Health Beyond Capitalism, *Health Care Under the Knife*, chapter 4.
41 David Squires and Chloe Anderson, *U.S. Health Care from a Global Perspective: Spending, Use of Services, Prices, and Health in 13 Countries* (New York: The Commonwealth Fund, 2015), www.commonwealthfund.org/publications/issue-briefs/2015/oct/us-health-care-global-perspective.
42 Samantha Artiga and Elizabeth Hinton, "Beyond Health Care: The Role of Social Determinants in Promoting Health and Health Equity," Henry J. Kaiser Family Foundation, May 2018, http://files.kff.org/attachment/issue-brief-beyond-health-care; Harry J. Heiman and Samantha Artiga, "Beyond Health Care: The Role of Social Determinants in Promoting Health and Health Equity," Henry J. Kaiser Family Foundation, November 2015, https://health.maryland.gov/healthenterprisezones/Documents/Kaiser%20Family%20Foundation%20Issue%20Brief.pdf; Raj Chetty, Michael Stepner, Sarah Abraham, et al., "The Association Between Income and Life Expectancy in the United States, 2001–2014," *JAMA 315* (2016): 1750–66, doi:10.1001/jama.2016.4226; Anne Case and Angus Deaton, "Rising Morbidity and Mortality in Midlife among White Non-Hispanic Americans in the 21st Century," *Proceedings of the National Academy of Sciences U S A* 112 (2015): 15078–83, www.pnas.org/content/112/49/15078.
43 For recent work at the intersection of militarism and social medicine, see: Howard Waitzkin, "Revolution Now: Teachings from the Global South for Revolutionaries in the Global North," *Monthly Review* 69, no. 6 (November 2017): 18–36; Howard Waitzkin, Mario Cruz, Bryant Shuey, Daniel Smithers, II, Laura Muncy, and Marylou Noble, "Military Personnel Who Seek Health and Mental Health Services Outside the Military," *Military Medicine* 183 (2018): e232–e240, doi:10.1093/milmed/usx051.
44 "2019 Was 2nd Hottest Year on Record for Earth Say NOAA, NASA," National Oceanic and Atmospheric Administration, January 15, 2020, https://www.noaa.gov/news/2019-was-2nd-hottest-year-on-record-for-earth-say-noaa-nasa.

45 Howard asked the same question during his medical residency, and the question remains to this day: Howard Waitzkin and Barbara Waterman, *The Exploitation of Illness in Capitalist Society* (Indianapolis: Bobbs-Merrill, 1974).
46 Waitzkin and the Working Group on Health beyond Capitalism, *Health Care Under the Knife*.
47 Fredric Jameson, "Future City," *New Left Review* 21 (May–June 2003): 65–79, https://newleftreview.org/II/21/fredric-jameson-future-city. Jameson actually said, "Someone once said that it is easier to imagine the end of the world than to imagine the end of capitalism. We can now revise that and witness the attempt to imagine capitalism by way of imagining the end of the world."
48 This section is adapted from Howard Waitzkin, *Rinky-Dink Revolution: Moving Beyond Capitalism by Withholding Consent, Creative Constructions, and Creative Destructions* (Ottawa: Daraja Press, 2020, and New York: Monthly Review Essays, 2020), https://darajapress.com/publication/rinky-dink-revolution-moving-beyond-capitalism-by-withholding-consent-creative-constructions-and-creative-destructions, https://mronline.org/2020/05/19/rinky-dink-revolution/.
49 Emma Goldman, *Anarchism and Other Essays* (New York: Mother Earth Publishing Association, 1911). These writings convey Goldman's views about the futility of voting; the precise quotation, widely attributed to Goldman, actually does not appear in her published writings.
50 Tommy Douglas, "Mouseland," www.youtube.com/watch?v=kdwySCMovHk. Douglas himself lived out his life as an attractive politician, frequently invoking class structure through the Mouseland metaphor but never moving the leftist Canadian New Democratic Party beyond efforts to reform capitalism. Still, the metaphor conveys the class-based, corrupt, and ineffective structure of bourgeois electoral democracy that must be transformed, rather than the appealing or revolting elected representatives of the moment.
51 Vladimir I. Lenin, *The State and Revolution* (New York: International Publishers, 1935), chapter 5, www.marxists.org/archive/lenin/works/1917/staterev/ch05.htm.
52 Karl Marx and Friedrich Engels, *Manifesto of the Communist Party* (New York: International Publishers, 1983), chapter 1, www.marxists.org/archive/marx/works/1848/communist-manifesto/ch01.htm. For instance, during the worldwide economic crisis of 2008, public-sector bailouts of the private sector created a type of socialism in the United States and other capitalist countries – public ownership to a substantial extent of the means of economic production and also of the system's key financial institutions (Jon Meacham, "We Are All Socialists Now," *Newsweek*, February 6, 2009, www.newsweek.com/we-are-all-socialists-now-82577). But it was a socialism for the rich, who then controlled even more wealth than they did before. By recent estimates, the concentration of wealth has increased in the United States to the point that the top 0.1 percent of the population controls as much wealth as the bottom 90 percent. Considering the world, as Oxfam has reported, eight men recently have controlled the same wealth as the bottom half of the world's population ("Just 8 Men Own Same Wealth as Half the World," January 15, 2017, www.oxfamamerica.org/press/just-8-men-own-same-wealth-as-half-the-world/, and "An Economy for the 99%," January 15, 2017, www.oxfamamerica.org/explore/research-publications/an-economy-for-the-99-percent/); six months later, five men controlled this amount of wealth (Paul Buchheit, "Now Five Men Own Almost as Much Wealth as Half the World's Population,

Nation of Change, June 12, 2017, www.nationofchange.org/2017/06/12/now-five-men-almost-much-wealth-half-worlds-population/.

53 Aaron Reeves, Martin McKee, and David Stuckler, "The Attack on Universal Health Coverage in Europe: Recession, Austerity and Unmet Needs," *European Journal of Public Health* 25, no. 3 (2015): 364–65; Vicente Navarro and Carles Muntaner, eds., *The Financial and Economic Crises and Their Impact on Health and Social Well-Being* (Amityville, New York: Baywood Publishing Company, Inc., 2014); Anna Maresso et al., eds., *Economic Crisis, Health Systems and Health in Europe: Country Experience* (Brussels: WHO Regional Office for Europe/European Observatory on Health Systems and Policies, 2015); Adam Gaffney and Carles Muntaner, "Austerity and Health Care," in Waitzkin and the Working Group for Health Beyond Capitalism, *Health Care Under the Knife*.

54 Waitzkin, *Medicine and Public Health at the End of Empire*, chapter 3, and *The Second Sickness*, chapter 2; Claus Offe, *Modernity and the State: East, West* (Cambridge, MA: MIT Press, 1996).

55 This legitimation function dates back to the initial traces of the welfare state in nineteenth-century Germany, as Chancellor Bismarck initiated the world's first national health program explicitly as a method to win support from the working class and to prevent more fundamental revolutionary action. The "national socialism" of Nazi Germany actually functioned as a version of the welfare state, as it implemented a strong public sector that provided unprecedented benefits for its Aryan population (the so-called *Volksgemeinschaft*), including affordable housing, accessible education, food security, and even health services. Similarly, in the midst of massive unrest and episodes of revolt in the United States during the mid-1960s, Medicare and Medicaid became a tactic to prevent socialization of the entire health care system as part of a struggle to transform the capitalist economic system. See, for instance: Theodore Marmor, *The Politics of Medicare*, Second Edition (Piscataway, NJ: Transaction Publishers, 2000); Piven and Cloward, *Regulating the Poor*.

56 The following websites give an overview of efforts to create a solidarity economy: https://neweconomy.net/members, https://ussen.org, http://solidarityeconomy.us, www.solidarityeconomy.coop, www.solidaritystl.org, https://cooperationjackson.org.

57 Consejo Nacional de Planificación, *Buen Vivir: Plan Nacional, 2013–2017* (Quito, Ecuador: Government of Ecuador, 2013), www.unicef.org/ecuador/Plan_Nacional_Buen_Vivir_2013-2017.pdf; Fernando Huanacuni Mamani, "BOLIVIA-Buen Vivir/Vivir Bien. Los 13 principios," Caminante del Sur, February 5, 2018, https://caminantedelsur.com/2018/02/05/bolivia-buen-vivir-vivir-bien-los-13-principios-por-fernando-huanacuni-mamani/; Chris Hartmann, "Buen Vivir (Living Well): Implications for Public Health in Latin America and Globally," University of Florida, April 11, 2018, http://epi.ufl.edu/onehealth/seminars/specialseminars/; "'Live Beautiful, Live Well' ('*Vivir Bonito, Vivir Bien*') in Nicaragua: Environmental Health Citizenship in a Post-Neoliberal Context," *Global Public Health* 14, no. 6–7 (2018): 923–38, doi:10.1080/17441692.2018.1506812; J. B. Spiegel, B. Ortiz Choukroun, A. Campaña, K. M. Boydell, J. Breilh & A. Yassi, "Social Transformation, Collective Health and Community-Based Arts: 'Buen Vivir' and Ecuador's Social Circus Programme," *Global Public Health* 14, no. 6–7 (2018): 899–922, doi: 10.1080/17441692.2018.1504102. Regarding mutual aid, the biologist Peter Kropotkin made important observations in the anarchist tradition; see *Mutual Aid* (Boston, MA: Extending Horizon Books, 1914), chapters 7 and 8.

58 For information about Cooperation Jackson's path-breaking efforts in Mississippi, see: Kali Akuno and Ajamu Nangwaya, *Jackson Rising* (Montreal, Canada: Daraja Press, 2017).
59 Again, the efforts of Cooperation Jackson offer helpful perspectives on sustainable food production and distribution: Akuno and Nangwaya, *Jackson Rising*.
60 For helpful discussions of the expropriation/robbery of nature as an inherent characteristic of the capitalist economic system, see: John Bellamy Foster and Brett Clark, "The Expropriation of Nature," *Monthly Review* 69, no. 10 (March 2018): 1–27; and "The Robbery of Nature," *Monthly Review* 70, no. 3 (July–August 2018): 1–20.
61 Dirk Notz and Julienne Stroeve, "Observed Arctic Sea-Ice Loss Directly Follows Anthropogenic CO_2 Emission," *Science* 54 (2016): 747–50.
62 For more on transition from the capitalist state to post-capitalist participatory governance, see István Mészáros, *Beyond Capital* (New York: Monthly Review Press, 2010), especially chapters 13, 19, and 20. Helpful discussions of the applications of Mészáros's work in Venezuela's Bolivarian Revolution, especially concerning the communal transition, appear in: John Bellamy Foster, "Chávez and the Communal State: On the Transition to Socialism in Venezuela," *Monthly Review* 66, no. 11 (April 2015): 1–17; Michael Lebowitz, *The Socialist Imperative* (New York: Monthly Review Press, 2015), chapters 5–6; and Marta Harnecker, *A World To Build* (New York: Monthly Review Press, 2015), chapters 7–9. A similar model of communal governance but with more anarchist roots has emerged in the autonomous region of Rojava in northern Syria, as part of the so-called Rojava Revolution. See, for instance, Michael Knapp, Anja Flach, and Ercan Ayboga, *Revolution in Rojava: Democratic Autonomy and Women's Liberation in Syrian Kurdistan* (London: Pluto Press, 2016), chapters 5–7, 11–13.
63 Especially because so many people in the United States have easy access to guns and because deep-seated violence based on racism and anti-communism are so much part of U.S. tradition, obtaining weapons for self-defense by the Black Panther Party, Puerto Rican independence groups, American Indian tribes, and others has happened as an understandable response. Those actions have led to repression by police and military forces, plus at least some policy reforms. See Piven and Cloward, *Regulating the Poor*.
64 Ernesto Che Guevara, "On Revolutionary Medicine," August 19, 1960, www.marxists.org/archive/guevara/1960/08/19.htm.
65 Erica Chenoweth and Maria J. Stephan, *Why Civil Resistance Works: The Strategic Logic of Nonviolent Conflict* (New York: Columbia University Press, 2012); Erica Chenoweth, "It May Only Take 3.5% of the Population to Topple a Dictator—with Civil Resistance," *The Guardian*, February 1, 2017, www.theguardian.com/commentisfree/2017/feb/01/worried-american-democracy-study-activist-techniques. If the relevant population of the United States, the world's third most populous country (total population 324,420,000), includes eligible voters (231,557,000), 5 percent would involve 11,578,000 nonviolently resisting individuals. If instead the relevant population includes registered voters who actually voted for president in November 2016 (138,885,000), fundamental change could happen through concerted nonviolent action by about seven million people.
66 Jenna Arnold, Kanisha Bond, Erica Chenoweth, and Jeremy Pressman, "These are the Four Largest Protests since Trump was Inaugurated," *Washington Post*, May 31, 2018, https://www.washingtonpost.com/news/monkey-cage/wp/2018/05/31/these-are-the-four-largest-protests-since-trump-was-inaugurated/; Kaveh Waddell, "The Exhausting Work of Tallying America's

Largest Protest," *The Atlantic*, January 23, 2017, https://www.theatlantic.com/technology/archive/2017/01/womens-march-protest-count/514166/.

67 Until the pipeline's completion, crude oil traveled in tank cars from Bakken to Patoka, mainly along the tracks of the Burlington Northern and Santa Fe (BNSF) Railway. Train accidents leading to environment destruction and injuries have happened along that route, including a derailment in Galena, Illinois, during 2015 that narrowly missed contaminating the nearby Mississippi River. Similar train accidents involving Bakken crude during 2015 contaminated a river in West Virginia and during 2013 killed 47 people in a Quebec town.

68 Such attempts to understand the vulnerability of pipelines to nonviolent interruption have emerged as an ongoing methodology in several countries, including Mexico, where milking of pipelines has become more common with the attempted privatization of Mexico's oil industry; see Carlos Navarro, "Fuel Thefts Increase Significantly in the Triángulo Rojo Region of Puebla State," Latin America Digital Beat, March 15, 2017, https://digitalrepository.unm.edu/sourcemex/6332/.

69 Actions targeting the infrastructure of corporate capitalism resemble the "roaming strikes" that have become a component of a resurgent labor movement. As Steve Early and others have pointed out, the elite leadership of the largely debilitated labor unions in the United States will not likely spearhead militant direct actions, for instance, a general strike. However, the militancy of nonunionized workers in Fast Food Forward, OUR Walmart, Warehouse Workers United, Warehouse Workers for Justice, Fight for 15, and many similar struggles can achieve powerful effects by slowing or stopping production through a roaming but escalating strategy. See Steve Early, *Save Our Unions: Dispatches from A Movement in Distress* (New York: Monthly Review Press, 2013). For more on the history of direct action in the United States, see L.A. Kauffman, *Direct Action and the Reinvention of American Radicalism* (New York: Verso, 2017), and for similar direct actions against the Dakota Access Pipeline in addition to Standing Rock, see "Meet the Two Catholic Workers Who Secretly Sabotaged the Dakota Access Pipeline to Halt Construction," *Democracy Now*, July 28, 2017, www.democracynow.org/2017/7/28/meet_the_two_catholic_workers_who.

70 "Physician Compensation Report 2019," *Medscape*, April 10, 2019, https://www.medscape.com/slideshow/2019-compensation-overview-6011286; Jonathan Rothwell, "Make Elites Compete: Why the 1% Earn So Much and What to Do about It," *Brookings Social Mobility Papers*," March 25, 2016, https://www.brookings.edu/research/make-elites-compete-why-the-1-earn-so-much-and-what-to-do-about-it/; "The Top 1 Percent: What Jobs Do They Have?" *New York Times*, January 15, 2012, https://archive.nytimes.com/www.nytimes.com/packages/html/newsgraphics/2012/0115-one-percent-occupations/.

71 War Resisters League, "Where Your Income Tax Money Really Goes," War Resisters League, Spring 2018–2020, https://www.warresisters.org/store/where-your-income-tax-money-really-goes-fy2021, www.warresisters.org/store/where-your-income-tax-money-really-goes-fy2019. For details of how to do tax resistance, see the helpful materials produced by the National War Tax Resistance Coordinating Committee, https://nwtrcc.org.

72 For only some items in the growing literature on the psychotherapeutic advantages of resistance and revolution, see: James Petras, "Neo-Liberalism, Popular Resistance and Mental Health," *The James Petras Website*, December 17, 2002, http://petras.lahaine.org/?p=109; Ignacio Martín-Baró, *Writings for a Liberation Psychology* (Cambridge, MA: Harvard University Press,

1994), chapter 1; Chitra Nagarajan, Shannon Harvey, Adam Ramsay, and Ezekiel Incorrigible, "Activists Talk Mental Health," *Transformation*, April 14, 2014, www.opendemocracy.net/transformation/chitra-nagarajan-shannon-harvey-adam-ramsay-ezekiel-incorrigible/activists-talk-menta; Carl Ratner, "Overcoming Pathological Normalcy: Mental Health Challenges in the Coming Transformation," in Waitzkin and the Working Group for Health Beyond Capitalism, *Health Care Under the Knife*; and of course Franz Fanon, *The Wretched of the Earth* (New York: Grove Press, 2004 [1961]).

73 For Peter Kropotkin's under-appreciated observations about the biological benefits of mutual aid: *Mutual Aid*, chapters 7 and 8.

Appendix

Organizations and Resources in Social Medicine and Collective Health

(This listing is a work in progress. The authors welcome suggestions that will improve the book's website, www.routledge.com/9781138685987 and later revisions. Please contact Howard Waitzkin: waitzkin@unm.edu.)		
Albert Einstein College of Medicine, Department of Family and Social Medicine, Montefiore Medical Center, Bronx, New York	http://www.einstein.yu.edu/departments/family-social-medicine/	The department's mission is "to promote the health of underserved communities, train future healthcare leaders, and advocate for social justice through collaborative primary care delivery, education, and research." This department has provided an important base within the United States for educational, research, and service programs in social medicine.
Allende Program in Social Medicine/ El Programa Allende en Medicina Social	http://allendeprogram.org	This small foundation encourages "activism, progressive research, and strategic analysis concerning contemporary health problems." A motivation for starting the program was a recognition that sources of support for this type of activity often are difficult to find. The program takes its name from Salvador Allende, physician and former president of Chile. Several chapters of this book describe Allende's pathbreaking work in social medicine.

(Continued)

American Medical Student Association (AMSA)	https://www.amsa.org	AMSA is the oldest and largest independent association of physicians-in-training in the United States. "At AMSA, activism is a way of life. Student idealism is transformed into meaningful public service, innovation and institutional change."
Asociación Latinoamericana de Medicina Social (ALAMES, Latin American Association of Social Medicine)	http://alames.org	Latin American social medicine takes a critical approach to political economy and health policy. ALAMES provides a base for thousands of scholars, activists, practitioners, researchers, and policy makers who pursue social medicine. Chapter 8 gives more information. Further details about teaching programs in Latin American social medicine are available from the authors (waitzkin@unm.edu).
Associação Brasileira de Saúde Coletiva (ABRASCO, Brazilian Association of Collective Health)	https://www.abrasco.org.br/site/	This organization provides a base for thousands of scholars, activists, practitioners, researchers, and policy makers in Brazil who pursue an approach similar to social medicine but emphasizing health rather than medicine, and collective organizing. Chapter 8 explains these distinctions and provides details.
Association of Clinicians for the Underserved (ACU)	http://clinicians.org	The ACU is a leading organization supporting U.S. safety net organizations. Their website is useful for tracking political developments in Washington and what is happening in community health centers. The ACU publishes a journal; see https://www.press.jhu.edu/journals/journal-health-care-poor-and-underserved.

Berkeley Center for Social Medicine, University of California, Berkeley	https://bcsm.berkeley.edu/about	The Berkeley Center for Social Medicine uses a multidisciplinary approach to health. The center focuses on social systems in a way that moves beyond the clinical level. It emphasizes social difference, health, and health care in the United States and internationally.
California Nurses Association/ National Nurses United	https://www.nationalnursesunited.org; https://www.nationalnursesunited.org/california-nurses-association	These organizations of nurses and their supporters have played an important role in the advocacy for improved access to services and a single-payer national health program in the United States. They see their role as advocates for transformative change in the U.S. health care system. Their work often applies principles and actions based on social medicine.
Civilian Medical Resources Network (CMRN)	https://civilianmedicalresources.net	CMRN is a national collaborative network of volunteer health and mental health professionals who provide medical and mental health services for U.S. active duty military personnel who cannot meet their needs within the military or the Veterans Administration. Social medicine influences CMRN's work.
Claudio Schuftan website	http://claudioschuftan.com	This website provides helpful materials about human rights and social medicine. Claudio Schuftan is a freelance public health consultant in Ho Chi Minh City, Vietnam, and an ex-adjunct associate professor in the Department of International Health at the Tulane School of Public Health in New Orleans, United States. He is a Chilean national and received his MD and pediatrics degree in his native country. Dr. Schuftan is one of the founding members of the People's Health Movement.

(Continued)

communityhealth.in	http://www.communityhealth.in/~commun26/wiki/index.php?title=Main_Page	This website is a collaboration to create "a comprehensive resource on community health and the Health For All movement in India. Contributors include health workers, researchers, activists, and others with an interest in community health."
Corporations and Health	https://corporationsandhealth.org/2009/07/08/researching-for-advocacy-the-industry-trade-press-as-a-resource-for-activists/	Run by researcher and professor Nick Freudenberg, this website (updated monthly) examines the effects of corporate practices on health.
CUNY School of Medicine, Community Health and Social Medicine Department	https://www.ccny.cuny.edu/csom/communityhealthandsocialmedicinedept	The school tailors its curriculum to prepare students as community-oriented primary care physicians who will serve in medically underserved areas. "This mission is achieved through the School's intensive three-year sequence of courses in Community Health and Social Medicine (CHASM), which include field placements in community medicine in partnership with community-based health centers and health-related programs in underserved areas of New York City."
Democracy Now! Healthcare	https://www.democracynow.org/topics/healthcare	This key progressive media source follows closely "the movement to reform the healthcare system in the United States. We have interviewed policy makers, doctors, patients, independent journalists, academics, single payer healthcare advocates, and filmmakers."

Doctors for Global Health (DGH)	http://www.dghonline.org/	DGH promotes health, education, and human rights throughout the world. It works with communities to establish long-lasting relationships and aims to address social conditions as a cause of adverse health outcomes.
Global Health Watch (GHW)	http://www.ghwatch.org/	GHW is an initiative of the People's Health Movement to prepare an "alternative World Health Report." It also organizes WHO Watch, an important initiative that seeks to insert a progressive voice into debates at the World Health Organization.
Harvard Medical School, Department of Global Health and Social Medicine, Boston, Massachusetts	https://ghsm.hms.harvard.edu	This department "applies social science and humanities research to constantly improve the practice of medicine, the delivery of treatment, and the development of health care policies locally and worldwide." One of its premises is that "diseases have social roots; attaining health at a population level requires the coordination of health policies with social policies."
Health Policy Advisory Center (Health/PAC) archives	http://www.healthpacbulletin.org	Health/PAC was an important activist health organization during the 1960s and 1970s. The Health/PAC Bulletin developed critical assessments of health institutions, the pharmaceutical industry, and insurance corporations. Health/PAC created the concept of the "medical industrial complex. This link gives readers access to all issues of the bulletin.

(Continued)

Health Care Renewal	https://hcrenewal.blogspot.com	This blog, written by Dr. Roy Poses, addresses "threats to health care's core values, especially those stemming from concentration and abuse of power" and advocates for "accountability, integrity, transparency, honesty and ethics in leadership and government."
The Healthcare Revolution	https://www.the-healthcarerevolution.org	Started by medical students, the Healthcare Revolution "provides a forum for progressive-minded individuals and students who are eager to work toward creating a more equal and just society in order to strengthen the health of communities." It explores and addresses "how individual and community health are eroded by: systemic racism, gender inequality, media control, economic inequality, and environmental exploitation."
Hesperian Health Guides	https://hesperian.org	Hesperian produces and shares easy-to-understand health information for people worldwide. The organization partners with community health workers, villagers, medical professionals, and others to develop, publish, and share information. The health guides span community health, women's health, children with disabilities, HIV, environmental health, and other topics useful in underserved areas.
International Journal of Health Services	https://journals.sagepub.com/home/joh	This journal publishes research studies and policy analyses with a critical, progressive, and international orientation. The journal frequently covers important themes in social medicine through articles written by scholars, practitioners, and activists based in many countries.

Jawaharlal Nehru University, Centre of Social Medicine and Community Health, New Delhi, India	http://csmch.tripod.com	The center's objective is "to understand the health problems and health needs of the Indian people with a view to find workable solutions for them in the existing social structure and to examine the social structure itself to delineate the structural constraints which limit the scope of health interventions."
Latin American Medical School/ Escuela Latinoamericana de Medicina (ELAM)	https://instituciones.sld.cu/elam/	ELAM provides free medical education in Cuba for thousands of students from underserved areas around the world. Students commit to returning to their home countries after graduation to provide care for underserved communities. More than 27,000 students have graduated, including some from underserved areas in the United States.
Medical Education Cooperation with Cuba (MEDICC)	http://medicc.org/ns/, http://www.mediccreview.org	MEDICC promotes health collaboration between Cuba and the United States and highlights "Cuba's public health contributions to global health equity and universal health." The organization publishes a journal, MEDICC Review, with articles about Cuban medical education, research, and services and also offers support for medical students and graduates who have attended the Latin American Medical School.
Medicine and Social Justice	https://medicinesocialjustice.blogspot.com	Dr. Josh Freeman, a leader in U.S. family medicine, writes this blog, where he includes helpful information for people working in social medicine. While focusing on issues of social justice, Dr. Freeman also comments on medical education, health reform, and global health.

(Continued)

Migrant Clinicians Network	https://www.migrantclinician.org	The network provides support, technical assistance, and professional development to clinicians in Federally Qualified Health Centers (FQHCs) and similar health care delivery sites, including case management for patients who face barriers to care due to migration. Perspectives from social medicine guide much of the network's efforts.
Monthly Review	https://monthlyreview.org	This independent socialist magazine is influential in analyses and struggles toward social change worldwide. The magazine and Monthly Review Press frequently publish articles and books pertinent to social medicine, mental health, and the "welfare state."
National Association of Community Health Centers	http://www.nachc.org	This association advocates and supports community-based health centers and the expansion of health care access for the medically underserved and uninsured. The purpose is to promote "efficient, high quality, comprehensive health care that is accessible, culturally and linguistically competent, community directed, and patient centered for all."
New England Journal of Medicine, Case Studies in Social Medicine	https://www.nejm.org/case-studies-in-social-medicine	"A series of Perspective articles that highlight the importance of social concepts and social context in clinical medicine. The series uses discussions of real clinical cases to translate theories and methods for understanding social processes into terms that can readily be used in medical education, clinical practice, and health system planning."

No Free Lunch	http://nofreelunch.org	This group's mission is "to encourage health care providers to practice medicine on the basis of scientific evidence rather than on the basis of pharmaceutical promotion." As health care providers, the leaders "believe that pharmaceutical promotion should not guide clinical practice. We discourage the acceptance of all gifts from industry by health care providers, trainees, and students. Our goal is improved patient care."
People's Health Movement (PHM)	https://phmovement.org	This global network brings together "grassroots health activists, civil society organizations, and academic institutions worldwide, especially from low and middle income countries. PHM maintains a presence in about 70 countries." Priorities include the People's Charter for Health, comprehensive primary health care, and addressing the social, environmental, and economic determinants of health.
Physicians for a National Health Program (PNHP)	https://pnhp.org	PNHP advocates a universal, comprehensive single-payer national health program. PNHP has more than 20,000 members and chapters across the United States and has taken a leading role in the single-payer proposal, "Improved Medicare for All." Its website contains helpful research findings and policy analyses pertinent to health activism and social medicine.
Public Health and Social Justice	https://phsj.org	This website, maintained by Dr. Martin Donohoe, offers hundreds of critical slide presentations covering everything from concierge medicine to the politics of gold, diamonds, and flowers.

(Continued)

Social Medicine Consortium (SMC)	http://www.socialmedicineconsortium.org	SMC is a collective of committed individuals, universities, and organizations "fighting for health equity through education, training, service and advocacy, with social medicine at its core." The organization seeks "diverse geographic, professional, racial, and class perspectives." One of the SMC's key projects is the Campaign Against Racism, which aims "to dismantle structural racism and its effects on health around the world – because racism kills...."
The Social Medicine Portal; *Social Medicine/ Medicina Social*	http://www.socialmedicine.org, http://www.socialmedicine.info	The portal's purpose is to link the diverse international community of people working in social medicine and health activism. Faculty members in the Department of Family and Social Medicine of the Albert Einstein College of Medicine/ Montefiore Medical Center in New York developed the portal. Collaborating with the Latin American Social Medicine Association (ALAMES), this group publishes an online bilingual (in English and Spanish), open-access academic journal, *Social Medicine/ Medicina Social*.
Socialist Caucus of the American Public Health Association (APHA)	https://www.apha.org/apha-communities/caucuses/socialist-caucus	The caucus "focuses on issues of importance to labor and social equity as they affect the health of workers." At its sessions during the APHA annual meeting, the caucus sponsors sessions that deal with important topics in social medicine.
Spirit of 1848 Caucus of the American Public Health Association (APHA)	https://www.apha.org/apha-communities/caucuses/spirit-of-1848-caucus	This caucus addresses "the link between social justice and public health." The tribute to 1848 refers to the creation of social medicine by Engels, Virchow, and other scholars and activists during that revolutionary historical period.

Organizations and Resources 275

		This caucus's sessions at APHA consider key topics in social medicine, and its active list serve provides extensive additional information and debate.
The Structural Competency Working Group	https://www.structcomp.org	This group, located in the San Francisco Bay Area, includes clinicians, scholars, public health professionals, students, educators, and other community members. Their goal is to help promote the training of health professionals in structural competency, which they define as "the capacity for health professionals to recognize and respond to health and illness as the downstream effects of broad social, political, and economic structures."
UCLA Center for Social Medicine and Humanities	https://hssm.semel.ucla.edu/	"We are a community of scholars focused on the historical and sociocultural contexts of health and disease as well as clinical and scientific practices." The Center includes a training program for postdoctoral fellows in social studies of medicine. Programs also focus on underserved populations with mental health problems.
University of California, San Francisco, Department of Anthropology, History and Social Medicine	http://dahsm.ucsf.edu	This department of the School of Medicine "provides training and research on the social and historical contexts that affect health. Our goal is to conduct research and prepare scholars for the complexities of medical and social science practice in an increasingly diverse and internationally linked world." The department runs doctoral programs in the History of Health Sciences and Medical Anthropology (joint with UC Berkeley).

(Continued)

University of New Mexico/ University of Guadalajara, Latin American Social Medicine Digital Archive	https:// digitalrepository. unm.edu/lasm_ hslic/, https:// digitalrepository. unm.edu/lasm/	This web-based project provides a database of structured abstracts summarizing classic and contemporary works in Latin American Social Medicine (LASM). The abstracts are available in the Spanish, Portuguese, and English languages. LASM offers important information about the social, economic, and cultural determinants of health with descriptions of organized responses to confront the problems. Originally, this information circulated mostly among interested professionals located in Latin America. The LASM database enhances access to this information worldwide.
University of North Carolina School of Medicine, Department of Social Medicine	https://www.med. unc.edu/socialmed/	The department is "committed to the promotion and provision of multidisciplinary education, leadership, service, research, and scholarship at the intersection of medicine and society. This includes focus on the social conditions and characteristics of patients and populations; causes of illness and contexts of medical care; the ethical and social contexts of biomedical clinical and research professionals and institutions; and questions of allocation, organization and financing of health resources including health law and policy."

Index

Note: **Bold** page numbers refer to tables and *Italic* page numbers refer to figures. Page numbers followed by "n" refer to endnotes.

abandonment 201
activism 55, 109, 116, 118, 173, 177, 180, 181, 224, 225, 227, 232, 237, 238, 243, 256
Affordable Care Act (ACA) 12, 19, 199, 204, 227, 229–31; *see also* Obamacare
African American 4, 10, 89, 90, 93–6, 237
agriculture and COVID-19 65–9
Aguas del Tunari 164–5
Aid for Families with Dependent Children (AFDC) 128
AIDS 18, 92, 141, 144, 145, 152, 154
Albert Einstein College of Medicine, Department of Family and Social Medicine 265
Allende Program in Social Medicine/ El Programa Allende en Medicina Social 265
Allende, Salvador 25, 26, *34*, 34–42, 48, 49, 79, 100, 163, 179, 181–5, 218, 225, 265
Alma Ata Declaration: primary health care for all, The 12–13
American Academy of Pediatrics 116
American Journal of Medical Sciences (Nott) 92–3
American Medical Association (AMA) 113, 116, 127, 133
American Medical Student Association (AMSA) 266
American Public Health Association (APHA) 134
American Recovery and Reinvestment Act 206

American Urological Association 95
Amin, Samir 234
AMLO *see* López Obrador, Andrés Manuel
Anderson, Elizabeth Milbank 121
Anderson, Matt 207
Andrews, John B. 132
aristocracy of labor 234
artificial diseases 31
artificial epidemics 9
asbestos (lung disease and cancer) 55–7
Asociación Latinoamericana de Medicina Social (ALAMES, Latin American Association of Social Medicine) 266
Associação Brasileira de Saúde Coletiva (ABRASCO, Brazilian Association of Collective Health) 266
Association of Clinicians for the Underserved (ACU) 266

Bagley, Sarah George 111
Balmaceda, José Manuel 179
Bartlett, Elisha 110–11
Bellevue–Yorkville 121–3
benzene 63
Berkeley Center for Social Medicine 267
Bethune, Norman 24
Betto, Frei 186
Biden, Joe 97
Bills of Mortality 7
Bismarck, Otto von 9, 18, 261n55
Black Panther Party 17
"the bloody week" 117

278 Index

Bolivia 153, 159, 160, 164–7, 232, 245, 251
Bolshevik movement 124, 132
brain disease (mercury poisoning) 60–2
Brazilian Association of Collective Health (Associação Brasileira de Saúde Coletiva, ABRASCO) 177
Bretton Woods accords 145–6
Brewster, Mary 119
Bright, John 8
British National Health Service 100
Brownson, Orestes 110–11
buen vivir 177, 180
Buffett, Warren 18
bureaucracy 178
Burlington Northern and Santa Fe (BNSF) Railway 252, 263n67
Burns, Mary 27
Bush, George W. 206

Calderón, Felipe 170, 171
California Nurses Association/National Nurses United 267
Canada 100
capitalism 25–8, 47–9, 53, 57, 71, 81, 88, 89, 93, 94, 142, 158, 173, 187, 193, 236–51, 253, 255
cardiac difficulties 122
Carnegie, Andrew 94, 142, *142*
Cartwright, Samuel 93
Cellular Pathology (Virchow) 30
Center on Budget and Policy Priorities 129
Centers for Disease Control and Prevention (CDC) 64, 66–7
Child Health Insurance Program (CHIP) 128
Chile 34–7, 40, 42, 159, 163, 178–83, 185, 186, 188–90, 192, 193
Chilean Medico-Social Reality, The (Allende) 34–5, 37, 41–2, 182–3
Chilean National Health Service 182
Chisso Corporation 60–2
chronic back injury 58
Civilian Medical Resources Network (CMRN) 214, 216, 217, 267
Civil Rights Act 94
civil service 100
Civil War 92, 126, 161, 163
Claudio Schuftan 267
Clinton, Bill 128, 230
Clinton, Hillary 87, 230

Coalition for the Defense of Water and Life (Coordinadora) 164–5
Cobden, Richard 8
Cochabamba 164–6
collateralized loan obligations (CLOs) 69–70
collective interviews 191
Colombia 150, 185, 186, 189, 192–3, 230, 232
colonialism 4, 140
Committee on the Costs of Medical Care (CCMC) 132–3
Communist Manifesto, The 41
community health centers (CHCs) 13, 14, 118–19, 121–2
communityhealth.in 268
Community-oriented primary care (COPC) 13–14
Condition of the Working Class in England in 1844, The (Engels) 27, 47, 59
Cooperation Jackson 249
Coordinadora 164–6
coronavirus disease 2019 (COVID-19) 2–6, 9, 20n4, 20n5, 50, 51, 64–8, 72, 77n45, 87, 90, 144–5, 150, 153, 156n11, 175n38, 205, 231, 237; and agriculture 65–9; collective health 177; laboratory in China 65; narrative of 69–71; tuberculosis and 25–6
Corporations and Health 268
Cuba 14, 15, 185, 186, 189, 235, 250
Cuban revolution 14, 185, 250
CUNY School of Medicine, Community Health and Social Medicine Department 268

Dakota Access Pipeline protest 251–5
Debs, Eugene V. 132
Declaration of Alma Ata 12
Decree 1024 162
Dellums, Ronald 235
democracy 118
Democracy Now! Healthcare 268
demystification 190
deprofessionalization 206
derived demand 11
dibromo-chloropropane (DBCP) 45
disaster capitalism 71, 238
Doctors for Global Health (DGH) 269
domestic violence 97
double agent 207, 213–14

Douglas, Tommy 244
DuBois, W. E. B. 93, 105n27
Duke, David 237

Ecuadoran group 192
Eisenhower, Dwight D. 134
elections 243–5
electoral democracy 167, 249
electronic medical record (EMR) system 206, 207
electronics production (leukemia and lymphoma) 62–4
El Salvador 160–3, 193
Engels, Friedrich 8, 9, 25–30, 27, 32, 34–7, 39–42, 43n8, 47–9, 59, 79, 100, 112, 190, 218, 225, 244, 274
epicenters 4
Epidemiology 101 70–1
Espejo, Eugenio 185

Farabundo Marti National Liberation Front (FMLN) 163
farmworkers 57–9, 60
fee-for-service system 234
FIRE sector of the global capitalist economy 234–5
Flexner, Abraham 94, 96
Flores, Francisco 162
food: independence 247; problem 246–7
four freedoms speech 10
Fowler, Liz 229–30
Fox, Vicente 167, 170, 171
Freire, Paulo 186
Fresh Air Fund 120
funding and services 51

GAF Corporation of New York 56
García, Juan César 186–7
gardening principles 247
Garret, Elizabeth 135n12
Gas War 166
Gates, Bill *144*
Gates Foundation 18, 66–8, 144–5, 153–4
Gates, Melinda *144*
Geiger, Jack 14, *16*
gender and sexism 95–9, **98**
General Agreement on Tariffs and Trade (GATT) 146, 147
generalized proletarianization 234
German Dispensary 113, 114, 118

GI Rights Hotline (GIRH) 215–16
global capitalist economic system 250–5
Global Health Watch (GHW) 269
global North 26, 43n7, 194n2, 250
global South 15, 26, 43n7, 177, 178, 191, 192, 194n2, 244, 250
global warming 42, 101, 239, 248
Goldman, Emma 119, 243
Goodman, Alan 90
Gorz, André 226
Gospel of Wealth, The (Carnegie) 142
Gramsci, Antonio 189, 224, 225
Great Depression 8, 69, 87, 199, 203, 244
Great Recession 129, 131
Guerin, Jules 7
Guevara, Ernesto Che 184, 250

hantavirus 1–5
Harvard Medical School, Department of Global Health and Social Medicine 269
Hatch, John *16*
HCA model 232
health care for all (HFA) 231–2
Health Care Renewal 270
Healthcare Revolution 270
health–illness 15, 53, 183, 191–2
Health Insurance Law (1883) 9
health maintenance organizations (HMOs) 204
Health Policy Advisory Center (Health/PAC) archives 269
hegemonic ideology 190
Heggie, Vanessa 96
Henry Street settlements 119–21, *120*
Hesperian Health Guides 270
homelessness 202
hookworm 143, 144, 150, 154
horizontal programs 18
House Un-American Activities Committee (HUAC) 133, 134
How the Other Half Lives (Riis) 119
Hunting Ground, The 97
hygienic interventions *(higienismo)* 183–4
hypertension and racism 90, *91*

imperialism 35, 40, 139–41, 155, 158–60, 187, 213, 225, 237, 245, 251
industrialization 8, 57, 109, 111, 112, 158
Industrial Revolution 7, 110

inequality 3–5, 9, 12, 14, 39, 40, 42, 48–51, 53, 64, 71, 79–81, *81, 84*, 85, 87–90, 92, 95, 99, 100, 153, 159, 169, 173, 192, 225, 237, 239, 241, 245, 253
injustice 94, 114, 237
intensive care unit (ICU) 46
international financial institutions and trade agreements 18, 67, 139, 141, 145–8, **149**, 151, 152, 189–92, 228, 229, 231
international health organizations 66–8, 139, 141, 150–4, 189
International Journal of Health Services (Navarro) 187, 270
International Monetary Fund (IMF) 66, 146, 152, 159, 231
International Safety Bureau 150, 151

Jacobi, Abraham 113–17, *114*
Jacobi, Mary Corrinna Putnam *116*, 116–18
Jameson, Fredric 239
Jawaharlal Nehru University, Centre of Social Medicine and Community Health 271
Johns Hopkins Center for Health Security 68
Johnson, Lyndon B. 10, 94, 128
Justo, Juan B. 183–4

Kerr, Lorin E. 134
Kleindeutschland 112–14, 119

labor movement 109–12, 115, 118, 182, 263n69
laissez-faire 8
Latin America 8, 15, 18, 26, 34, 49, 79, 140, 154, 158–60, 177–8, 215, 225, 231, 232, 245, 251–5; Chile and Allende 181–3; history 180–1; Max Westenhöfer and 180–1; political repression 188–9; productivity and danger 178–80; public health 183–5; 1960s and later 185–8; social medicine groups 191–3; theory, method, and debate 189–91
Latin American Association of Social Medicine (Asociación Latinomericana de Medicina Social, ALAMES) 177
Latin American Medical School/ Escuela Latinoamericana de Medicina (ELAM) 271

Latin American social medicine (LASM) 15–16, 177–8, 180, 184–7, 189–91, 193, 276
Laurell, Asa Cristina 167–73, 175n38, 191
lax regulations 50
lazy man's disease 143
Legitimate Government of Mexico 170
legitimation function of State 245
Lenin, Vladimir 244
leukemia 62–4
little Germany 112–18
liver cancer 54–5
López Obrador, Andrés Manuel 167, 168, 170–3, 175n38
lopezobradorista ("López-Obrador-ist") movement 170, 171
Lowell, Francis Cabot 109–11
lung disease and cancer 55–7
lymphoma 62–4

McCain, John 227
McCarthy, Joseph 133
McCaskill, Claire 97
McKinlay, John B. 48
magic bullet approach 67, 144–5, 152–3
malaria 18, 143–5, 150, 152–4
managed care 144, 192, 204–10, 212–14, 216, 218, 231–2
managed care organizations (MCOs) 204, 205, 207–9, 216
Manchester Liberalism 8
Mao Zedong 66
market orientation 19
markets and competition 229
Marmor, Theodore R. 125–7
Martín-Baró, Ignacio 193
Marx, Karl 47, 81, 85–6, 88–9, 113, 189–90, 206, 244
Medicaid 10, 45, 95, 127–8, 200, 208, 233
medical and public health services **149**
Medical Committee for Human Rights (MCHR) 17
Medical Education Cooperation with Cuba (MEDICC) 271
medical encounter 199, 207, 210, 212–13, 218
medical industrial complex (MIC) 11, 21n22
medical loss ratio (MLR) 228
Medically Indigent Adult (MIA) program 200

Medical Reform (Virchow) 9
Medicare 10–11, 95, 127–8, 208, 228–9, 232–3
medications, access to **149**
Medicine and Social Justice 271
medico-social program 39
melting pot 119
mental health 3, 80–1, 190, 192, 213–15, 217–18, 225, 248–9, 254–6
mercury poisoning 60–2
mesothelioma 56
Mexico 1, 4, 45, 67, 160, 167, 169–73, 185, 189–92, 203, 231–2
Mexico City 167, 169–70, 187
Mexico City Government (MCG) 169
Migrant Clinicians Network 272
Milbank, Albert G. 121
Milbank Memorial Fund 121
militarism 51, 71, 79, 213, 217–18, 225, 237–8, 241, 255
Minamata Disease 60–2
mixed approach 230
mixed capitalist–socialist societies 48
mixed private–public systems 231
Mohawk–Brighton 124
Monroe, James 158
Monthly Review 272
Morales, Evo 165–7
mortality 4, 7, 15, 24, 28–9, 32, 35, 36, 39–40, 51, 53, 70, 80, *82, 84,* 85, 89–90, 95, 99–100, 102n3, 111, 120, 123, 150, 181, 182, 192, 236
Morton, Samuel 92
Movement for National Regeneration (Movimiento Regeneración Nacional, MORENA) 172, 192
multi-method approach 191–2
Municipal Medical and Hospital Services Act 133
Muntaner, Carles 86
Mutual Exchange of Work units (MEOWs) 246–7

nanny state 10
National Association for the Advancement of Colored People (NAACP) 121
National Association of Community Health Centers 272
national health insurance (NHI) 132–3, 235–6

national health program (NHP) 100, 185, 206, 214, 225, 227–36, 244–5, 249, 255
national health service (NHS) 235
National Social Unit Organization (NSUO) 124–5
Navajo Nation 1, 3–4, 19n1
Navarro, Vicente 83, 155 n.4, 187
neocolonialism 140
neoliberalism 18, 159, 166, 171, 173, 227–8, 233–4, 236, 245
neoliberal retreat from Alma Ata, The 18–19
New England Journal of Medicine 272
New models of health care in the United States during the 1960s and 1970s 16–17
New York Milk Committee 121
Nicaragua 160, 186
Ninety miles from Miami: the Cuban health system 14–15
No Free Lunch 273
non-reformist praxis 236–8
non-reformist reforms 226–7
nontariff barriers to trade 146
North American Free Trade Agreement (NAFTA) 148, 172
Nott, Josiah 92–3

Obama, Barack 97, 148, 206, 227, 230, 233
Obamacare 12, 19, 200, 202, 227–36
occupational and environmental health **149**
Occupational Safety and Health Research Institute 63
Odets, Clifford 199
1 1/2 centuries of forgetting and remembering the social origins of illness 49
Organic mercury 60

Paine, Thomas 126
Pan American Health Organization (PAHO) 151, 179, 186–7
Paredes, Ricardo 185
Paris Commune 117
Party of National Action (Partido de Acción Nacional, PAN) 167, 170–1
Party of the Democratic Revolution (Partido de la Revolución Democrática, PRD) 167, 170–1

patient–doctor communication 210–13, 218
patient–doctor relationship 204–10, 213
Pedagogy of the Oppressed (Freire) 186
People's Health Movement (PHM) 273
Perry, Thomas 134
personal dignity 204
philanthrocapitalism 19, 66
philanthropy 139, 141–5, 154
Phillips, Wilbur C. 123–5
Physicians for a National Health Program (PNHP) 232–3, 235–6, 273
Piketty, Thomas 88, 99
Piven, Frances Fox 129
plastic industry (liver cancer) 54–5
Plekhanov, Georgi 7
political economic systems 25–6, 36, 42, 43n4, 53, 64, 71, 79, 94
political economy 34, 36, 38, 43n4, 94
political repression 109, 188–9
polyvinyl chloride (PVC) 54, 55
Popular Insurance Program (Seguro Popular) 170
population health 3, 4, 6–12, 15, 25, 31, 35, 36, 38, 42, 46, 51, 53, 60, 64, 66, 70–1, 79–81, 87–90, 93–4, 100, 110, 119, 121, 123, 125–6, 131, 144, 162, 164, 166–7, 169–70, 173, 182–3, 185, 192, 204, 213, 217, 225, 227–8, 230–2, 237–9, 248, 250–1, 253, 261n52
post-traumatic stress disorder (PTSD) 213, 216–18
poverty 2, 4–7, 39, 48, 53, 64, 71, 80–1, 85, 88–9, 92, 99, 115, 119, 128–31, 146, 152–4, 159, 178, 184, 185, 192, 200, 202, 225, 227, 236, 241, 245, 248
praxis 189, 224–5; contradictions of reform 225–7; health and illness 236–55; health and mental health 255–6; NHP 227–36; non-reformist 236–8
premature deaths 39, 201
Prison Notebooks (Gramsci) 225
private insurance 12, 144, 171, 201, 202, 227–8, 230–3, 236
privatization 18, 70, 125, 146, 158–60, 171, 173, 179, 190–2, 217, 225, 231, 263n68; in El Salvador 160–3; water in Bolivia 164–7
Program of Free Health Care and Drugs 169

Progressive Era 118–23, 130–1
proletarianization 205–6
protest 251–5
provider organizations (PPOs) 204
public health: Latin America 183–5; nursing 119
Public Health and Social Justice 273
public–private partnerships 144

race and racism 89–90, *91*, 92–5
racial capitalism 94, 237
racial differences 92–3, 95
racism 51
Reagan, Ronald 10, 18, 127, 151, 228
La Realidad Médico-Social Chilena see *Chilean Medico-Social Reality, The* (Allende)
Recabarren, Luis Emilio 181–2
Red Scare 124, 132–4
reformist reforms 226–7
Report of a General Plan for the Promotion of Public and Personal Health 112
Report of the Commission on Macroeconomics and Health: Investing in Health for Economic Development 152–3
Report on Macroeconomics and Health 154
Republican Nationalist Alliance (Alianza Republicana Nacionalista, ARENA) 161
Revolutionary Institutional Party (Partido Revolucionario Institucional, PRI) 171
revolving door 229, 230
Rickettsia 5
Rico, Puerto 140
Riis, Jacob 119
rinky-dink revolution 240–2
Robin Hood Tax 88
Rockefeller Foundation 142–4, 154, 185
Rockefeller, John D. 142–5, *143*, 154, 185
Rodriguez, Arturo S. 59
Rodríguez, María Isabel 163, 187, 188
Roe v. Wade (1973) 96
Rojava Revolution 262n62
Romney, Mitt 227, 230
Roosevelt, Franklin D. 10, 126–8
Roosevelt, Theodore 10, 130–1
Rosen, George 8, 123, 134

Sachs, Jeffrey 152–3
safety and quality: of food **149**; of products **149**
Salvadoran Institute of Social Security (Instituto Salvadoreño del Seguro Social, ISSS) 161
Salvadoran Institute of Social Security (Sindicato de Trabajadores del ISSS, STISS) 161, 162
Salvadoran Institute of Social Security (Sindicato Médico de Trabajadores del ISSS, SIMETRISS) 161, 162
Samsung 63–4
Sánchez Cerén, Salvador 163
Sánchez de Lozada, Gonzalo 166
Seidel, Emil 123
self-insurance 9
Servicio Municipal de Agua Potable y Alcantarillado (SEMAPA) 164, 166
severe acute respiratory syndrome (SARS) 2–3, 66, 150
sexual harassment 97–9, **98**
Shattuck, Lemuel 111–12, 114
shock therapy 152
short hoe 58–60
Sidney and Emily Kark's model *13*, 13–14
Sigerist, Henry E. 134
Silva Renard, Roberto 181
single mother 130–1
single-payer approach 232–3
Smithfield Foods 67–8, 76 n.32
social capital 99
social change 117–18
social class and classism 80–1, *81–6*, 83, 85, 86–9, 100, 102n8
social contradictions 32, 40, 47–8, 53–4, 58, 64, 72, 227, 232, 256
social determinants of health (SDOH) 26, 49–54, **50**, 79, 80, 99
social determination 79; gender and sexism 95–9, **98**; health and illness 236–55; origins 99–101; race and racism 89–90, *91*, 92–5; social class and classism 80–1, *81–6*, 83, 85–9; social determinants and 48–51, **50**, **52**, 53–4
social imperialism 140
social insurance 125–34
Socialist Caucus of the American Public Health Association (APHA) 274
Socialist Labor Party 131–2

Socialist Party of America 131–2
social medicine 3, 5, 9, 12–17, *13*, 24–7, 29, 30, 34, 42, 48, 51, 53, 54, 64, 86, 94, 100, 139, 141, 155, 158–60, 163, 166–7, 224–7, 232, 238–45, 247–8, 250–4; critical 19; Latin America (*see* Latin America); levels of analysis 72; medical encounter (*see* medical encounter); Mexico City and Mexico 167–73; organizations and resources 265–76; praxis, health and mental health 255–6; roots of 7–8; strength of 47; United States (*see* United States)
Social Medicine Consortium (SMC) 274
Social Medicine Portal 43n5
The Social Medicine Portal; *Social Medicine/ Medicina Social* 274
social pathologies 100–1
social reform 114–15
social security system 126–7, 231
socio-medical reality 48
solidarity economy 242, 245–50, 255
Spirit of 1848 Caucus of the American Public Health Association (APHA) 274–5
Stamler, Jeremiah 134
state socialism 9
Stoeckle, John D. 48
Structural Competency Working Group, The 275
structural racism 51, 92–4, 100
Suárez, Pablo Arturo 185

Tajer, Debora 15
TANF-to-poverty ratio (TPR) 129
tarifazo 164
tariff barriers to trade 146
tax cuts 50
Temporary Assistance for Needy Families (TANF) 128–9
Thatcher, Margaret 10, 18, 228
Tobin, James 88
Torres, Camilo 186
Trans-Atlantic Free Trade Agreement (TAFTA) 147–8
Trans-Pacific Partnership (TPP) 147–8
trauma 90, 192, 213
Tren Maya 172
Truman, Harry S. 134
Trump, Donald 59, 81, 87, 99, 147, 237, 243

tuberculosis 18, 24, 28, 31, 35–7, 43n2, 64, 80, 90, 116, 122, 133, 144, 145, 152, 154, 182, 202; and COVID-19 25–6
typhus in Upper Silesia 5–7, 28, 30–3, 36, 41, 64

UCLA Center for Social Medicine and Humanities 275
underdevelopment of health 140
Unemployment Insurance (UI) 130–1
United Farm Workers (UFW) organization 59
United Kingdom 18, 83, 100, 141, 146, 228
United Nations Educational, Scientific, and Cultural Organization (UNESCO) 151
United States 1, 2, 8, 10–19, 24, 36, 45, 46, 50, 56–7, 62, 65–8, 70, 71, 80, 83–5, 87, 89, 90, 92–4, 96, 97, 99, 100, 109, 140–1, 146, 147, 151, 153, 158–60, 167, 186, 191, 199–202, 204, 206, 215, 217, 224–5, 227–8, 230–8, 245, 250–1, 253; industrialization 109–12; little Germany 112–18; Progressive Era 118–23; social insurance 125–34; Wilbur C. Phillips and 123–5
United States exceptionalism 125
universal health coverage (UHC) 231–2
University of California, San Francisco, Department of Anthropology, History and Social Medicine 275
University of New Mexico (UNM) Hospital 1
University of New Mexico/ University of Guadalajara, Latin American Social Medicine Digital Archive 276
University of North Carolina School of Medicine, Department of Social Medicine 276
Upper Silesia 5–7, 31, 36, 41, 64
U.S. Environmental Protection Agency 56
U.S. Occupational Safety and Health Administration 54
usos y costumbres (uses and customs) 164

Vermont Asbestos Company (VAC) 56–7
Vermont Asbestos Group (VAG) 57

Vermont Occupational Safety and Health Administration 56
vertical programs 18
Vietnam War 17, 216
violence 42, 79, 90, 97, 99, 186, 189, 192–3, 216, 218, 237, 249–50
Virchow, Rudolf 5–7, 9, 19, 25–6, *30*, 30–4, 36, 39–42, 48–9, 64, 79, 100, 113–14, 180–2, 185, 191, 218, 225
Virchow's triad 30
Volksgemeinschaft 261n55

Waiting for Lefty (Odets) 199
Waitzkin, Howard 75n20, 200, 203, 207, 209
Wald, Lillian 119–21
Walsh, Julia A. 18
Walter Reed Army Medical Center 216
Waltham System 109
Warren, Kenneth S. 18
Washington consensus 146
water, privatization of 164–7
Water War 164, 166
Weber, Max 83, 85, 178
Westenhöfer, Max 34, 180–2
Whitehall study 100
White, Paul Dudley 134
women's health movement 95–7, 99
Women's Medical Association 117
working class 115
World Bank 15, 66, 144, 146, 151–4, 159–62, 164, 190, 228, 230–1
World Development Report: Investing in Health 152
World Economic Forum 68
World Health Organization (WHO) 12, 18, 49, **50**, 51, 64, 66, 67, 99, 145, 151–4, 179
World Trade Organization (WTO) 146–8, 153

yellow fever 143, 150, 154

Zapata, Emiliano 172, 173
Zapatista Army of National Liberation (Ejercito Zapatista de Liberación Nacional, EZLN) 172, 192
Zapatista revolutionary movement 160, 172
ZDoggMD 206
Zika virus 66, 145

9781138685987